EVERYDAY SUPER FOOD

JAMIE OLIVER

MICHAEL JOSEPH
an imprint of
PENGUIN BOOKS

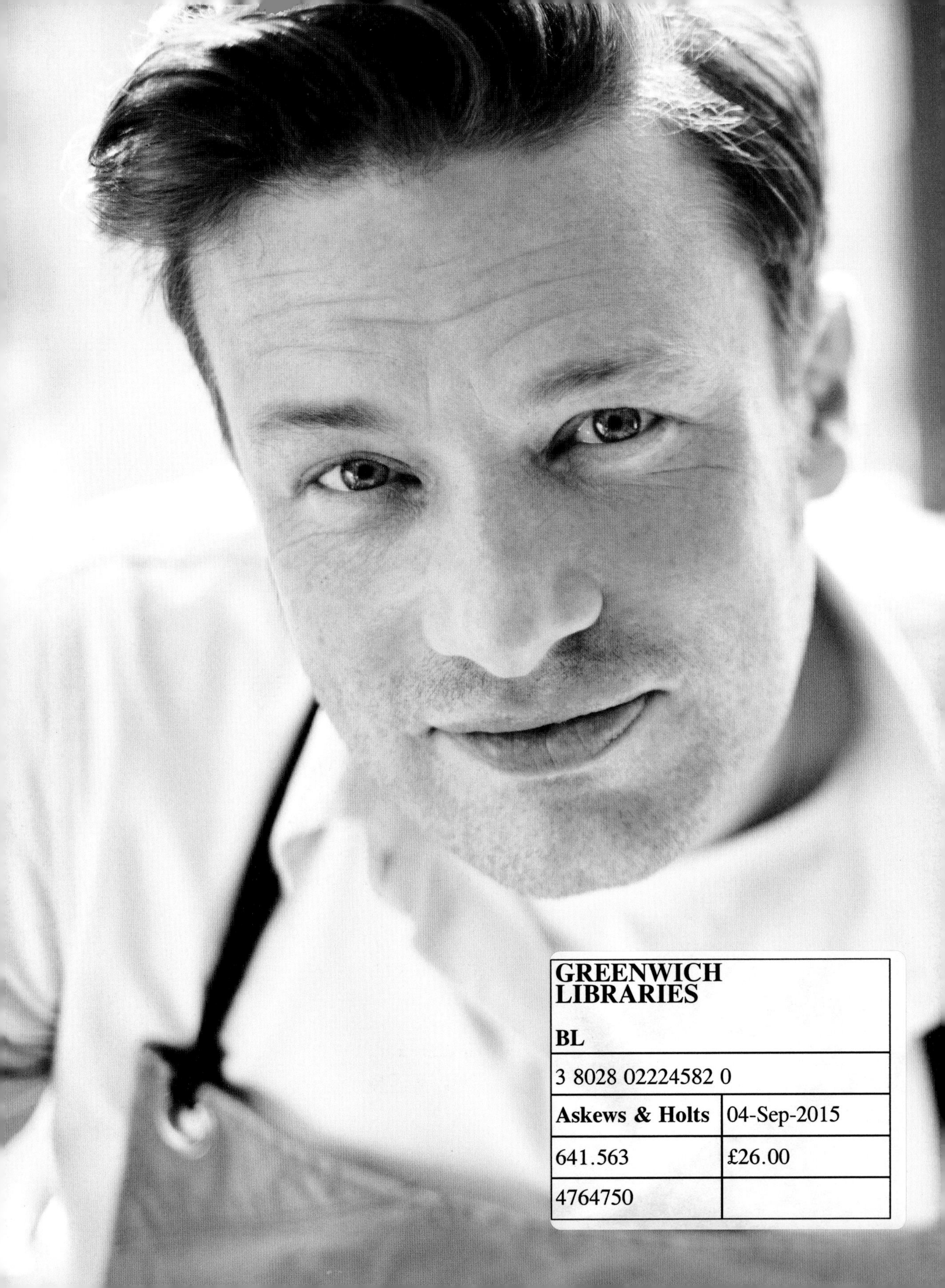

ALSO BY JAMIE OLIVER

The Naked Chef
The Return of the Naked Chef
Happy Days with the Naked Chef
Jamie's Kitchen
Jamie's Dinners
Jamie's Italy
Cook with Jamie
Jamie at Home
Jamie's Ministry of Food
Jamie's America
Jamie Does . . .
Jamie's 30-Minute Meals
Jamie's Great Britain
Jamie's 15-Minute Meals
Save with Jamie
Jamie's Comfort Food

FOOD PHOTOGRAPHY
Jamie Oliver

OTHER PHOTOGRAPHY
Paul Stuart
Freddie Claire

DESIGN
Superfantastic
wearesuperfantastic.com

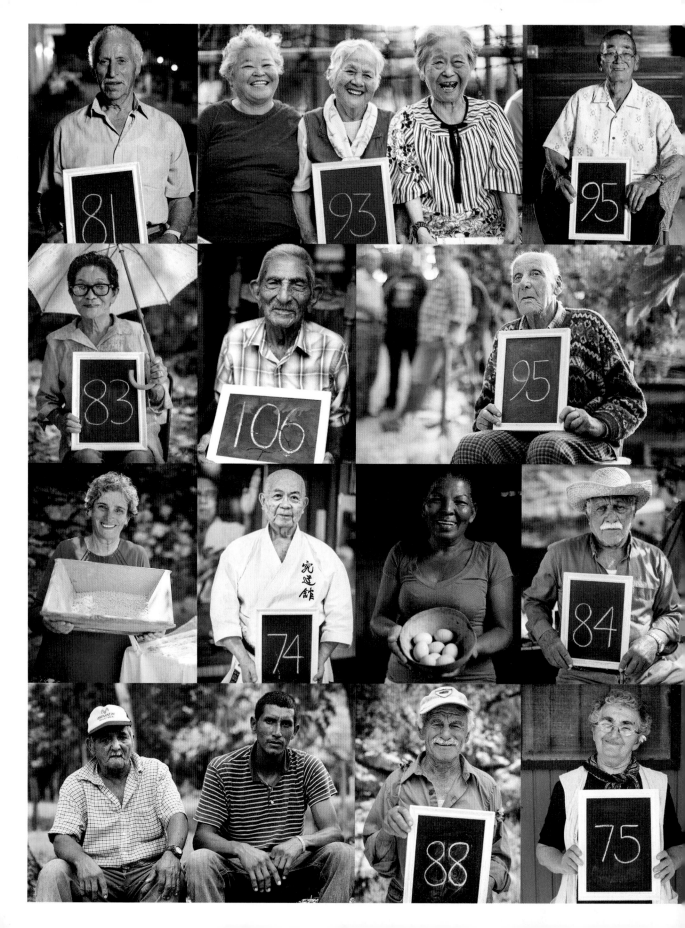

DEDICATION

This book is dedicated to my amazing food and nutrition teams, all the recipe testers, all the incredible doctors, scientists and professors, and of course, all the wonderful, old but still amazingly active people, in some of the healthiest places on the planet, who I've met on the epic journey of creating this book.

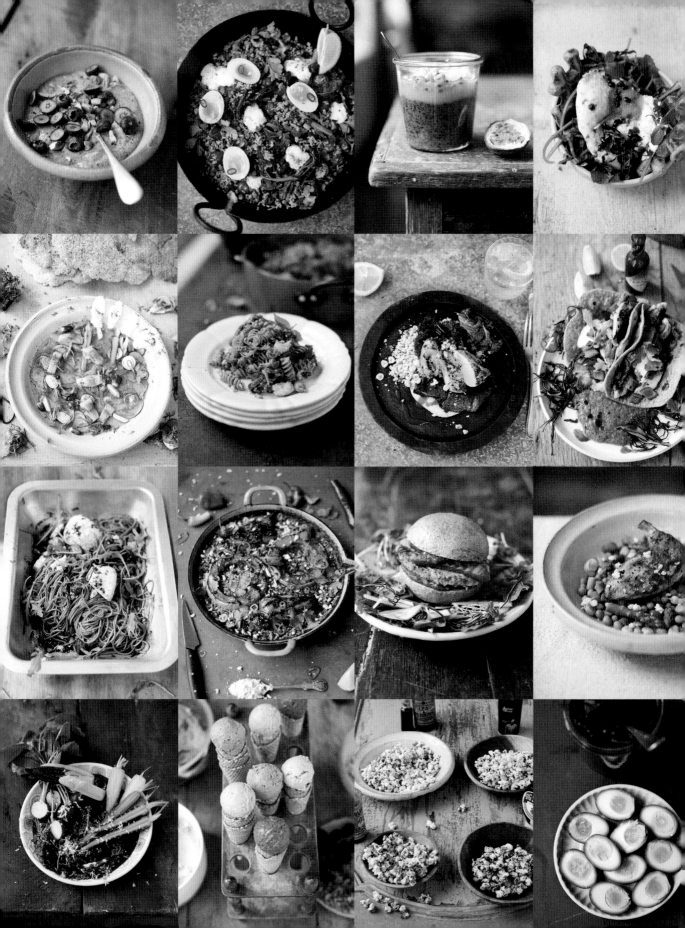

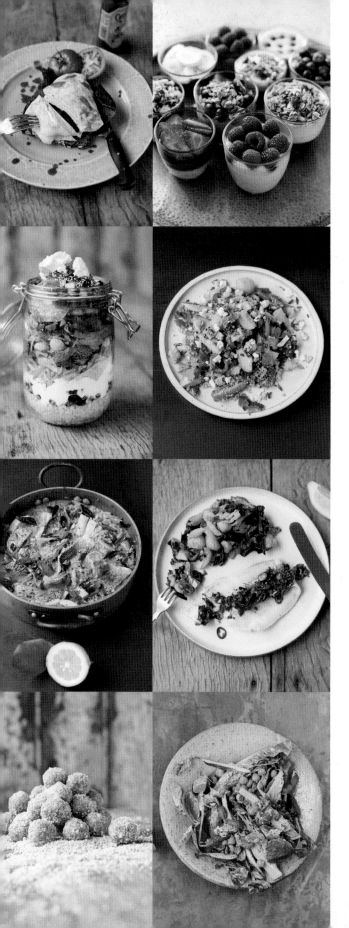

CONTENTS

INTRODUCTION ···················· 8

BREAKFAST ···················· 14

LUNCH ···················· 84

DINNER ···················· 154

SNACKS & DRINKS ···················· 224

LIVE WELL ···················· 258

MY PHILOSOPHY IN THIS BOOK
THE BALANCED PLATE ···················· 260

ILLUSTRIOUS VEG & FRUIT ···················· 262

CELEBRATING GOOD CARBOHYDRATES ······ 266

THE POWER OF PROTEIN ···················· 268

FAT IS ESSENTIAL ···················· 272

DIPPING INTO DAIRY ···················· 274

DRINK WATER & THRIVE ···················· 278

ALCOHOL ···················· 280

VOTE FOR ORGANIC FOOD ···················· 284

REVOLUTIONIZE SHOPPING ···················· 286

THE BASICS OF SLEEP ···················· 290

DO YOU WANT TO LIVE
TO BE 100 YEARS OLD? ···················· 292

INDEX ···················· 298

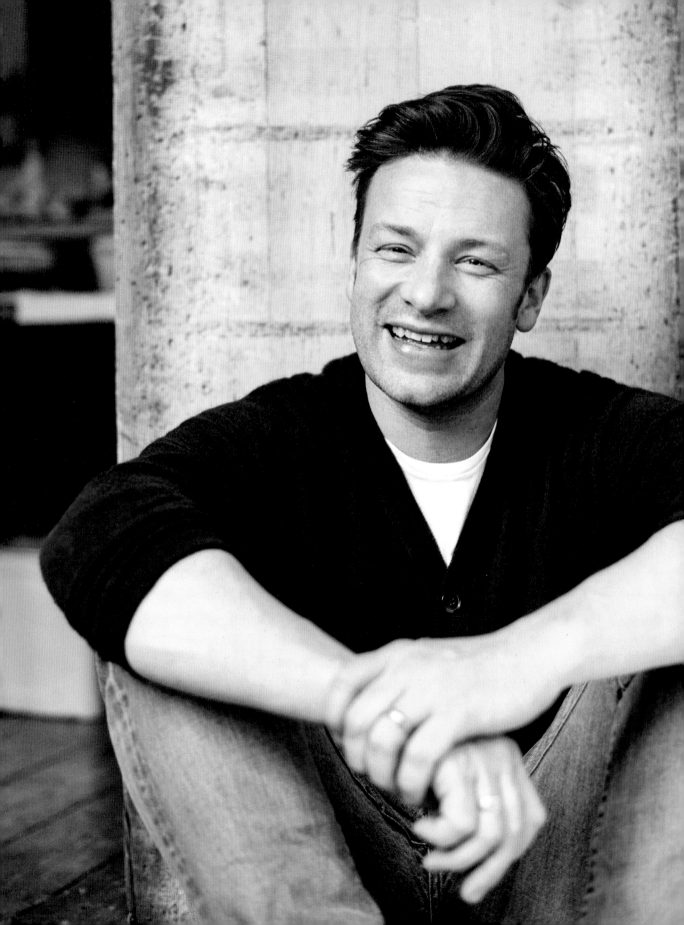

HEALTHY & HAPPY

First of all, thank you for picking up this book and welcome to my *Everyday Super Food*. The ultimate promise in these pages is that every recipe choice is a good choice. Quite simply, I wanted to create a super-safe place celebrating delicious, nutritious, achievable meals that will help you cook your way to a healthier, happier, more productive life.

By the time you read this, I will have reached my fortieth birthday. About 18 months ago, nudging ever closer to it, this upcoming milestone made me pause and look at life slightly differently. I'll be honest: it's taken me on a bit of a personal journey as far as my health is concerned. We all have very different lives – mine is particularly peculiar and I love it – but regardless of our individual circumstances, I think most of us want to achieve and support a happy, healthy family at home; be the best we can be at work; maintain good friendships; continue to experience new things; and have lots of laughs along the way. There's certainly no one-size-fits-all answer and getting it wrong sometimes is all part of the journey. But, in order to give yourself the best chance, good personal health needs to be your utmost priority. So, my philosophy in this book is to help you get it right on the food front, most of the time.

If you pick up just a handful of ideas from this book, you'll start thinking differently about food

I want this book to be a gateway to a more understanding and open relationship with food, as something to feed, fuel, fix and nourish you, but also as medicine. I want to give you knowledge and a better understanding of food and how to put a balanced meal together. I know it's a cliché, but knowledge really is power – that's what I want you to take from this book. I'm not saying you have to eat from it every day, nor for the rest of your life, but I hope it will arm you with the tools to make the right choices, allowing you to duck and dive at your own pace, mixing up these meals with some naughty days and a few treats – I'm not sure a sustainable healthy relationship with food is achievable without them. Personally, I'm using this book Monday to Thursday/Friday, then hitting up *Comfort Food* at the weekend.

My philosophy in this book is to help you get it right on the food front, most of the time

I believe my job with this book was to go out, learn from some of the best health and nutrition experts out there – doctors, scientists, professors – and travel to some of the healthiest places in the world, absorb as much info as possible, then express the most relevant stuff back to you. So that's exactly what I've done, combined with my 30 years of cooking in order to create these yummy recipes, as well as sharing some bite-sized nuggets of super-useful info that will be relevant to you in your everyday life. I've been bartering and bantering with my nutrition team to ensure that the recipes and ideas are exciting, fun, new and delicious, and that each one embraces the food groups and different ingredients super-rich in nutrients, vitamins and minerals that work together in a complementary way. Every recipe reflects the balanced plate philosophy and appropriate portion control to ensure you're getting the right amount of food (see page 260). And you really can eat a super-healthy meal and be satisfied – the recipe testers have been surprised at just how generous some of the portions are!

So, no matter which recipe you choose from each chapter – and there's at least 30 breakfasts, 30 lunches, and 30 dinners – it will first and foremost tickle your taste buds and fill you up, but you can also be sure it will fit within a daily structure of calories that will stand you in really good stead (less than 400 calories for breakfast and under 600 each for lunch and dinner, leaving you with plenty spare for snacks and drinks – see page 261).

And you know what, this book won't break the bank either. My team have costed up all the meals, using the supermarkets, as well as local butchers and fishmongers, and on average it's coming out at just £2.50 per portion at 2015 prices. I don't know about you, but for the health investment you're making by cooking from this book, for me, that's a total bargain.

Whether you use the book faithfully for every meal, or dip in and out of it to supplement other meal choices, my hope is that it will deliver on being that solid source you can always rely on. I wanted to show you what good really looks like for breakfast, lunch and dinner, plus some exciting snack and drink ideas, so you have a real understanding not just of how to balance your plate, but of how to balance your day, week and month too.

If you pick up just a handful of ideas from this book, you'll start thinking differently about food and the power it has to directly affect you both physically and mentally, inspiring positive changes not only in the way you eat, but hopefully in the eating habits of the people around you as well. Food is there to be appreciated, shared and enjoyed, and healthy, nourishing food should be colourful, delicious and, most importantly, fun.

The ultimate promise in these pages is that every recipe choice is a good choice

Rigorous recipe testing has, as usual, been at the heart of the development of this book because I want you to have success at home, every single time. With such a focus on nutrition, the process of writing it has been very different for me. Quite honestly, it's changed the way I work and how I approach putting a plate of food together. The book has become more of a natural diary for me, and this has meant that I've also photographed all the food myself, as the recipes have often taken time to shape and perfect. What you see in these pages is a real reflection of the journey I've been on and I'm really proud of this book – a lot has gone into it.

Embrace the book, enjoy it, use it as often as you like, cook for your loved ones, but most importantly, I hope it will capture your curiosity and fuel an interest in getting things right when it comes to food, in a way that really works for you. Good luck.

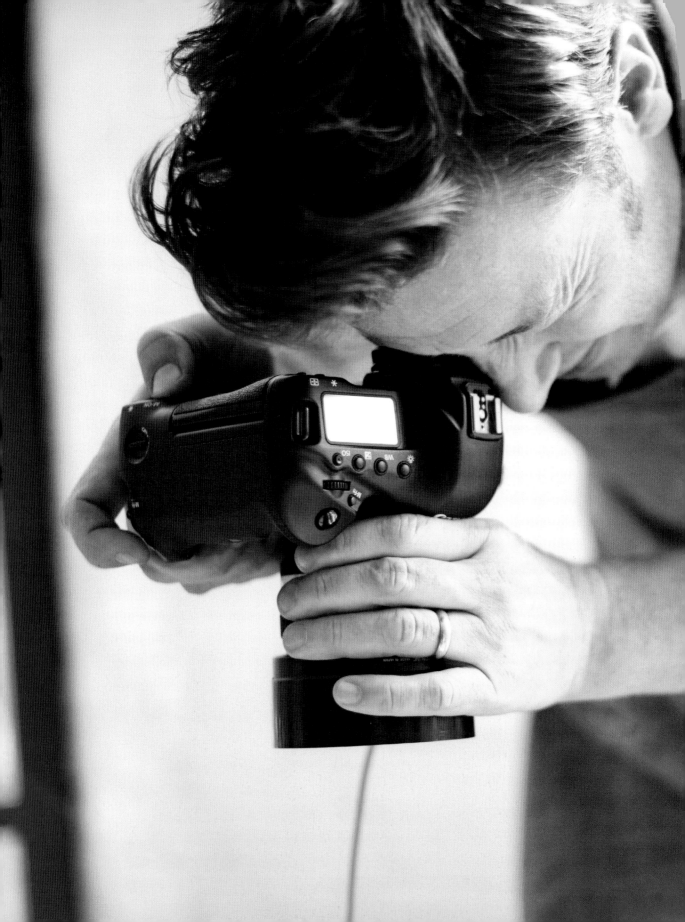

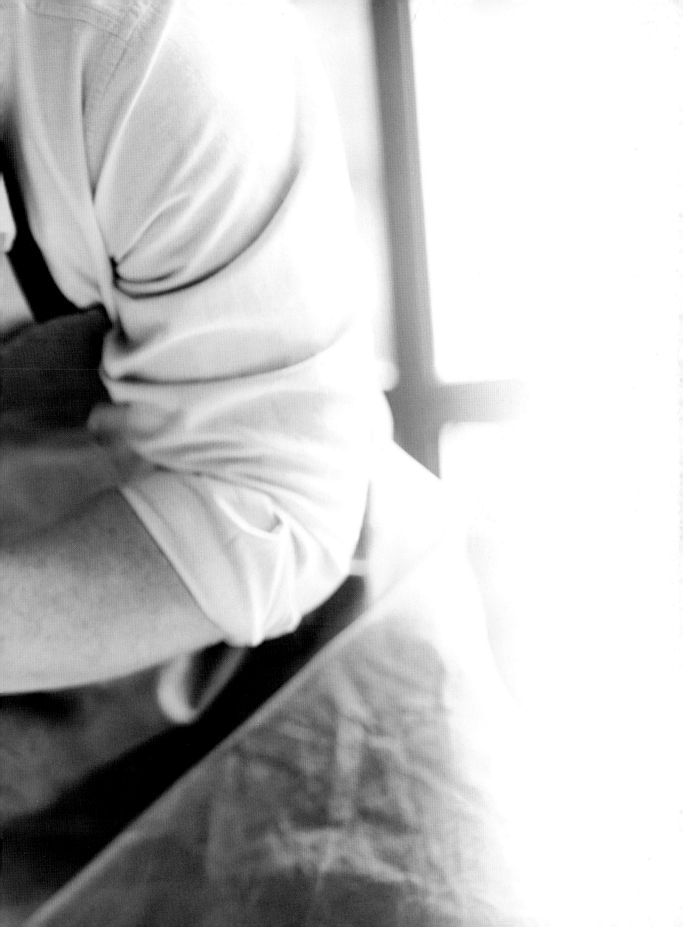

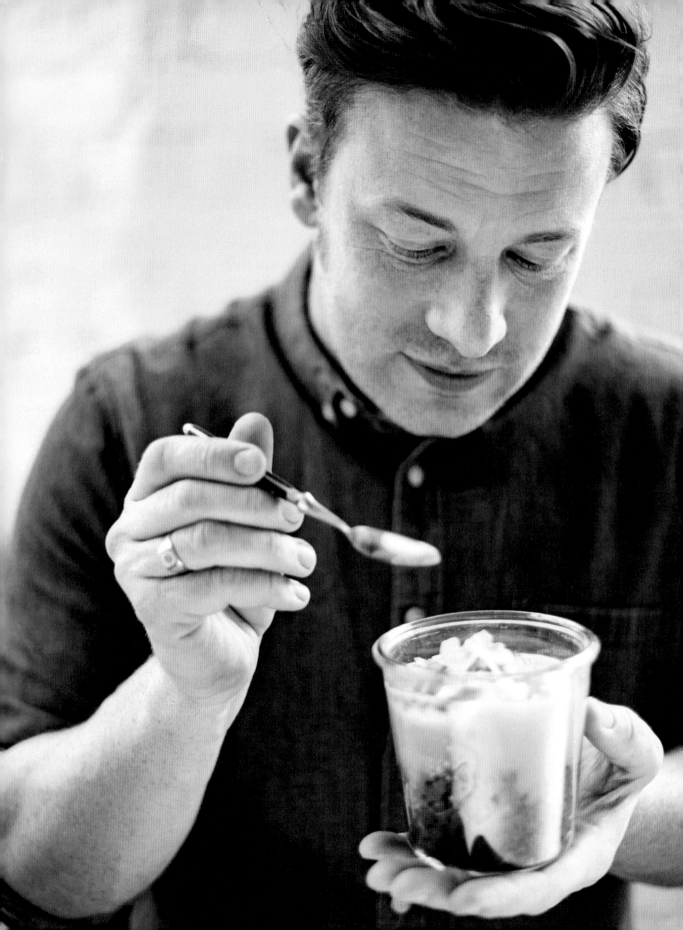

BREAKFAST

Enriching our bodies at breakfast with tasty, nutritious food that'll help us kick off the day in the best way we can is something we should all embrace. I think a lot of us have been brainwashed into believing we only have time to pour milk over cereal, but that's not true! In this game-changer of a chapter you'll find a whole host of super-quick dishes; batches of incredible things you can make up in advance to serve you well each morning, fitting easily into your normal busy routine; as well as simple ideas for lazier mornings and weekend brunches. All the recipes have a nice mix of the food groups and are less than 400 calories per portion. I hope you love them as much as I do.

BAKED EGGS IN POPPED BEANS
CHERRY TOMATOES, RICOTTA ON TOAST

— Mighty cannellini beans are a great source of protein, high in fibre, and contain vitamin C
as well as magnesium, a mineral that helps our muscles to function properly —

SERVES 2

250g mixed-colour ripe
    cherry tomatoes

½ a lemon

extra virgin olive oil

4 sprigs of fresh basil

1 x 400g tin of cannellini beans

1 good pinch of fennel seeds

2 large eggs

2 slices of seeded wholemeal
    bread

2 heaped teaspoons ricotta
    cheese

optional: thick balsamic vinegar

optional: hot chilli sauce

Halve the tomatoes, place in a bowl and toss with the lemon juice, 1 tablespoon of oil and a pinch of sea salt. Pick, tear and toss in the basil leaves (reserving the smaller ones for garnish), then leave aside to macerate for a few minutes.

Meanwhile, place a large non-stick frying pan on a high heat. Drain the beans and put into the hot pan with the fennel seeds and a pinch of black pepper. Leave for 5 minutes, shaking occasionally – you want them to char and pop open, bursting their skins. Pour the macerated tomatoes into the pan with 100ml of water, season, then leave to bubble away vigorously for 1 minute. Crack in an egg on each side, then cover with a lid, plate or tin foil, reduce to a medium-low heat and slow-cook for 3 to 4 minutes for nice soft eggs, or longer if you prefer. Meanwhile, toast the bread.

Divide the ricotta and spread over the two pieces of hot toast, then serve on the side of the baked eggs in beans. Sprinkle the reserved baby basil leaves over the top and tuck right in. Nice finished with a drizzle of balsamic vinegar and/or a drizzle of hot chilli sauce. Delicious.

CALORIES	FAT	SAT FAT	PROTEIN	CARBS	SUGAR	FIBRE	20 MINUTES
399kcal	15.7g	3.6g	22g	40.7g	5.8g	12.6g	

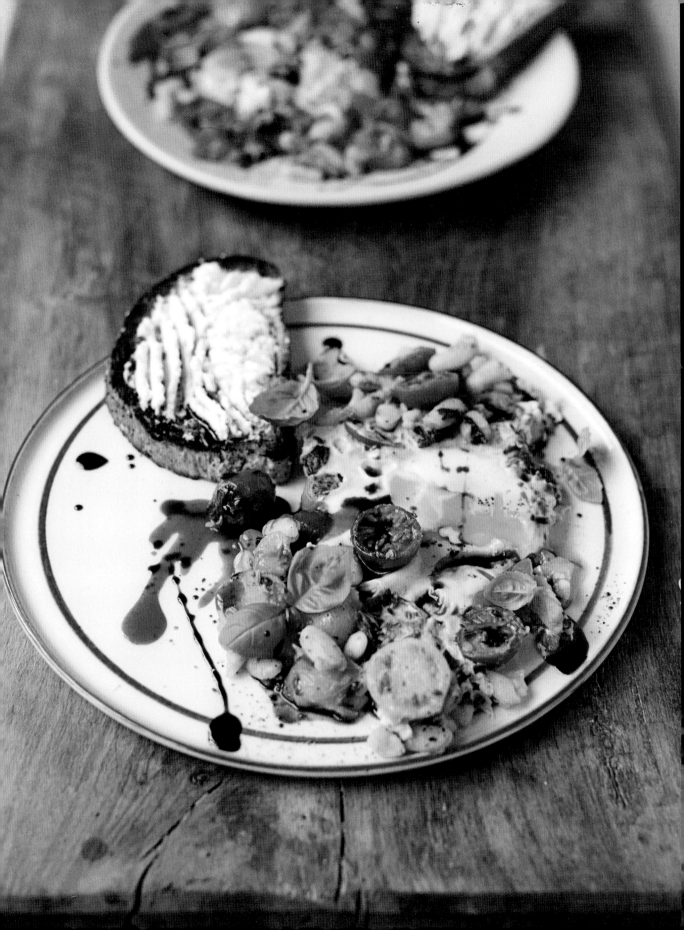

AWESOME GRANOLA DUST
NUTS, SEEDS, OATS & FRUIT GALORE

— Mornings will be amazingly fast and convenient with this epic megamix of brilliant
ingredients, giving us loads of nutritional benefits from the nuts, seeds, oats and fruit —

MAKES 32 PORTIONS

1kg porridge oats

250g unsalted mixed nuts, such
as walnuts, Brazils, hazelnuts,
pecans, pistachios, cashews

100g mixed seeds, such as
chia, poppy, sunflower,
sesame, linseed, pumpkin

250g mixed dried fruit, such as
blueberries, cranberries,
sour cherries, mango,
apricots, figs, sultanas

3 tablespoons quality cocoa
powder

1 tablespoon freshly ground
coffee

1 large orange

Me and my wife get really frustrated about how so many – in fact most – breakfast cereals are full of added sugar, and nutritionally aren't the best start to the day. So, with my nutrition team, I developed this delicious recipe for us all to enjoy – make a big batch and it'll last a couple of weeks (or more!). Turn the page for loads of fantastic ways we use it – we love it!

Preheat the oven to 180°C/350°F/gas 4. Place the oats, nuts and seeds in your largest roasting tray. Toss together and roast for 15 minutes, stirring halfway. Stir the dried fruit, cocoa and coffee into the mix, finely grate over the orange zest, then, in batches, simply blitz to a rough powder in a food processor, tipping it into a large airtight jar as you go for safekeeping.

To serve, you can have loads of fun – the simplest way is 50g of granola dust per person, either with cold cow's, goat's, soya, nut or oat milk or 2 tablespoons of natural yoghurt, and a handful of fresh fruit (80g is one of our 5-a-day).

You can make porridge using **50g of granola dust** to **200ml of milk**, then top with fresh fruit, and this ratio also works for a smoothie – I like to chuck **1 ripe banana** and **1 handful of frozen raspberries** into the mix too. It's even a great base for pancakes – simply beat **2 heaped tablespoons of granola dust** with **1 heaped tablespoon of wholemeal self-raising flour, 1 mashed banana** and **1 egg**, then cook as normal. And in winter, try a hot drink – heat **25g of granola dust** with **200ml of your favourite milk** to your desired consistency.

CALORIES	FAT	SAT FAT	PROTEIN	CARBS	SUGAR	FIBRE	25 MINUTES
400kcal	14.7g	3.8g	14.7g	52.1g	32.2g	8.2g	

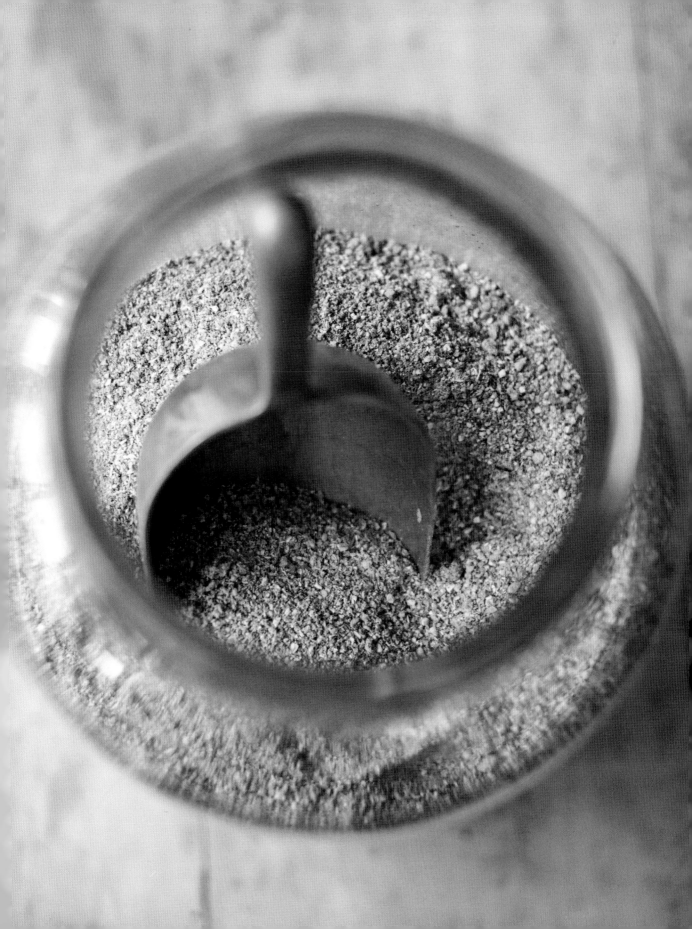

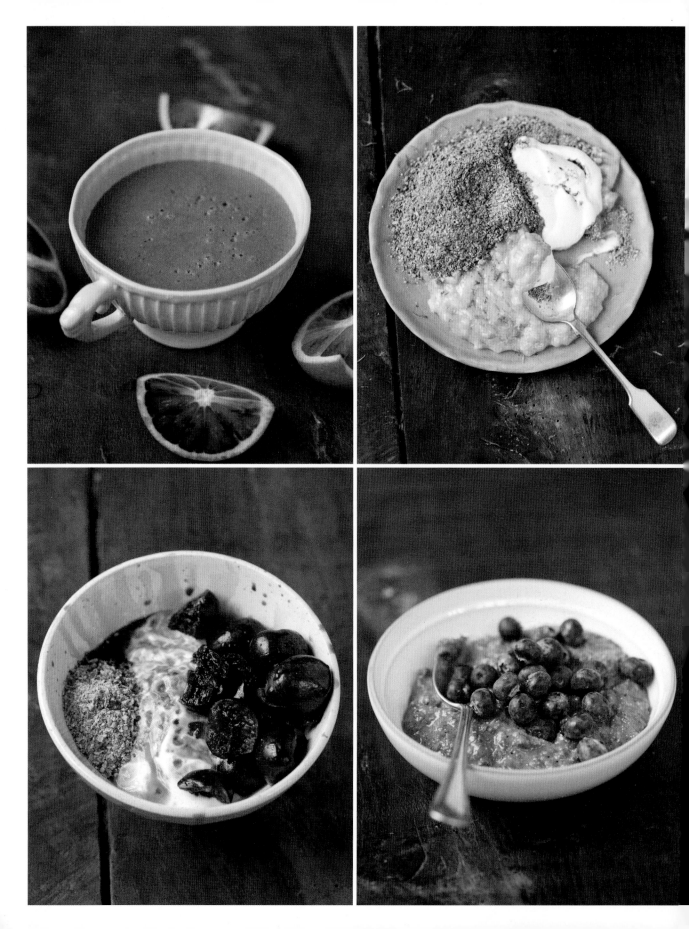

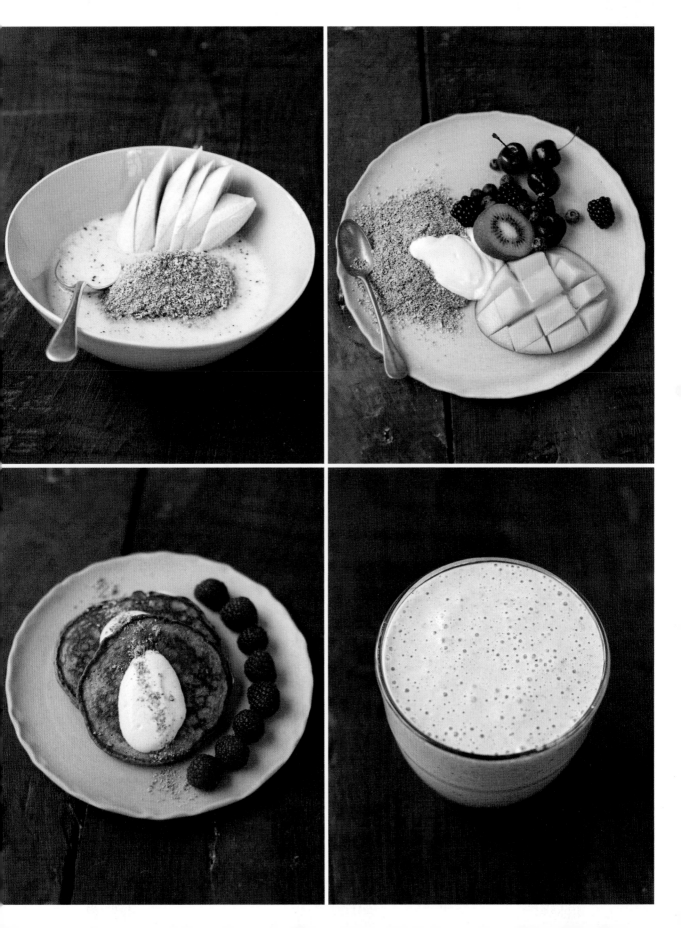

MAGIC POACHED EGG
SMASHED AVO & SEEDED TOAST

— Our brains love protein in the morning, and eggs are a fantastic, affordable source that —
are quick to cook. With a kick of chilli, this dish will wake us up and lift our spirits

SERVES 2

olive oil

½–1 fresh red chilli

2 large eggs

2 ripe tomatoes

extra virgin olive oil

¼ of a small red onion

1 lime

½ a ripe avocado

2 thick slices of seeded
   wholemeal bread

4 sprigs of fresh coriander

Lay a 30cm sheet of good-quality clingfilm flat on a work surface and rub with a little olive oil. Finely slice half the chilli (deseed it if you like) and scatter in the centre of the sheet, then carefully crack an egg on top. Pull in the sides of the clingfilm and, importantly, gently squeeze out any air around the egg. Tie a knot in the clingfilm to secure the egg snugly inside. Repeat with the remaining chilli and the second egg, then put the parcels to one side. Place a pan of water on a medium heat and bring to a simmer.

Use a small sharp knife to remove the core from the tomatoes, then drop them into the simmering water for just 40 seconds. Remove to cold water, then peel and chop into eighths, discarding the seedy centre. Place in a bowl with 1 teaspoon of extra virgin olive oil. Peel and coarsely grate in the onion, mix together, then season to taste with sea salt, black pepper and half the lime juice. Poach the eggs in the simmering water for around 6 minutes for soft-boiled, or until cooked to your liking.

Meanwhile, peel, destone and smash up the avo with the remaining lime juice and season to perfection. Toast the bread, then divide and spread the smashed avo on it like butter, and spoon over the dressed tomato. Unwrap your eggs and place them proudly on top, then finish with the coriander leaves.

CALORIES	FAT	SAT FAT	PROTEIN	CARBS	SUGAR	FIBRE	
258kcal	13.9g	3.2g	12.6g	23g	5.1g	5g	10 MINUTES

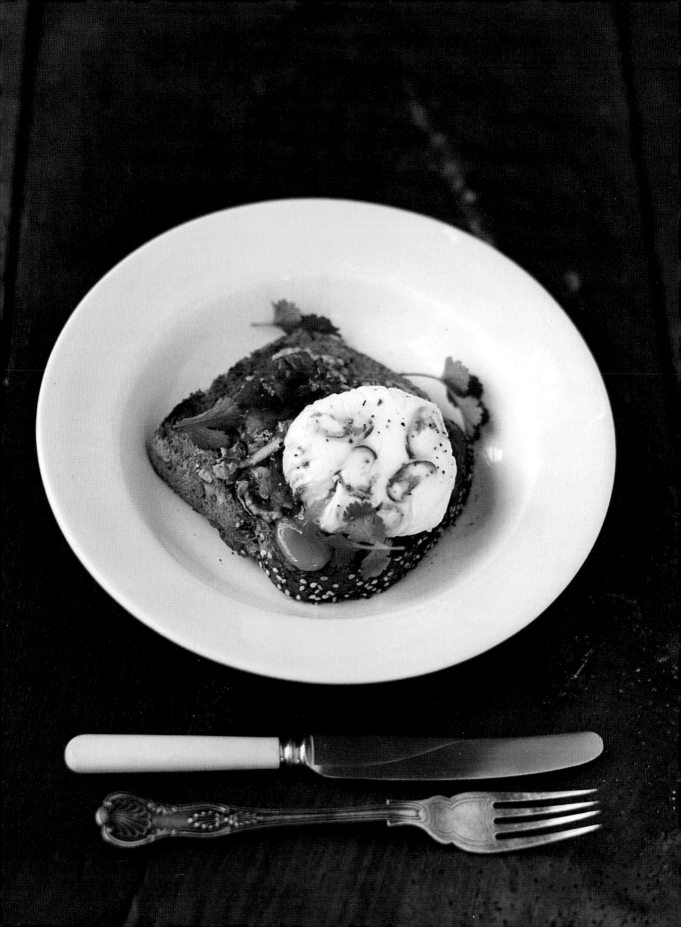

SMOOTHIE PANCAKES
BERRIES, BANANA, YOGHURT & NUTS

_ The high-fibre wholemeal flour in these super-pancakes will help keep us full till _
lunch, plus we get one of our 5-a-day and a nice vitamin C boost from the fruit

MAKES 4 PORTIONS

320g blueberries or raspberries

1 ripe banana

170ml semi-skimmed milk

1 large egg

250g wholemeal self-raising flour

4 tablespoons natural yoghurt

ground cinnamon

30g mixed unsalted chopped
    nuts, such as walnuts, pecans,
    hazelnuts

manuka honey

Blitz half the blueberries or raspberries, the peeled banana, milk, egg and flour in a blender to make a smoothie pancake batter. Tip into a bowl and fold in the remaining berries. Place a large non-stick frying pan on a medium–high heat. Once hot, put your batter into the pan to make large pancakes or little ones, whichever you fancy. Either way, cook for a couple of minutes on each side, or until crisp and golden. Sometimes I flip them for an additional 30 seconds on each brown side to ensure they get super-crispy. Serve as and when they're ready, while you get on with more.

To serve, I like to slice my pancakes in half so you can see all that lovely fruit, like in the picture. Top with a dollop of yoghurt, a sprinkling of cinnamon and a scattering of toasted nuts, then finish with a little drizzle of honey.

....
: ⌐⌐ ⌐⌐⌐ ⌐ade the pancake batter, you can cook it right away or pop :
: it into t⌐ ⌐ ⌐ge to keep for up to 3 days, to use each morning. :
....

CALORIES	FAT	SAT FAT	PROTEIN	CARBS	SUGAR	FIBRE	20 MINUTES
357kcal	10g	2.2g	13.3g	54.9g	17g	8.9g	

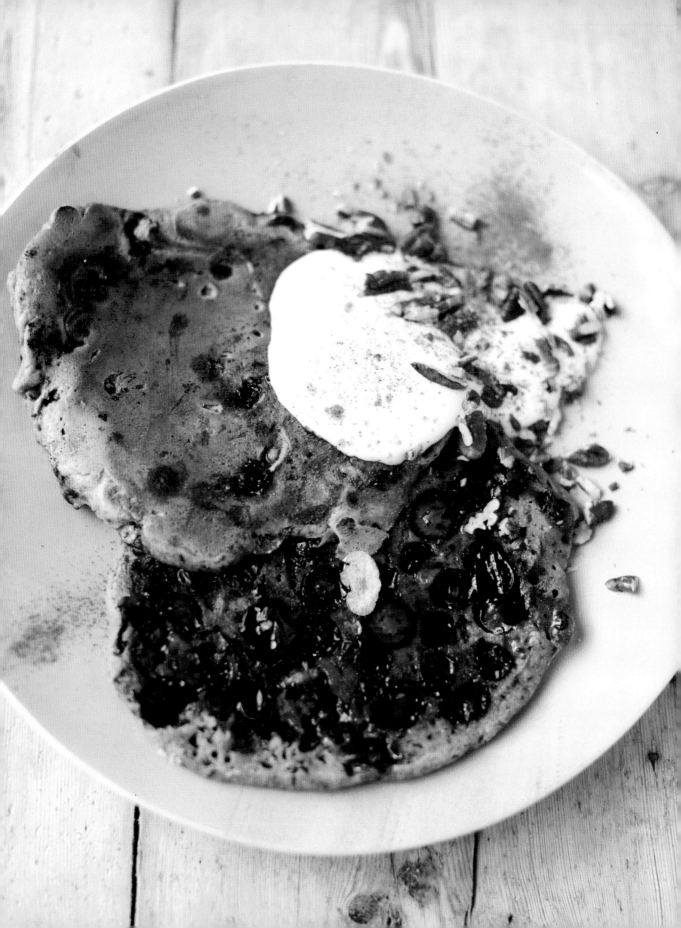

MEXICAN PAN-COOKED BREKKIE
EGGS, BEANS, TOMATOES, MUSHROOMS

— Wonderful little black beans are the highest-protein bean, so are great for brekkie, especially if we exercise in the morning as protein helps our muscles to repair —

SERVES 2

olive oil

2 ripe mixed-colour tomatoes

6 chestnut mushrooms

2 large eggs

½ x 400g tin of black beans

Worcestershire sauce

1 wholemeal tortilla

2 tablespoons cottage cheese

2 sprigs of fresh coriander

Tabasco chipotle sauce

Put a 25cm frying pan on a medium heat with 2 teaspoons of oil. Halve the tomatoes and add cut side down. Slice the rim and stalk off the mushrooms, exposing the whole inside, and place face down in the pan (keep the trimmings for another day). Cook for 6 to 7 minutes, gently twiddling the tomatoes and mushrooms in the oil and turning only when beautifully golden.

Reduce the heat to low and crack the eggs into the pan, angling it so the whites completely coat the base to create a yummy eggy plate. Working fairly quickly, drain the beans and toss with a splash of Worcestershire sauce, then scatter into the pan. Sprinkle with a pinch of sea salt and black pepper from a height, then cover the pan with a lid, plate or tin foil and leave for about 2 minutes, or until the eggs are cooked to your liking.

Meanwhile, warm the tortilla in a dry pan for just 1 minute, then slice into 1cm strips for dipping. Serve the breakfast straight from the pan or slide it onto a sharing plate. Add dollops of cottage cheese, pick and sprinkle over the coriander leaves and finish with a drizzle of Tabasco chipotle sauce.

CALORIES	FAT	SAT FAT	PROTEIN	CARBS	SUGAR	FIBRE	15 MINUTES
324kcal	13.1g	3.7g	20g	25.7g	4.7g	14.1g	

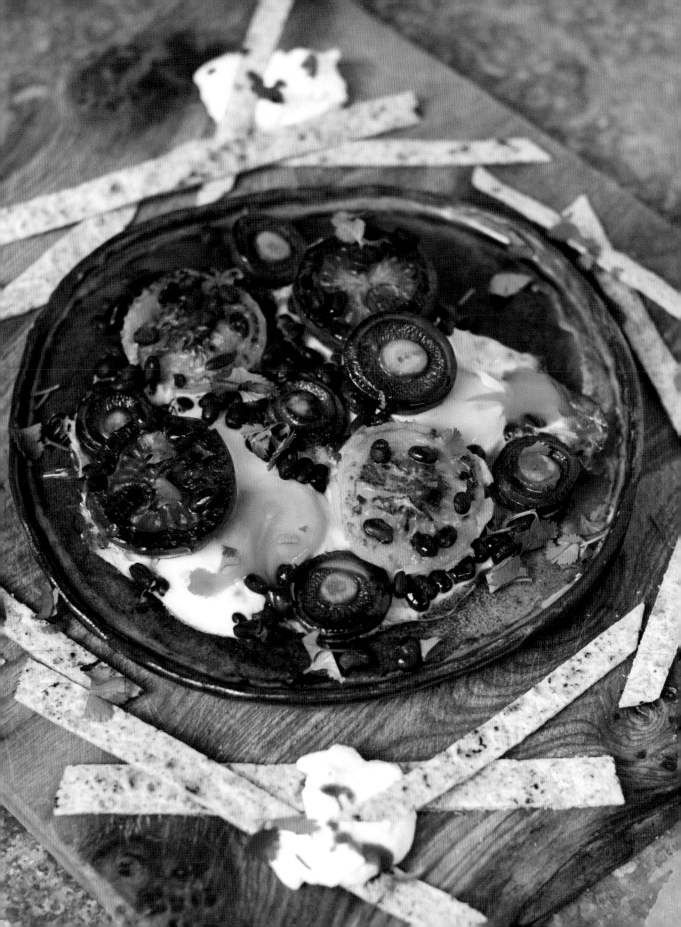

BLACK RICE PUDDING
MANGO, LIME, PASSION FRUIT & COCONUT

Hazelnut milk contains vitamin B12, helping us to think properly and stay alert, while hazelnuts are super-high in vitamin E, protecting our cells against damage

MAKES 4 JARS

200g black rice

1 ripe mango

1 lime

1 tablespoon blanched hazelnuts

1 tablespoon coconut flakes

2 ripe bananas

200ml hazelnut milk

1 tablespoon vanilla extract

optional: manuka honey

4 heaped tablespoons natural
   yoghurt

2 wrinkly passion fruit

Cook the black rice according to the packet instructions, overcooking it slightly so it's plump and sticky, then drain and cool. Meanwhile, peel and destone the mango, blitz the flesh in a blender with the lime juice until smooth, and pour into a bowl. Separately, toast the hazelnuts and coconut in a dry frying pan until lightly golden, then bash up in a pestle and mortar.

Peel the bananas and tear into the blender, then blitz with the hazelnut milk, vanilla extract and two-thirds of the black rice – depending on the sweetness of your bananas, you could also add a teaspoon of honey. Once smooth, stir that back through the rest of the rice – this will give you great texture and colour. Divide between four nice jars or bowls. Spoon over the blitzed mango, squeeze half a passion fruit over each one, then delicately spoon over the yoghurt and sprinkle with the hazelnuts and coconut.

> I make these on a Sunday night and rack them up in the fridge, ready and waiting to be enjoyed with no effort in the days that follow.

CALORIES	FAT	SAT FAT	PROTEIN	CARBS	SUGAR	FIBRE	
277kcal	6.2g	2.5g	6.5g	48.4g	11.4g	5.2g	50 MINUTES

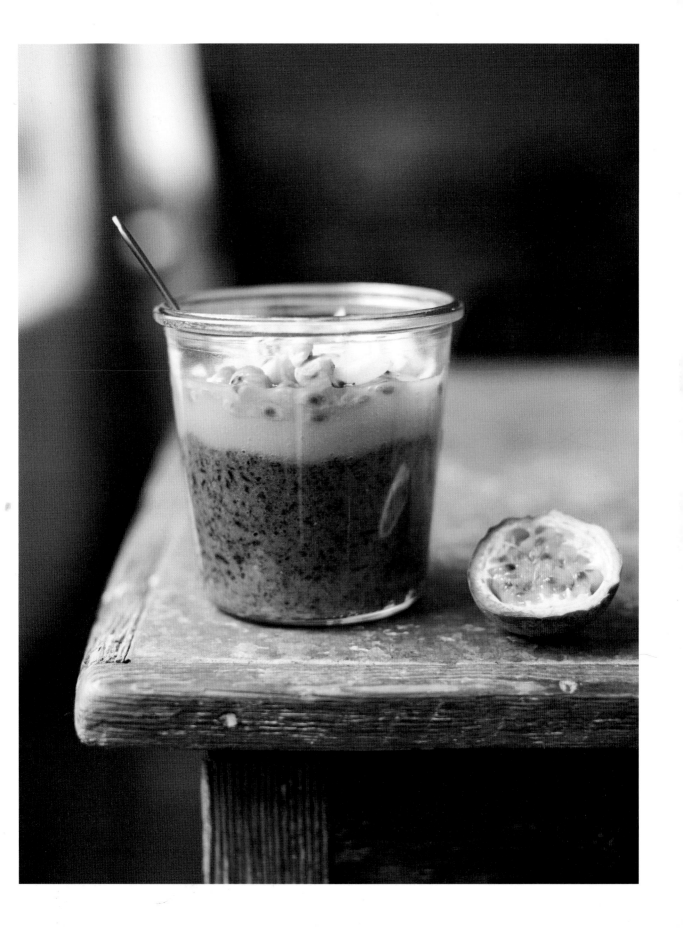

FIGGY BANANA BREAD
BLOOD ORANGE & NUT BUTTER

Full of healthy ingredients, this beautiful bread uses nutrient-packed wholemeal flour, nuts, seeds and good oil, utilizing the natural sweetness of figs, rather than adding sugar

SERVES 12

250g dried figs

75ml cold-pressed rapeseed oil

125g natural yoghurt

1 tablespoon vanilla extract

4 ripe bananas

2 large eggs

150g wholemeal self-raising flour

1 heaped teaspoon baking powder

100g ground almonds

1 tablespoon poppy seeds

½ teaspoon ground turmeric

1 eating apple

50g whole almonds

Preheat the oven to 180°C/350°F/gas 4. Line a 25cm ovenproof frying pan or tin with a scrunched sheet of wet greaseproof paper. Place 200g of figs in a food processor with the oil, yoghurt, vanilla extract, peeled bananas and eggs, then blitz until smooth. Add the flour, baking powder, ground almonds, poppy seeds and turmeric and pulse until just combined, but don't overwork the mixture. Coarsely grate and stir in the apple.

Spoon the mixture into the prepared pan and spread out evenly. Tear over the remaining figs, pushing them in slightly, then chop the almonds and scatter over. Bake for 35 to 40 minutes, or until golden, cooked through and an inserted skewer comes out clean. Transfer to a wire rack to cool a little.

I like to serve each portion with 1 tablespoon of nut butter (see page 242), 1 tablespoon of natural yoghurt and some wedges of blood orange. Store any extra portions in an airtight container, where it will keep for 2 to 3 days.

CALORIES	FAT	SAT FAT	PROTEIN	CARBS	SUGAR	FIBRE	50 MINUTES
250kcal	15.8g	1.7g	7.5g	29g	20.3g	4g	

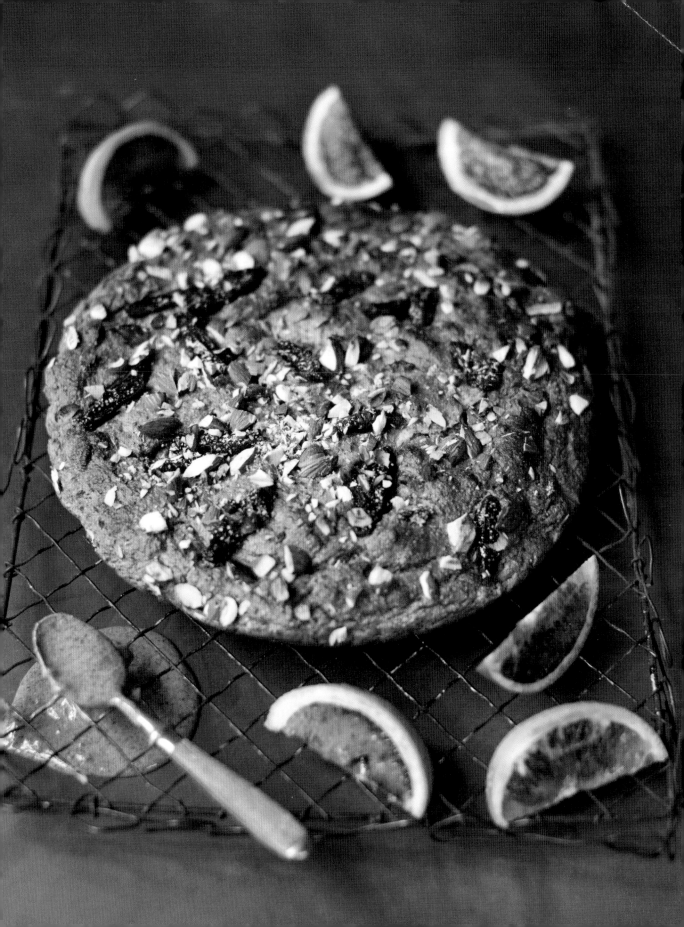

SILKEN OMELETTE
SPINACH, TOMATO, PARMESAN & RYE

— Rye bread is super-high in fibre, as well as the mineral manganese, which protects the —
tissue connecting our organs as well as our bones, keeping us strong and healthy

SERVES 1

1 small slice of rye bread

olive oil

2 large eggs

5g Parmesan cheese

1 handful of baby spinach

hot chilli sauce

1 beautifully ripe tomato

This omelette cooks really quickly in a hot pan. The heat of the pan is our friend – it prevents the omelette from sticking. At the same time, we don't want to colour the omelette – it really takes no time to cook at all. So, pop the rye bread on to toast. Place a 30cm non-stick frying pan on a high heat with a drizzle of oil, then wipe it around and out with kitchen paper.

When the pan's hot, beat the eggs in a bowl for 10 seconds, then pour into the pan and swirl around two or three times to cover the base. Evenly grate the cheese over the egg from a height, then turn the heat off. By the time you've done that, the omelette will be cooked. Use a rubber spatula to gently ease it away from the edges and fold it in half – then I like to roll it up a few times, or fold it into quarters or eighths. If folding and rolling causes you any problems just think badly folded handkerchief and you'll achieve that lovely texture. Pile the spinach onto your toast and top with the omelette and a few drips of chilli sauce. Slice the tomato, sprinkle with a little sea salt, and enjoy on the side.

Feel free to add some torn fresh herbs, such as oregano, flat-leaf parsley or basil, to your eggs too if you fancy, or to use any other good hard cheese.

CALORIES	FAT	SAT FAT	PROTEIN	CARBS	SUGAR	FIBRE	10 MINUTES
259kcal	14.8g	4g	19.3g	14.6g	3.5g	2.6g	

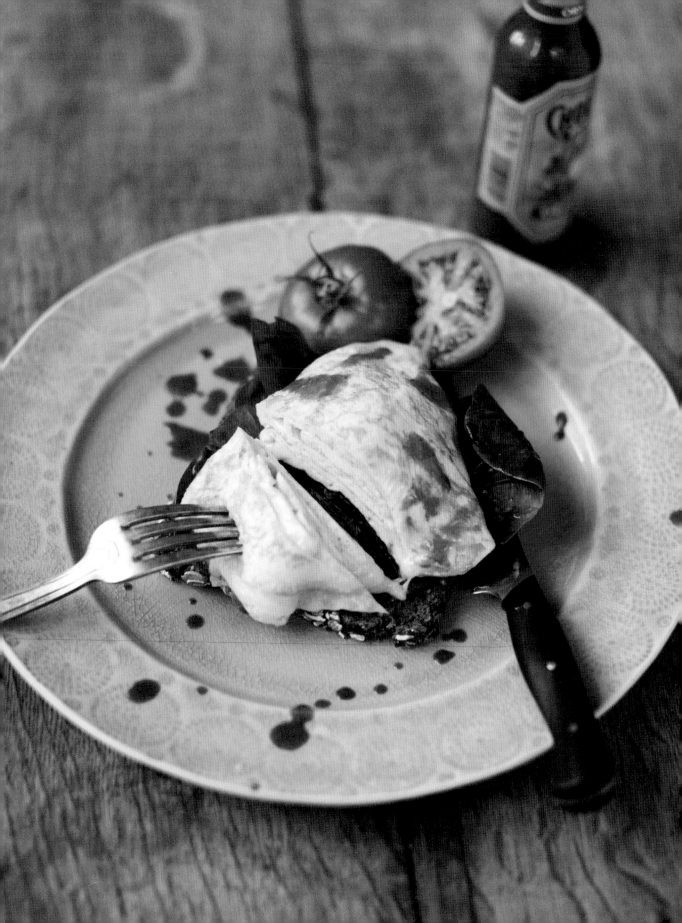

PRETTY FRUIT POTS
TRENDY CHIA & NUT MILK

_ Chia seeds are pretty cool if you flavour them well. They're really high in protein _
and fibre, and a source of magnesium, for strong and healthy bones and teeth

MAKES 10 POTS

4 small bananas (400g)

1 teaspoon vanilla extract

600ml chilled hazelnut or
    unsweetened almond milk

120g chia seeds

300g frozen fruit, such as mango
    or mixed berries

½ a lime

Peel and tear 3 bananas into a blender. Add the vanilla extract and 300ml of milk, then blitz until smooth. Pour into a jug, and stir in half the chia seeds. Divide between ten pots or cups, then pop into the fridge to start setting.

Meanwhile, tip your chosen frozen fruit (it's really nice to ring the changes and mix things up each time you make these) into the blender, peel and tear in the remaining banana, and add the remaining 300ml of milk and the lime juice. Blitz until smooth, then decant into the jug and stir through the remaining chia seeds. Divide between your ten pots or cups, pouring it in gently over the back of a spoon so you get a nice line where the two flavours meet. Return to the fridge and they'll be good to go in a couple of hours.

> These pretty pots are great for up to 3 days after you've made them. Each morning you can top them with any fresh fruit, granola or toasted nuts you've got, so have fun with it, and enjoy this happy colourful brekkie.

CALORIES	FAT	SAT FAT	PROTEIN	CARBS	SUGAR	FIBRE	15 MINUTES
117kcal	4.9g	0.6g	3.2g	14.7g	11.9g	6g	PLUS CHILLING

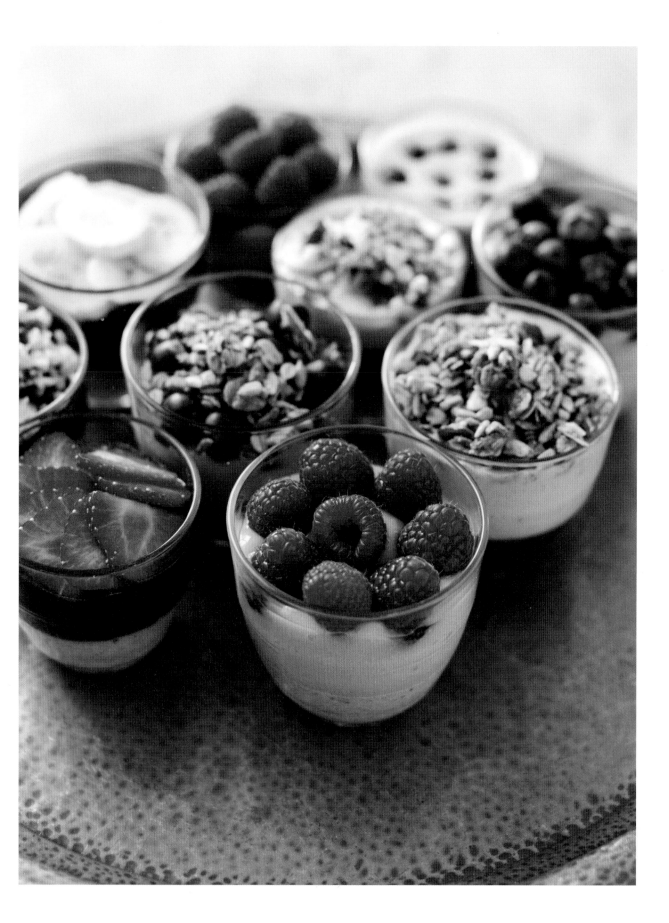

PROTEIN PORRIDGE
BLENDED OATS, SEEDS, NUTS & QUINOA

— Protein is a macronutrient that helps keep our appetites at bay – this lovely megamix of oats, seeds, nuts and brilliant quinoa will ensure we're getting a lovely morning protein boost —

MAKES 14 PORTIONS

400g porridge oats

100g linseeds

50g shelled walnuts

50g shelled pistachios

50g whole almonds

50g regular, black or red quinoa

2 teaspoons vanilla extract

3 tablespoons malted powder,
   such as Horlicks or Ovaltine

FOR EACH PORTION

150ml of your favourite milk,
   such as cow's, goat's, soya, nut
   or oat

80g seasonal berries, such
   as blueberries, raspberries,
   blackberries

1 heaped teaspoon mixed
   unsalted chopped nuts

Make up a batch of this protein porridge powder and it'll easily keep for a couple of weeks, making mornings a breeze. Just cook up, and enjoy.

In a blender, simply blitz the oats, linseeds and all the nuts, the quinoa, vanilla extract and malted powder until fine and combined, giving it a shake and working in batches if you need to. Decant the porridge powder into an airtight jar or tin, and keep covered, ready to use whenever you like.

When you want a portion, simply place 50g of protein porridge mixture in a small pan with 150ml of your favourite milk. Stir regularly for 3 minutes on a medium–low heat, or until thickened to your desired consistency.

I like to mash up half my fruit with a fork and stir it through the porridge to give it colour, flavour and natural sweetness, then serve the rest sprinkled on top with the nuts – toast them first, if you like, for extra flavour. Yum.

CALORIES	FAT	SAT FAT	PROTEIN	CARBS	SUGAR	FIBRE	
347kcal	17.4g	3.4g	14.4g	32g	13.2g	7.7g	20 MINUTES

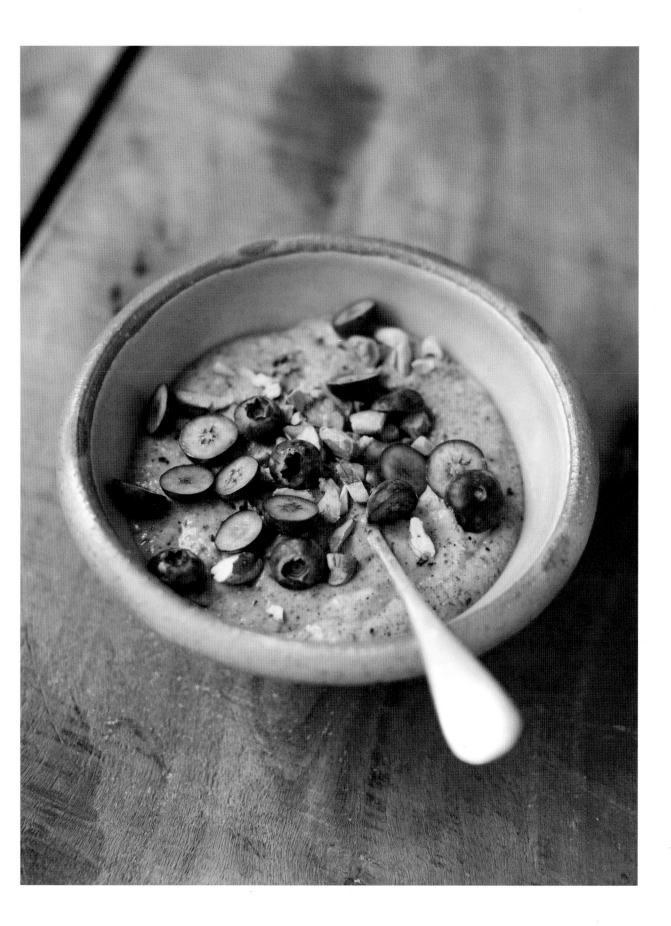

VEGEREE NOT KEDGEREE
SPICED RICE, VEG, EGGS & YOGHURT

Using veg instead of fish starts us off with two of our 5-a-day, plus all the nutrients that go with them, and the egg provides good protein to help us feel fuller for longer

SERVES 2

150g brown basmati rice

2 large eggs

4 chestnut mushrooms

3cm piece of ginger

1 fresh red chilli

½ a bunch of fresh coriander (15g)

2 spring onions

olive oil

medium curry powder

100g ripe cherry tomatoes

100g frozen peas

100g baby spinach

1 lemon

2 heaped tablespoons fat-free natural yoghurt

Cook the rice in a pan of boiling salted water according to the packet instructions, adding the eggs to the pan to soft-boil for the last 6 minutes.

Meanwhile, place a large non-stick frying pan on a medium-high heat. Quarter the mushrooms and place in the dry pan, stirring occasionally, while you peel the ginger and deseed the chilli. Saving a few slices of chilli for garnish, finely chop the rest with the ginger, half the coriander leaves and all the stalks. Trim and slice the spring onions. Push the mushrooms to one side of the pan, then add 1 tablespoon of oil, the chopped ginger, chilli, coriander and spring onions, and 1½ heaped teaspoons of curry powder. Stir-fry for 2 minutes, while you halve and add the tomatoes, followed by the peas and spinach. Drain and add the rice. Toss, stir regularly and fry for 4 minutes, then squeeze in half the lemon juice and season to perfection.

Briefly hold the eggs under cold running water until cool enough to handle, then peel, halve and dot in and around the vegeree. Spoon over the yoghurt, sprinkle with the reserved chilli and coriander leaves, add an extra pinch of curry powder and serve right away, with lemon wedges for squeezing over.

CALORIES	FAT	SAT FAT	PROTEIN	CARBS	SUGAR	FIBRE	30 MINUTES
400kcal	9.5g	2.2g	16.3g	67.2g	6.8g	5.5g	

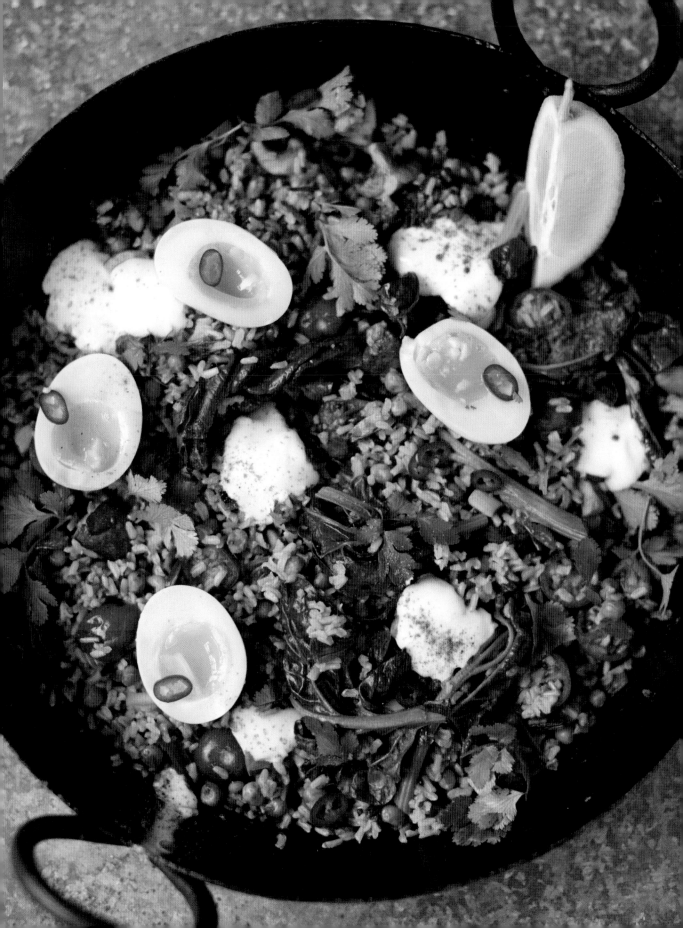

FRUIT SOUPS
YOGHURT & GRANOLA DUST

— Think of this as a smoothie in a bowl and you'll absolutely love it. Chia seeds are super-high in fibre, a macronutrient that helps keep us regular and keeps our bowels nice and healthy —

ALL SERVE 1

MINT & KIWI

In a blender, blitz **8 fresh mint leaves, 2 peeled kiwi fruit, 1 handful of baby spinach, 2 heaped tablespoons of chia seeds** and 1 regular mug of boiling water (250ml) until smooth, sweetening with a little **runny honey**, if you like. Decant into a bowl, and top with **1 heaped tablespoon of natural yoghurt, 1 handful of granola dust** (see page 18) and some **fresh fruit**. Serve straight away or chill, if you prefer.

BASIL & STRAWBERRY

In a blender, blitz **8 fresh basil leaves, 100g of hulled strawberries, 1 teaspoon of balsamic vinegar, 2 heaped tablespoons of chia seeds** and 1 regular mug of boiling water (250ml) until smooth, sweetening with a little **runny honey**, if you like. Decant into a bowl, and top with **1 heaped tablespoon of natural yoghurt, 1 handful of granola dust** (see page 18) and some **fresh fruit**. Serve straight away or chill, if you prefer.

NETTLE TEA & BLACKBERRY

Make **1 mug of nettle tea** (250ml). Once brewed, strain into a blender and blitz with **100g of blackberries** and **2 heaped tablespoons of chia seeds** until smooth, sweetening with a little **runny honey**, if you like. Decant into a bowl, and top with **1 heaped tablespoon of natural yoghurt, 1 handful of granola dust** (see page 18) and some **fresh fruit**. Serve straight away or chill, if you prefer.

GINGER TEA & MANGO

Make **1 mug of ginger tea** (250ml). Once brewed, strain into a blender and blitz with **100g of frozen mango, ½ a level teaspoon of ground turmeric**, the **juice of ½ a lime** and **2 heaped tablespoons of chia seeds** until smooth, sweetening with a little **runny honey**, if you like. Decant into a bowl, and top with **1 heaped tablespoon of natural yoghurt, 1 handful of granola dust** (see page 18) and some **fresh fruit**. Serve straight away or chill, if you prefer.

CALORIES	FAT	SAT FAT	PROTEIN	CARBS	SUGAR	FIBRE	5 MINUTES
375kcal	18.1g	2.5g	14.1g	36.1g	23.5g	19.6g	

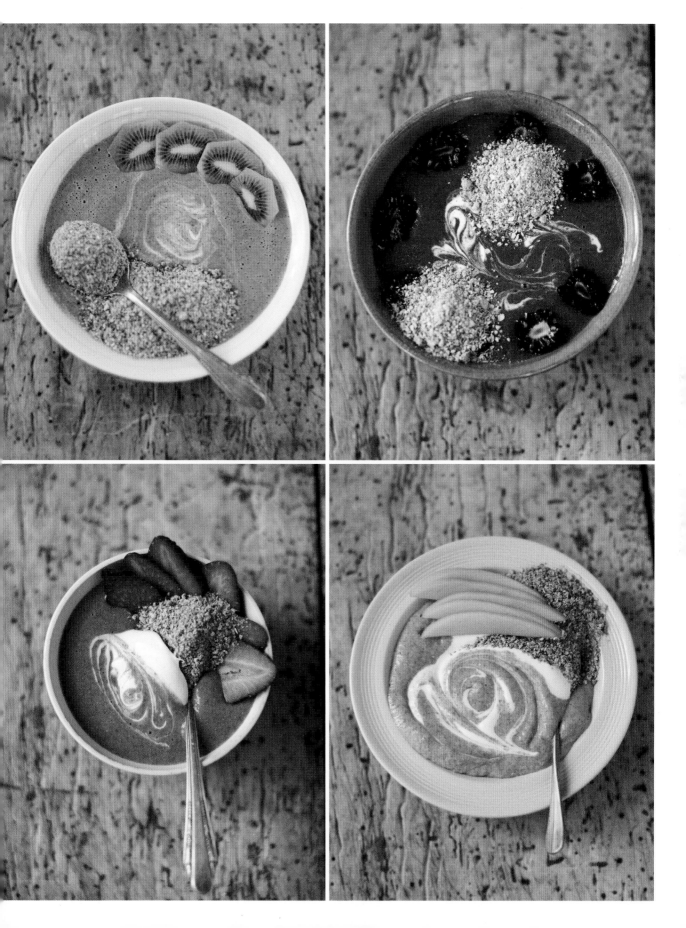

HARISSA WAFFLES
SESAME FRIED EGGS & CARROT SALAD

There's lots of goodness in these waffles – wholemeal flour gives fibre to fill us up and keep pre-lunch hunger pangs at bay, while milk provides an all-important hit of calcium

SERVES 2

100g wholemeal self-raising flour

1 tablespoon poppy seeds

2 teaspoons harissa

3 large eggs

100ml semi-skimmed milk

sesame oil

sesame seeds

1 large carrot

50g baby spinach

1 pomegranate

2 sprigs of fresh mint

2 tablespoons fat-free natural yoghurt

hot chilli sauce

Preheat your waffle iron. In a bowl, mix the flour, poppy seeds, harissa and 1 egg together, then gradually add the milk, whisking until combined, and season with sea salt and black pepper. Brush the waffle iron with a minimal amount of sesame oil, then sprinkle half a teaspoon of sesame seeds into each side, followed by a quarter of your waffle mixture each side – I make two small waffles, rather than one big one, per person by only part-filling each mould, giving you the ability to make a waffle sandwich later! Cook the waffles for a few minutes, or until golden, fluffy and cooked through.

Meanwhile, peel and matchstick the carrot, ideally on a mandolin (use the guard!), place in a bowl, then finely slice and add the spinach. Halve the pomegranate, then, holding one half cut side down in your fingers, bash the back with a spoon so the seeds tumble into the bowl. Squeeze the other half through your fingers so the juice dresses the salad. Toss together, then pick and tear over the mint leaves. Drizzle a small non-stick frying pan on a medium heat with oil, then wipe around and out with kitchen paper. Crack in 1 of the remaining eggs, sprinkle with a pinch of sesame seeds, then cover the pan to set the top of the egg and cook to your liking.

Serve the waffles with half the salad, the sesame fried egg, a dollop of yoghurt and a good shake of chilli sauce, then get on with your second portion.

CALORIES	FAT	SAT FAT	PROTEIN	CARBS	SUGAR	FIBRE	
366kcal	15g	3.7g	23g	41.5g	11.4g	8.4g	25 MINUTES

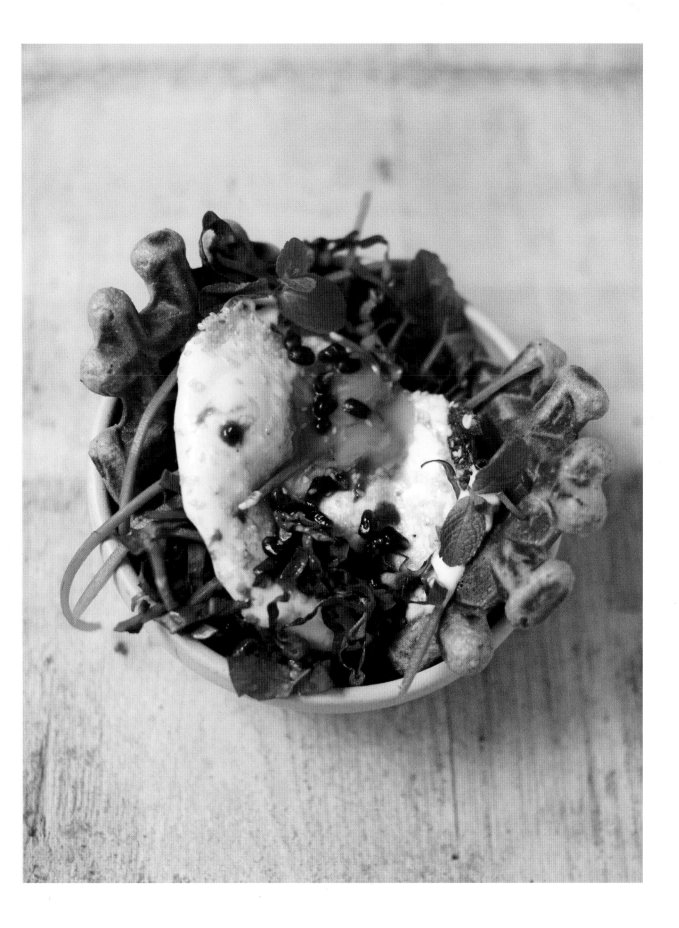

RYE SODA BREAD
SUPER-FAST, SUPER-EASY

_ Rye flour is high in lots of essential nutrients, especially phosphorus. Adding oats to _
the equation really ups the fibre content of the loaf too – it's a real all-rounder

SERVES 6

250g wholemeal flour, plus extra
for dusting

100g rye flour

50g porridge oats

1 teaspoon bicarbonate of soda

1 large egg

1 x 300ml tub of buttermilk
or natural yoghurt

This bread is delicious hot from the oven – it requires no proving in the making, and there are lots of wonderful ways to enjoy it. Preheat the oven to 190°C/375°F/gas 5. Place both flours, the oats, bicarbonate of soda and 1 level teaspoon of sea salt in a large bowl and mix together. In a separate bowl, whisk the egg and buttermilk or yoghurt together, then use a fork to stir the egg mixture into the flour. Once it starts to come together, use your lightly floured clean hands to pat and bring the dough together.

Shape the dough into a round ball and place on a lightly floured baking tray, dusting the top lightly with flour, too. Use your hands to flatten the dough into a disc, roughly 3cm deep. Score a cross or star into the top with a knife, about ½cm deep, then bake in the centre of the oven for 40 to 45 minutes, or until a firm crust has formed and it sounds hollow when tapped on the bottom.

Transfer to a wire cooling rack, and serve slightly warm. As you'd expect, this is great with all your favourite toppings. For lots of ideas, see page 70.

CALORIES	FAT	SAT FAT	PROTEIN	CARBS	SUGAR	FIBRE	50 MINUTES
248kcal	3.3g	0.7g	10.4g	46.5g	3.5g	6.5g	

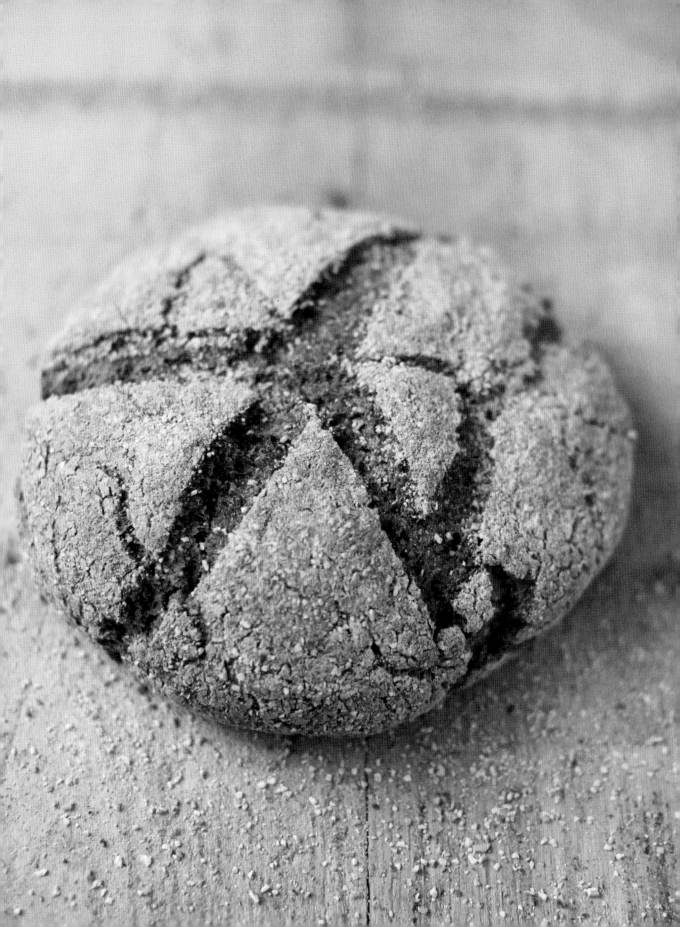

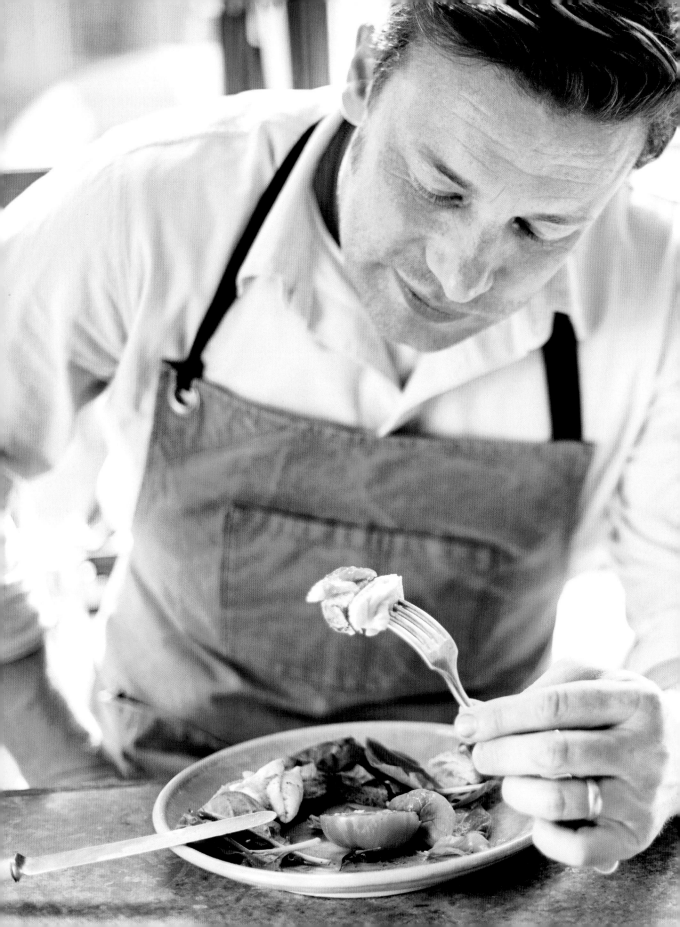

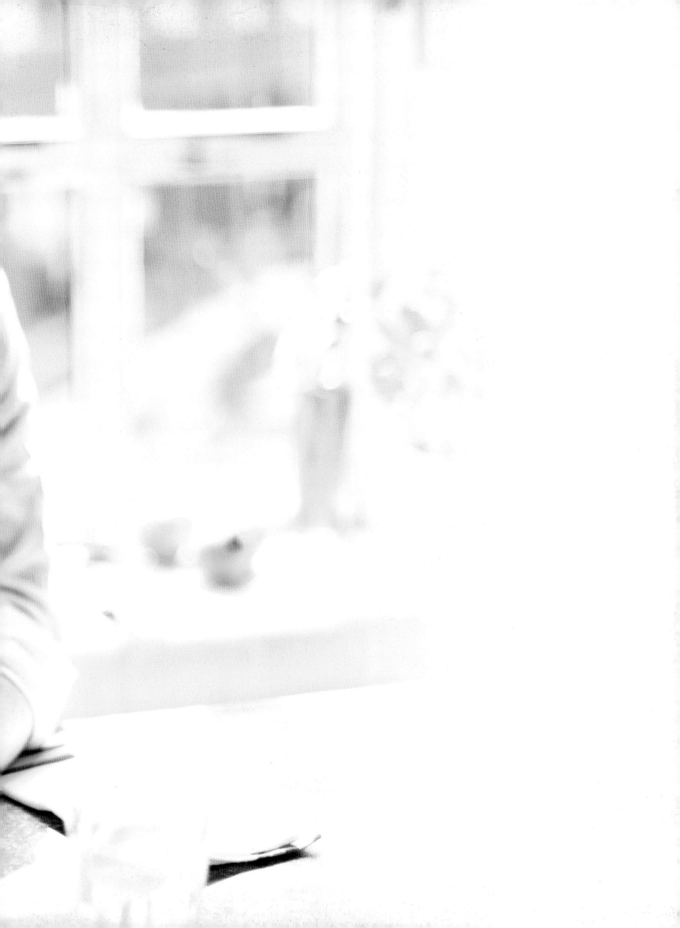

PERFECT PORRIDGE BARS
NUTS, SEEDS, FRUIT & SPICES

— These portable bars are packed with lots of complementary nutritious ingredients, such as iron-rich dried apricots, which the vitamin C in the orange helps us to absorb —

MAKES 12 PORTIONS

100g unsalted mixed nuts, such as walnuts, Brazils, hazelnuts, pecans, pistachios, cashews

50g mixed seeds, such as chia, poppy, sunflower, sesame, linseed, pumpkin

100g mixed dried fruit, such as blueberries, cranberries, sour cherries, mango, apricots, figs, sultanas

1 heaped teaspoon ground ginger

½ teaspoon ground turmeric

1 orange

2 ripe bananas

1 tablespoon runny honey

175g porridge oats

10g oat bran

Preheat the oven to 190°C/375°F/gas 5. In a food processor, pulse the nuts, seeds, dried fruit and spices with the finely grated orange zest, then tip into a bowl. Peel the orange then blitz the segments to a pulp with the peeled bananas in the processor. Pour the mixture into a measuring jug, add the honey and top up to 500ml total volume with water. Pour into a large pan on a medium-high heat and just bring to the boil, then use a rubber spatula to stir in the oats, bran and blitzed nut mixture. Keep stirring, beating and mashing over the heat for 5 minutes, or until the oats start releasing their starch and the mixture becomes gluey.

Transfer to a non-stick 25cm square baking tin. Spread it out and, to help you later, score your twelve bar portions into the top. Bake at the bottom of the oven for 45 to 50 minutes, or until golden and set. Leave to cool in the tray for 10 minutes, then transfer to a wire rack.

> Store your porridge bars in an airtight container in the fridge for up to 3 days. For a balanced brekkie, enjoy with fresh fruit and a glass of milk.

CALORIES	FAT	SAT FAT	PROTEIN	CARBS	SUGAR	FIBRE	1 HOUR
171kcal	9g	1.2g	4.4g	20.8g	11.6g	3.6g	

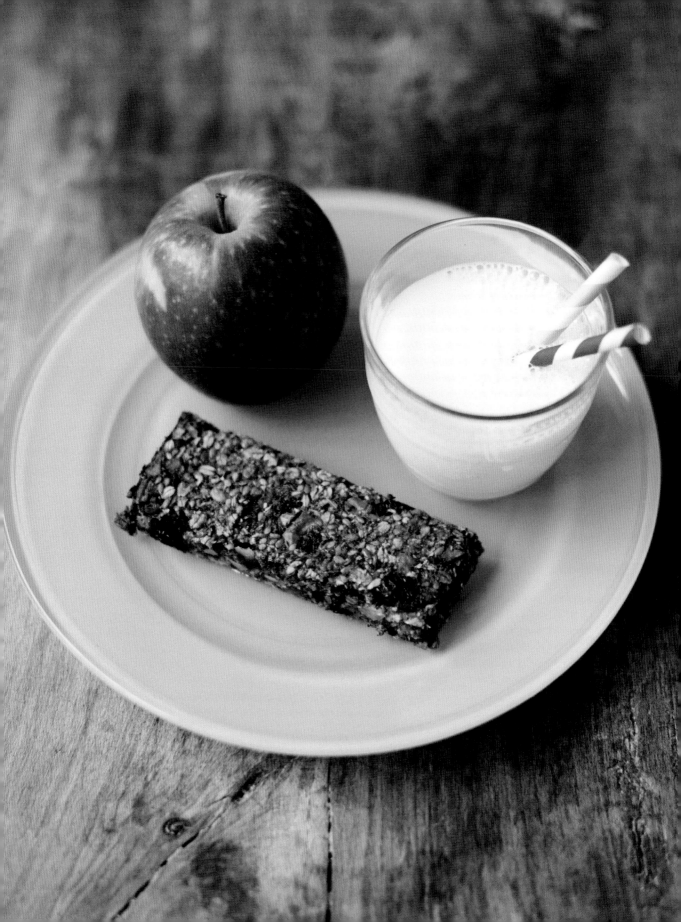

BREAKFAST POPOVERS
CHEESE, HAM, MUSHROOM & TOMATO

__ As well as being super-quick and tasty, cottage cheese, eggs and ham all give us satiating __
protein, helping our muscles to repair and recover and helping to keep us full till lunch

SERVES 2

1 heaped tablespoon wholemeal
self-raising flour

1 large egg

2 heaped tablespoons cottage
cheese

1 slice of quality smoked ham

1 ripe plum tomato

2 chestnut mushrooms

15g Parmesan cheese

hot chilli sauce

2 tablespoons natural yoghurt

2 handfuls of rocket

½ a lemon

Place the flour in a bowl and beat well with the egg and cottage cheese. Finely chop the ham, tomato and mushrooms, and stir through the mixture with a good pinch of sea salt and black pepper. Put a large non-stick frying pan on a medium-low heat. Once hot, put heaped spoonfuls of the mixture into the pan to give you six popovers. Leave them to get nicely golden for a few minutes, then flip over and gently flatten to 1cm thick with a palette knife.

Once golden on both sides, remove the popovers from the pan for a moment, then turn the heat off. Finely grate the Parmesan into the pan to melt. Place the popovers on top, wait for the Parmesan to sizzle and go golden from the residual heat of the pan, then use your palette knife to gently push the cheese towards each popover. Once the crispy popovers can be easily prised away from the pan with your palette knife, bang them out on to a board.

Swirl some chilli sauce through the yoghurt, toss the rocket in a squeeze of lemon juice and serve both on the side, then enjoy!

CALORIES	FAT	SAT FAT	PROTEIN	CARBS	SUGAR	FIBRE	10 MINUTES
189kcal	9g	4g	15.1g	11.8g	4.3g	2.5g	

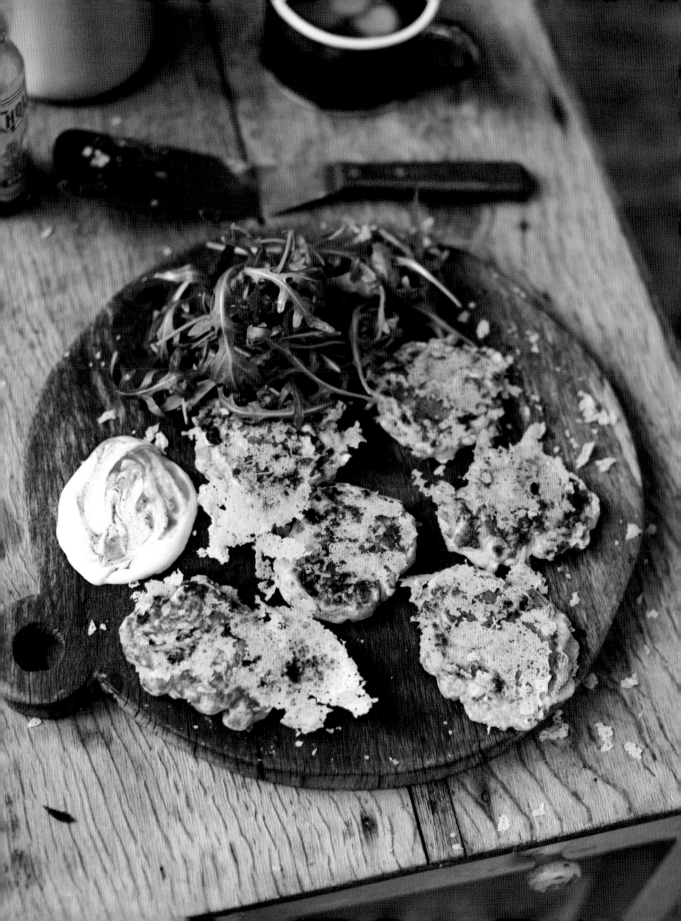

BERRY POCKET EGGY BREAD
PISTACHIOS, YOGHURT, HONEY & CINNAMON

— Crunchy pistachios are super-high in the mineral chloride, which our bodies need to make hydrochloric acid in the stomach, in turn aiding good digestion and keeping our gut happy —

SERVES 2

2 large eggs

1 small ripe banana

ground nutmeg

ground cinnamon

2 thick slices of seeded
   wholemeal bread

150g raspberries

olive oil

20g shelled pistachios

4 heaped tablespoons fat-free
   natural yoghurt

manuka honey

In a blender, blitz the eggs, peeled banana, and 1 pinch each of nutmeg and cinnamon until smooth, then pour into a wide shallow bowl. Cut your bread 2½cm thick, then cut a slit into the longest side of each slice and wiggle your knife inside to make a pocket. Use your finger to stuff the raspberries inside – pack as many in as you can, but be gentle so you don't tear the bread. Lay in the eggy mixture and gently squash the bread so it soaks up the eggs.

Meanwhile, put a large non-stick frying pan on a medium-low heat with 1 teaspoon of oil, then wipe it around and out with kitchen paper. Pour half the excess egg mixture into one side of the pan, then place a piece of soaked bread on top to give it a lovely pancake layer. Repeat with the rest of the mixture and the other slice alongside it. Cook for 3 to 4 minutes, or until golden, then confidently flip over to cook for the same amount of time. Meanwhile, smash up the pistachios in a pestle and mortar – toast them first, if you like.

Serve the eggy bread dolloped with yoghurt, sprinkled with pistachios and an extra pinch of cinnamon and drizzled with a little honey.

CALORIES	FAT	SAT FAT	PROTEIN	CARBS	SUGAR	FIBRE	15 MINUTES
344kcal	14.4g	3.1g	18.8g	38.2g	17.4g	6.7g	

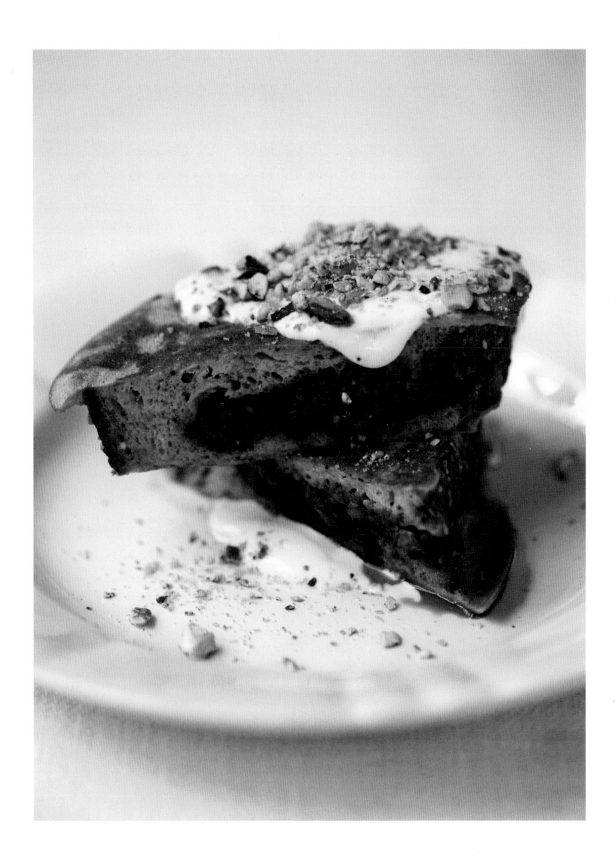

RAINBOW OPEN WRAP
SALAD, FETA & SPICED CRISPY BEANS

— Packed with a massive four of our 5-a-day, this also heroes black-eyed beans, which are full of protein, iron and B vitamins, especially folic acid, important for any expectant mothers —

SERVES 2

½ x 400g tin of black-eyed beans

sweet smoked paprika

4 heaped tablespoons natural yoghurt

½ a bunch of fresh coriander (15g)

2 limes

¼ of a small cucumber

1 small carrot

¼ of a small red cabbage (150g)

1 ripe tomato

¼ of an iceberg lettuce

1 fresh red chilli

2 spelt or wholewheat flatbreads

20g feta cheese

Drain the beans well, toss with a good pinch of paprika, tip them into a large non-stick frying pan on a high heat and simply leave to crisp up for around 10 minutes, or until they crackle and pop, then remove to a plate.

Meanwhile, in a blender blitz up the yoghurt, half the coriander leaves and all the stalks, and the juice of 1 lime to make a simple, clean dressing, then taste and season to perfection. Run your fork lengthways down the cucumber to create grooves, then finely slice along with the carrot, cabbage, tomato, iceberg and chilli (deseed if you like), either by hand with good knife skills, or ideally, for really beautiful results, on a mandolin (use the guard!).

Just warm the flatbreads in the empty frying pan for 20 seconds to make them flexible, then divide the veg between them and top with the crispy beans, a good drizzle of the dressing and a crumbling of feta. Pick over the remaining coriander leaves and add an extra squeeze of lime juice if you like, to taste. Roll them up and tuck in – they're a messy eat, but totally delicious. And as great as these are on their own, they're equally brilliant with a little leftover grilled or roasted meat thrown into the mix.

CALORIES	FAT	SAT FAT	PROTEIN	CARBS	SUGAR	FIBRE	15 MINUTES
313kcal	8.9g	3g	15.9g	37.2g	10.8g	16.5g	

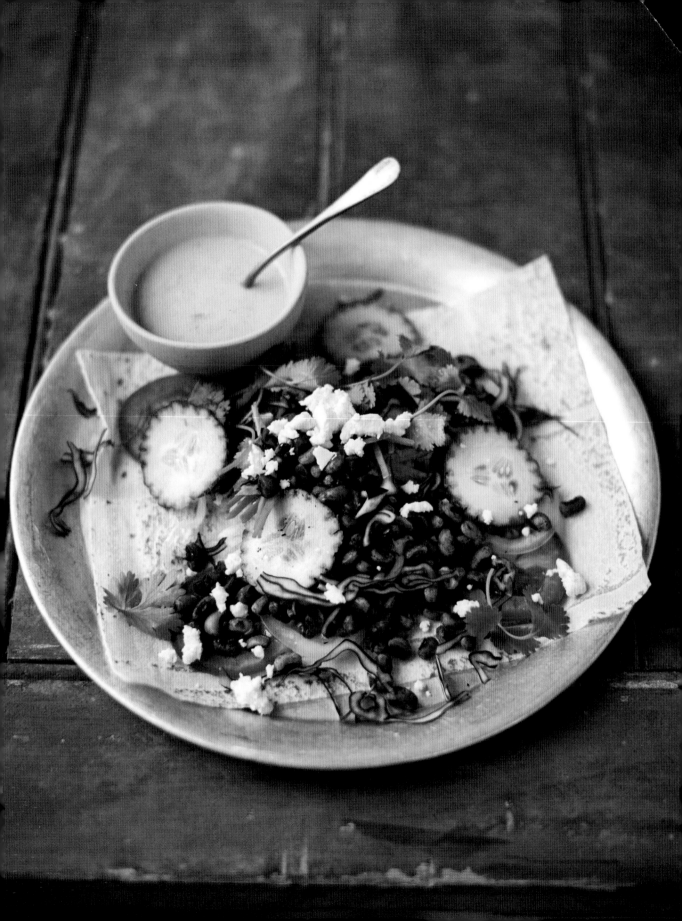

SCRAMBLED EGGS – PART ONE

Eggs are amazing – just two eggs give us over a day's worth of vitamin B12, which helps our bodies to produce red blood cells, keeping us awake and alert, perfect for the morning

BOTH SERVE 1

SMOKED SALMON & SPRING ONION EGGS

Pop **1 small slice of sourdough bread** on to toast. Trim **1 spring onion** and finely slice it with **25g of smoked salmon**. Beat **2 large eggs** with 1 pinch of black pepper, then fold through the sliced spring onion and smoked salmon. Put a small non-stick frying pan on a medium heat and wipe with a piece of oiled kitchen paper. Pour the egg mixture into the pan, and stir every 10 seconds with a rubber spatula until you've got beautiful silky strips of cooked egg, surrounded by softer, custardy egg. Serve on the toast, with **1 wedge of lemon** for squeezing over.

CALORIES	FAT	SAT FAT	PROTEIN	CARBS	SUGAR	FIBRE	5 TO 10 MINUTES
315kcal	15g	3.9g	25.1g	20.8g	2.2g	1.3g	

SPINACH, PARMESAN & CHILLI EGGS

Pop **1 small slice of seeded wholemeal bread** on to toast. Put a small non-stick frying pan on a medium heat and wipe with a piece of oiled kitchen paper. Finely chop **1 handful of baby spinach** and add to the pan to wilt, while you beat **2 large eggs** with 1 small pinch of sea salt and black pepper. Pour the eggs into the pan, finely grate in **5g of Parmesan cheese**, and stir every 10 seconds with a rubber spatula until you've got beautiful silky strips of cooked egg, surrounded by softer, custardy egg. Serve on the toast, with some sliced **fresh red chilli** on top.

CALORIES	FAT	SAT FAT	PROTEIN	CARBS	SUGAR	FIBRE	5 TO 10 MINUTES
300kcal	15.2g	4g	22.6g	17.6g	3.1g	3.2g	

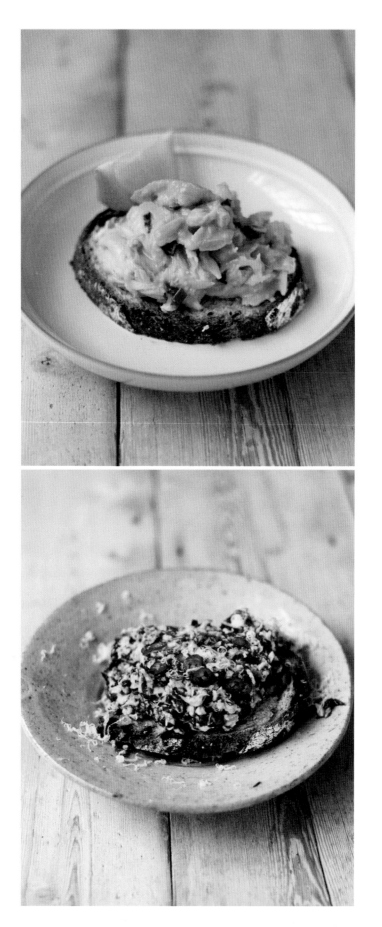

SCRAMBLED EGGS - PART TWO

As well as B_{12}, eggs provide a source of nearly all the other B vitamins, plus vitamin D, phosphorus, iodine, selenium and protein – what a nutritional powerhouse!

BOTH SERVE 1

TOMATO, CHEESE & BASIL EGGS

Pop **1 small slice of rye bread** on to toast. Put a small non-stick frying pan on a medium heat and wipe with a piece of oiled kitchen paper. Chop **2 ripe tomatoes**, then add to the pan with 1 small pinch of sea salt and black pepper and cook for 5 minutes. Beat **2 large eggs** in a bowl and tear in **8 fresh basil leaves**. Push the thick tomato sauce aside and melt a **5g slice of cheese** on top. Pour the eggs into the pan and stir every 10 seconds with a rubber spatula until you've got beautiful silky strips of cooked egg, surrounded by softer, custardy egg. Fold through the cheesy tomatoes and serve on the toast.

CALORIES	FAT	SAT FAT	PROTEIN	CARBS	SUGAR	FIBRE	5 TO 10 MINUTES
270kcal	13.3g	4g	21.3g	18.1g	6.3g	3.4g	

MUSHROOM & MARMITE EGGS

Pop **1 small slice of seeded wholemeal bread** on to toast. Put a small non-stick frying pan on a medium heat and wipe with a piece of oiled kitchen paper. Slice **1 handful of button mushrooms**, then add to the pan with **1 teaspoon of Marmite** and a splash of water. Cook for a few minutes while you beat **2 large eggs** with 1 pinch of black pepper. Pour the eggs into the pan and stir every 10 seconds with a rubber spatula until you've got beautiful silky strips of cooked egg, surrounded by softer, custardy egg. Serve on the toast, sprinkled with **1 pinch of cayenne pepper**.

CALORIES	FAT	SAT FAT	PROTEIN	CARBS	SUGAR	FIBRE	5 TO 10 MINUTES
265kcal	12.3g	3.3g	22.4g	18.2g	1.7g	3.7g	

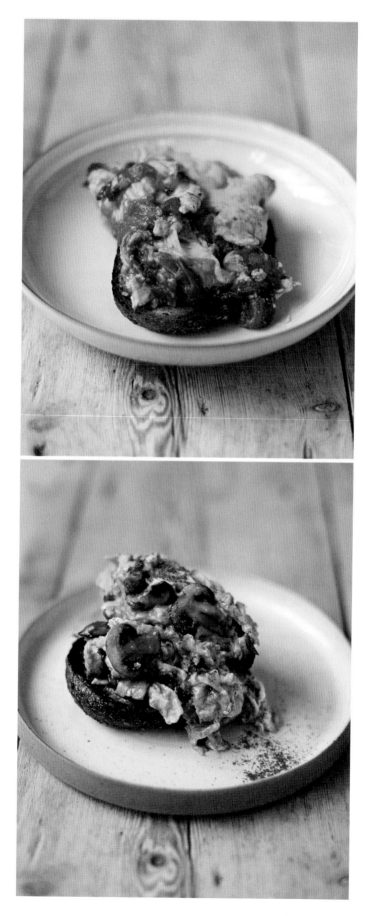

QUICK HOMEMADE TORTILLA
SCALDED VEG, CHILLI, CHEESE & AVO

Making quick, delicious wraps like this using wholemeal flour is super-easy and provides us with a great source of fibre to keep those mid-morning hunger pangs at bay

SERVES 2

extra virgin olive oil

white wine vinegar

6 spears of asparagus

6 spears of sprouting broccoli

2 ripe tomatoes

½ a ripe avocado

1 lime

80g wholemeal self-raising flour, plus extra for dusting

2 heaped tablespoons cottage cheese

hot chilli sauce

Mix 1 teaspoon each of oil and vinegar with a pinch of sea salt and black pepper in a large bowl. Put a large frying pan on a high heat. Rinse the asparagus and broccoli, then trim off the tougher ends and split the spears lengthways (other seasonal greens are great too, so embrace the best that the season has to offer). Place in the hot pan – the moisture from rinsing them will briefly steam the veg before they start to scald and char – turn halfway. Halve the tomatoes across the middle and add to the pan cut side down. Leave it all for 5 minutes, or until gnarly and on the edge of catching, removing and tossing in the bowl of dressing as and when they're done.

Peel and destone the avocado, smash up in a pestle and mortar until smooth, then muddle in the lime juice and season to perfection. To make your tortillas, simply mix the flour with 50ml of water and a pinch of salt until you have a smooth, pliable dough. On a lightly floured surface, roll out one half until 3mm thick and about 20cm in diameter, then cook through and char on one side only in a hot frying pan, so the top bubbles up, and repeat when done, I like to rest them over a rolling pin to give a natural curve to hold your filling.

Serve each tortilla loaded up with scalded veg. Spoon over the smashed avo and cottage cheese, and finish with a drizzle of chilli sauce.

CALORIES	FAT	SAT FAT	PROTEIN	CARBS	SUGAR	FIBRE	20 MINUTES
235kcal	8.4g	1.7g	10.2g	31.4g	6g	7.4g	

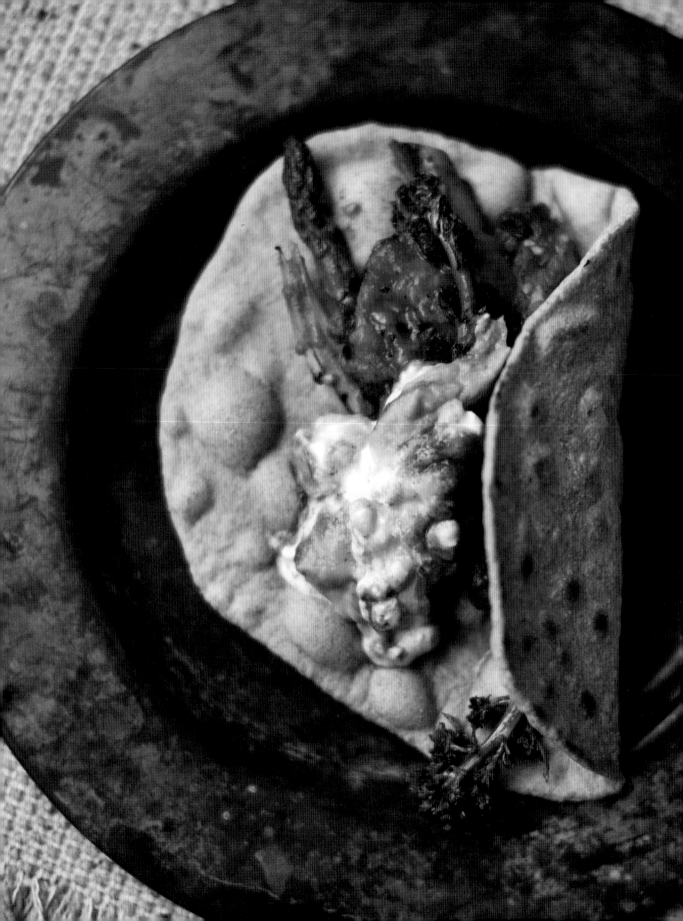

TOASTED OATS
MANGO, BLUEBERRIES & YOGHURT

_ Oats fill us up and act as a slow-burning fuel, so are a perfect start to the day. They're high in _
fibre, and the minerals phosphorus and magnesium, keeping our bones strong and healthy

SERVES 1

1 handful of porridge oats (50g)

1 level teaspoon fennel seeds

1 heaped teaspoon coconut flakes

2 heaped tablespoons natural
  yoghurt

1 small handful of blueberries

optional: rose water

1 small ripe mango

½ a banana

½ a lime

optional: manuka honey

Put the oats into a small frying pan on a medium heat with the fennel seeds and coconut and toast until lightly golden and smelling delicious, tossing regularly. Tip into your bowl and spoon the yoghurt on top.

Return the pan to the heat. Place the blueberries in with a good splash of water and a few drips of rose water (if using), which will add an incredible perfumed flavour. Simply boil for a couple of minutes until the berries burst and you have a loose sauce, then spoon over the yoghurt.

Slice one of the cheeks off the mango and cut a criss-cross pattern into the flesh, making sure you don't go all the way through, then turn it inside out so all the pieces pop up into a mango hedgehog (keep the rest of the mango for another day). Peel and slice the banana, then dress both mango and banana with a squeeze of lime juice. Add to your bowl and tuck right in. Great as it is, or if you like you can drizzle 1 teaspoon of honey over the top before serving.

CALORIES	FAT	SAT FAT	PROTEIN	CARBS	SUGAR	FIBRE	
329kcal	8.3g	3.4g	9.1g	53.5g	19.7g	8.5g	10 MINUTES

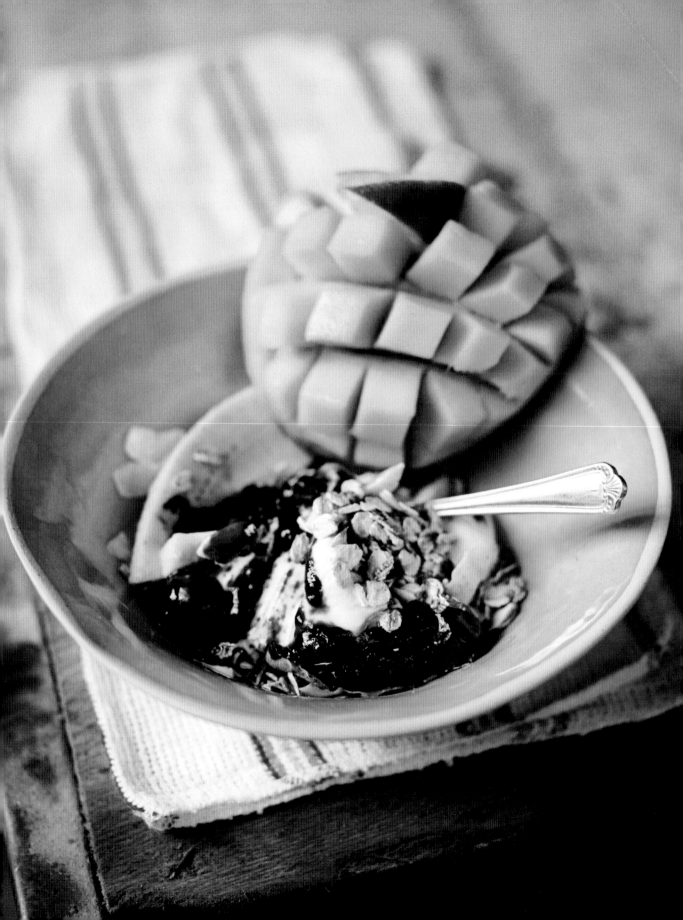

SWEET POTATO MUFFINS
CHILLI, CHEESE & SEEDS

Super sweet potatoes give us vitamin C, helping to protect our cells from damage caused by stress. The eggs, cheese and seeds also give protein, to help keep us feeling full till lunch

MAKES 6 PORTIONS

olive oil

600g sweet potatoes or
½ a butternut squash

4 spring onions

1–2 fresh red chillies

6 large eggs

3 tablespoons cottage cheese

250g wholemeal self-raising flour

50g Parmesan cheese

1 tablespoon sunflower seeds

1 tablespoon poppy seeds

Preheat the oven to 180°C/350°F/gas 4. Line a 12-hole muffin tin with paper cases or 15cm folded squares of greaseproof paper, then lightly wipe each one with oiled kitchen paper. Peel the sweet potatoes or squash and coarsely grate into a large bowl. Trim the spring onions, then finely slice with the chilli and add to the bowl, reserving half the chilli to one side. Crack in the eggs, add the cottage cheese and flour, then finely grate in most of the Parmesan and season with sea salt and black pepper. Mix until nicely combined.

Evenly divide the muffin mixture between the cases. Sprinkle over the sunflower and poppy seeds, then dot over the reserved slices of chilli. Use the remaining Parmesan to give a light dusting of cheese over each one, then bake at the bottom of the oven for 45 to 50 minutes (if using squash, it'll be a bit quicker – check after 35 minutes), or until golden and set.

These are amazing served warm 5 minutes after taking them out of the oven, and good kept in the fridge for a couple of days. Enjoy 2 muffins per portion.

> I like to make the muffin mixture and divide it up the night before, ready to bake fresh in the morning – that way you can even bake off portions as and when you want to eat them.

CALORIES	FAT	SAT FAT	PROTEIN	CARBS	SUGAR	FIBRE	1 HOUR
366kcal	12.5g	3.9g	18.2g	49.2g	7.1g	6.5g	

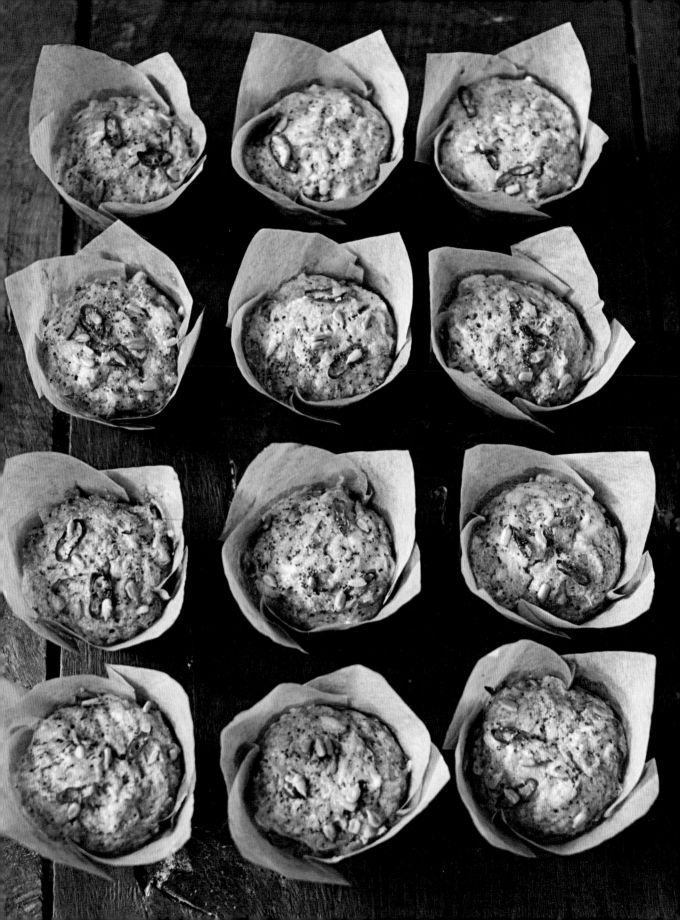

EPIC FRUIT SALAD
DELICIOUS NATURAL JUICES

— I've used a little extra virgin olive oil here so that our body absorbs all of the essential fat-soluble vitamins, such as vitamin E, found in these fruits, plus we get two of our 5-a-day —

MAKES 10 PORTIONS

2 wrinkly passion fruit

2 clementines

2 limes

½ a bunch of fresh mint (15g)

1 tablespoon cold-pressed
   extra virgin olive oil

1 teaspoon balsamic vinegar

1 ripe pineapple

1 ripe mango

2 ripe peaches

250g strawberries

200g blueberries

150g blackberries

Make a big batch of this delicious fruit salad to keep in the fridge and see you through a few days. This is an easy way to eat the good stuff.

Get yourself a big bowl that will fit happily in the fridge. Halve the passion fruit, then spoon the juicy centres into the bowl and squeeze in all the citrus juice. Pick and finely slice the mint leaves, add along with the oil and balsamic vinegar (trust me) and mix together. This will give extra flavour to your fruits, and the acid will stop any discolouring, but feel free to have fun and mix things up by adding flavours such as ginger, lemongrass, fresh basil, lemon balm, vanilla, tinned lychees or even prunes to accent the juices brilliantly.

Now for your fruit – quite simply just prep and cut it all up into random bite-sized pieces that are a pleasure to eat. Avoid using any bruised fruit – that's best frozen for use in smoothies. Add the fruit to the bowl as you prep it, then simply toss it all in the juices, cover and keep in the fridge until needed.

The combo listed here is one of my favourites, but other great fruit that's resilient enough to hold up includes grapes, melon (but not watermelon), pears, plums and papaya. Garnish-friendly fruit tends to be softer, such as bananas, raspberries and soft berries, watermelon and kiwi fruit – feel free to add this each time you take a serving to boost your fruit intake further, and remember, eating the rainbow is a wonderful thing. Serve with yoghurt or cottage cheese, and toasted nuts and seeds or granola dust (page 18).

CALORIES	FAT	SAT FAT	PROTEIN	CARBS	SUGAR	FIBRE	20 MINUTES
73kcal	1.5g	0.2g	1.1g	14.3g	13.3g	2.5g	

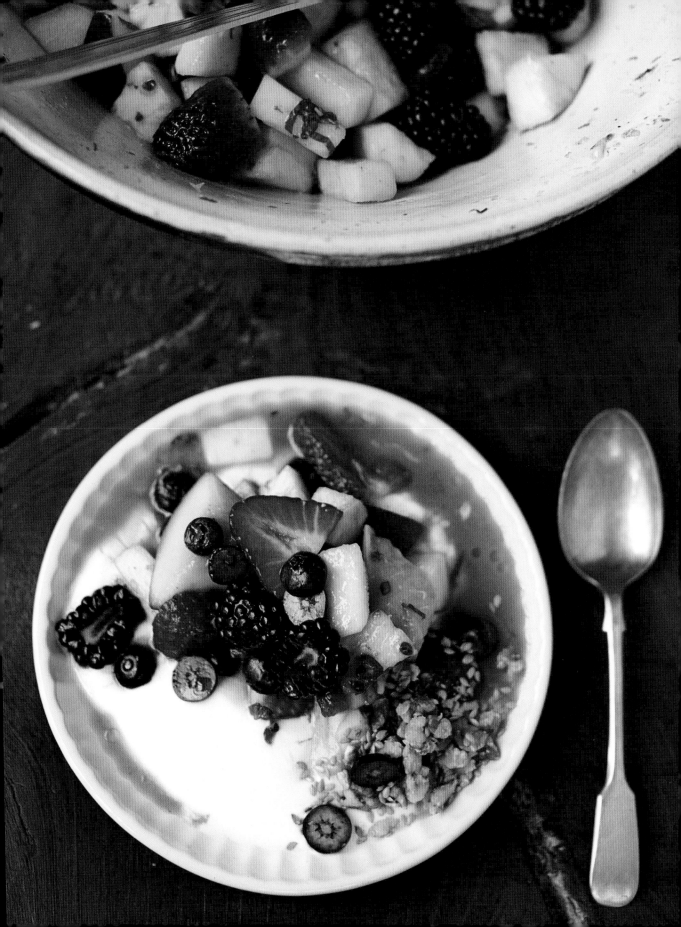

SUPER-FOOD PROTEIN LOAF
WHEAT-FREE, GLUTEN-FREE & TASTY

— For all you morning gym-goers this healthy protein bread is a great portable breakfast that will help with muscle repair and growth – for yummy topping ideas simply turn the page —

MAKES 14 PORTIONS

1 x 7g sachet of dried yeast

4 tablespoons extra virgin olive oil

250g gram flour

100g ground almonds

50g linseeds

100g mixed seeds, such as chia, poppy, sunflower, sesame, pumpkin

1 sprig of fresh rosemary

4 large eggs

optional: 3 teaspoons Marmite

Preheat the oven to 190°C/375°F/gas 5. Line a 1.5-litre loaf tin with greaseproof paper. Fill a jug with 375ml of lukewarm water, add the yeast and oil, then mix with a fork until combined and leave aside for 5 minutes.

Pile the flour, ground almonds and all the seeds into a large bowl with a pinch of sea salt and make a well in the middle. Pick, finely chop and add the rosemary leaves. Crack in the eggs, add the Marmite (if using – simply leave it out for a gluten-free friendly loaf) and beat together, then pour in the yeast mixture. Whisking as you go, gradually bring in the flour from the outside until combined – it'll be more like a batter than a dough. Pour into the prepared tin and smooth out nice and evenly on top.

Now you've got two choices – bake it straight away and it'll puff up a bit more and taste fantastic, or cover and place it in the fridge overnight and allow some slightly more complex sour flavours to develop. Both are brilliant, just different. To bake, place in the middle of the oven for 45 minutes, or until golden, cooked through and an inserted skewer comes out clean. Transfer to a wire rack to cool for at least 20 minutes before eating, then serve.

> This bread is good fresh for a couple of days, and delicious toasted for a few days after that. You could even use any leftovers to make croutons.

CALORIES	FAT	SAT FAT	PROTEIN	CARBS	SUGAR	FIBRE	1 HOUR PLUS COOLING
213kcal	14.5g	2g	10g	10.2g	0.9g	5.1g	

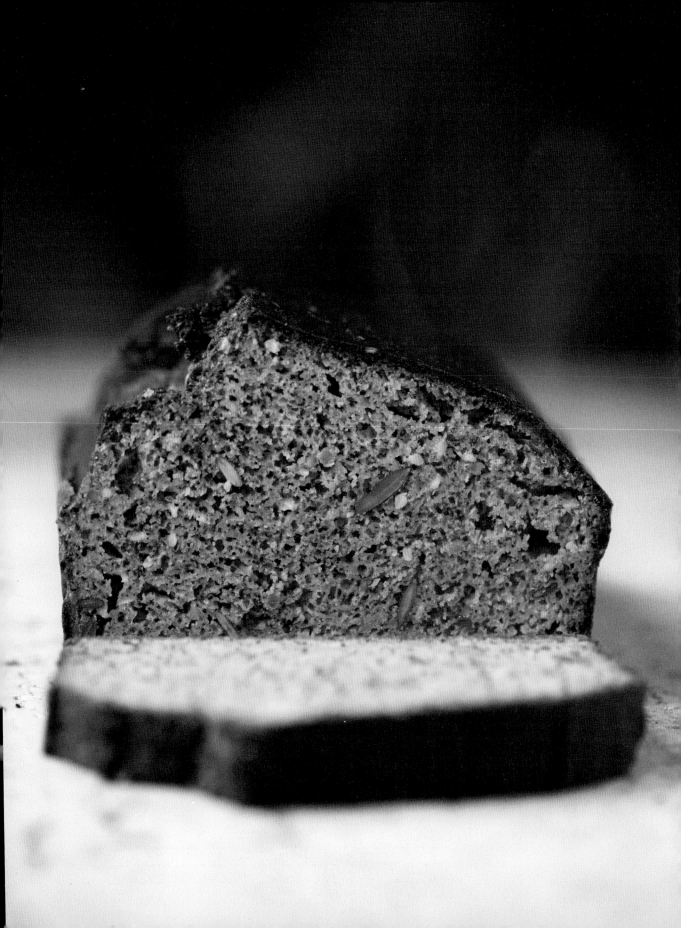

SUPER-FOOD PROTEIN LOAF
TOPPING IDEAS GALORE

This page is all about giving you loads of colourful inspiration for tasty topping combos that'll fill you with goodness – choose your favourites and tuck in

1. Chopped hard-boiled egg, yoghurt, paprika & cress

2. Ripe beef tomatoes, Swiss cheese & black pepper

3. Skinny cream cheese, ripe cherry tomatoes & fresh basil

4. Cottage cheese, soft-boiled egg, paprika & spring onions

5. Wilted spinach & cottage cheese

6. Squashed beetroot, natural yoghurt & balsamic

7. Grated cucumber & cottage cheese with smoked salmon

8. Skinny cream cheese, cherries & cinnamon

9. Skinny cream cheese, cucumber & hot chilli sauce

10. Skinny cream cheese, lemony grilled asparagus, fresh mint & chilli

11. Natural yoghurt, banana & cinnamon

12. Fried egg, natural yoghurt, ripe cherry tomatoes & curry powder

13. Avocado, cottage cheese & Tabasco chipotle sauce

14. Houmous, pomegranate seeds & rocket

15. Marmite, ripe avocado & natural yoghurt

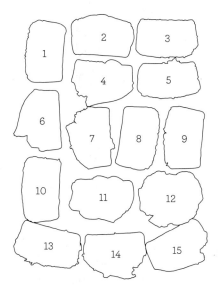

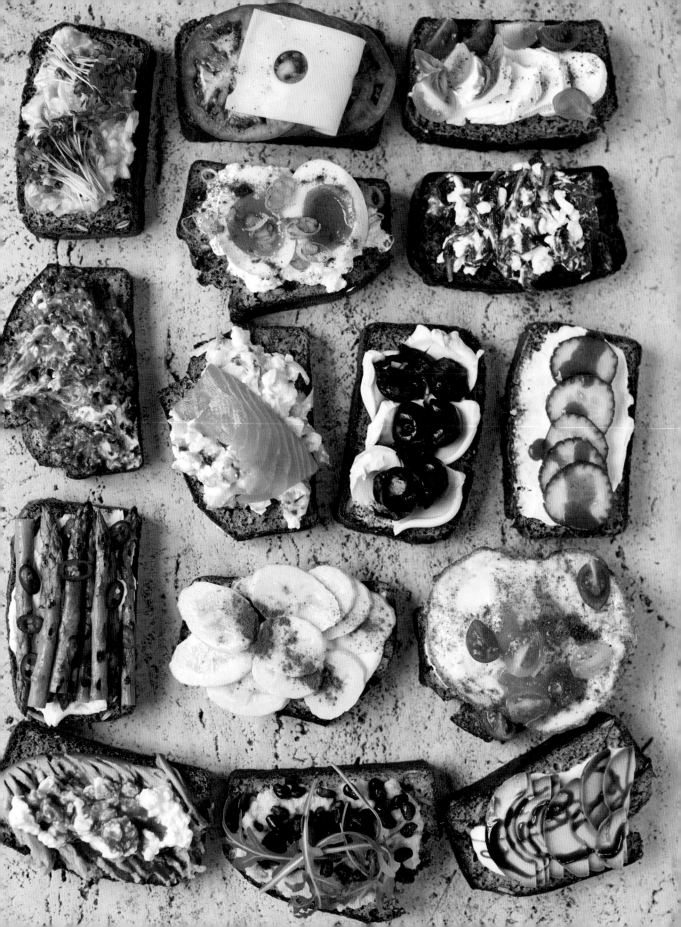

POST-GYM SUPER SALAD
CHICKEN, QUINOA & LOADSA VEG

— Lean chicken and quinoa are excellent protein sources post-exercise, when protein promotes muscle growth by repairing damage – for optimal benefit eat within 50 minutes of exercising —

SERVES 1

60g regular, black or red quinoa

¼ of a small cucumber

¼ of a small iceberg lettuce

½ a small carrot

½ an eating apple

1 ripe tomato

½–1 fresh red chilli

2 sprigs of fresh mint

1 small handful of baby spinach

1 lime

1 heaped tablespoon natural yoghurt

1 teaspoon hot chilli sauce

80g leftover cooked skinless chicken breast

½ a punnet of cress

Cook the quinoa according to the packet instructions, then drain (if you have the opportunity to cook up a batch of quinoa in advance to keep in the fridge ready for this dish, it will save time here).

Get yourself a large chopping board and roughly chop the cucumber, lettuce, carrot, apple and tomato. Finely chop the chilli (deseed if you like), pick over the mint leaves, and add the spinach to the story. Squeeze over the lime juice and spoon over the yoghurt. Drizzle over the chilli sauce, then chop and mix everything together until nice and fine, so all the flavours combine.

Mix in the quinoa, shred up and add the chicken, then have a taste and season to perfection with sea salt, black pepper and a little more chilli or lime juice, if you think it needs it. Serve in a bowl, or even a wrap if you're on the go, with the cress sprinkled on the top – delicious.

CALORIES	FAT	SAT FAT	PROTEIN	CARBS	SUGAR	FIBRE	30 MINUTES
400kcal	6.8g	1.5g	38.1g	49.6g	19.3g	4.3g	

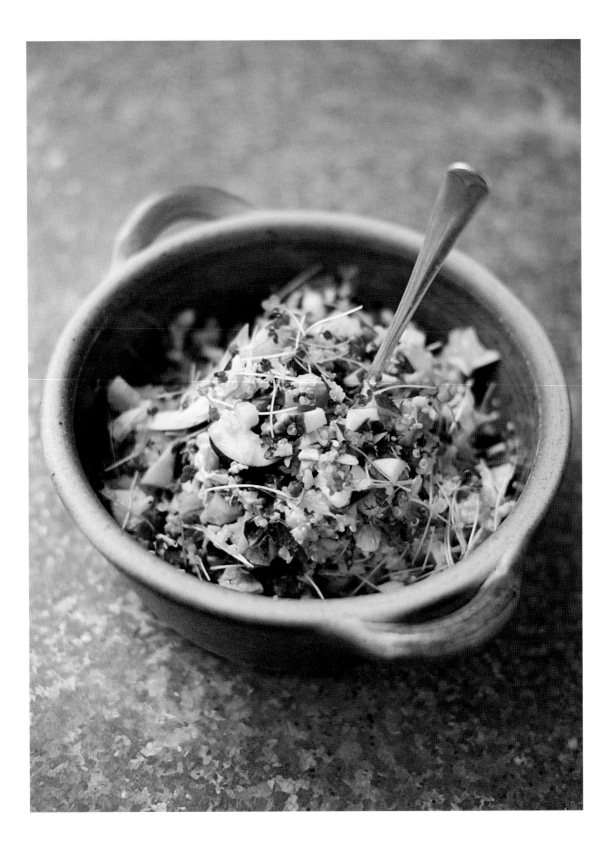

HEALTHY CHEESE & CORN PANCAKES
SMOKY BACON & CARAMELIZED BANANA

___ Cottage cheese is a great twist to this batter, making the pancakes super-light and fluffy, ___
and as well as being lower in fat than all other cheeses it's also super-high in protein

SERVES 4

1 x 340g tin of sweetcorn

6 spring onions

1 fresh red chilli

2 large eggs

200g cottage cheese

150g wholemeal self-raising flour

50ml semi-skimmed milk

olive oil

4 rashers of smoked streaky
  bacon

4 small bananas

optional: Tabasco jalapeño sauce

Tip the sweetcorn into a bowl, juice and all. Trim the spring onions and finely slice with the chilli (deseed if you like), then add to the bowl along with the eggs, cottage cheese and flour. Mix together, then gradually loosen with the milk to a thick but oozy batter. Lightly season with sea salt and black pepper.

I like to cook and serve 2 pancakes at a time so each person gets a lovely hot plate of food. Put a large non-stick frying pan on a medium heat and wipe with a piece of oiled kitchen paper. Place 1 rasher of bacon in the pan and as soon as it starts to release its smoky fat, wiggle that around the pan. Add 2 small ladles of batter to one side and flatten them slightly. Peel 1 banana and cut into four chunky slices at an angle. Add them to the pan to caramelize, turning when golden. Once the pancakes are golden on the bottom, flip them over to cook on the other side. Finessing your temperature control so that everything is ready at the same time is an art – just tweak the temperature to help you out until you get your groove.

Get your first lucky customer seated at the table and serve their pancakes with the banana, bacon and Tabasco (I'm loving the green jalapeño one here) for drizzling, if they fancy it, while you crack on with the next portion.

CALORIES	FAT	SAT FAT	PROTEIN	CARBS	SUGAR	FIBRE	30 MINUTES
400kcal	10.7g	4g	18.2g	59.9g	23.8g	6.6g	

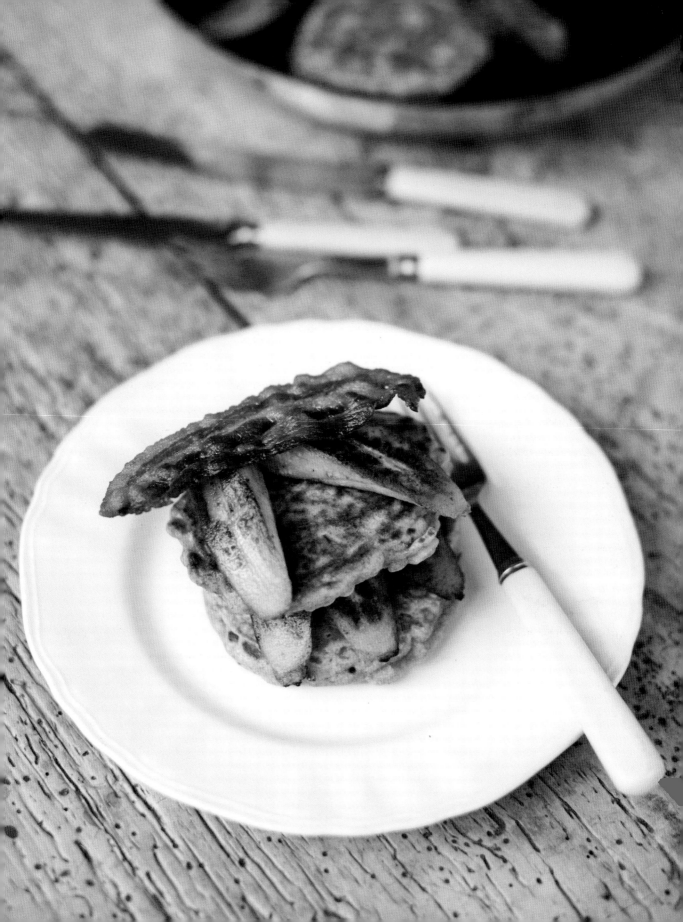

SEXY STEWED PRUNES
TOAST, BANANA, YOGHURT, ALMONDS

— Prunes are a fantastic source of fibre, hence their reputation for keeping us regular! —
Paired with yoghurt, this brekkie will also help keep our gut bacteria healthy

MAKES 6 PORTIONS

2 x 400g tins of prunes in
  natural juice

2 Earl Grey teabags

1 pinch of ground cloves

2cm piece of ginger

FOR EACH PORTION

1 thick slice of seeded
  wholemeal bread

1 tablespoon flaked almonds

½ a banana

1 heaped tablespoon Greek
  yoghurt

Drain the prune juice into a pan. Add the teabags and cloves, then peel, finely chop and add the ginger. Place over a medium heat to bubble and thicken for 7 minutes, while you squeeze the stones out of the prunes. When the time's up, remove and discard the teabags and stir the prunes into the sticky syrup.

For each portion, I pop a slice of bread on to toast while I lightly toast the almonds in a dry frying pan on a medium heat. Slice up the banana and smash it onto your toast with a fork. Spoon over the yoghurt, add 1 heaped tablespoon of hot or cold stewed prunes, scatter over the almonds and devour.

> What I love about these delicious, easy stewed prunes is that you can simply make and serve them warm for a crowd, or you can make a batch at the weekend to enjoy throughout the week. They're good kept in the fridge for up to 1 week.

CALORIES	FAT	SAT FAT	PROTEIN	CARBS	SUGAR	FIBRE	20 MINUTES
362kcal	9.3g	2.2g	12g	61.2g	40.1g	7.2g	

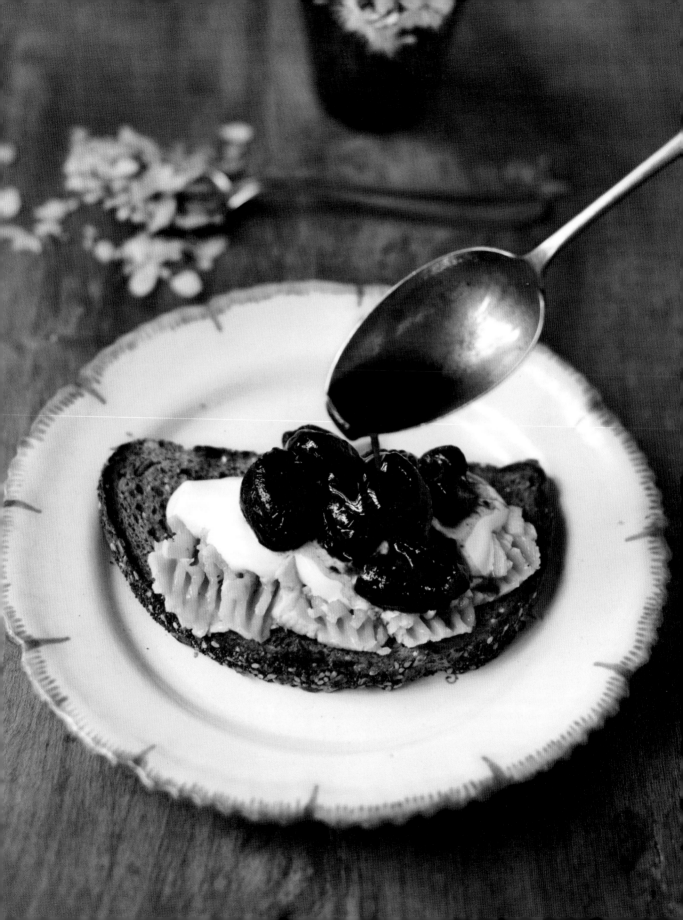

MY BIRCHER MUESLI
FRUIT, NUTS, YOGHURT & SEEDS

This recipe is full of goodness. It's super-high in fibre, and contains one portion of our 5-a-day plus a super sprinkling of nuts and seeds – a perfect portable start to the day

MAKES 10 PORTIONS

100g dried apricots

1 litre cow's or nut milk

2 ripe bananas

1 orange

1 fresh bay leaf

1 vanilla pod

500g porridge oats

FOR EACH PORTION

2 tablespoons natural yoghurt

½ an eating apple or pear

1 teaspoon mixed unsalted nuts

1 teaspoon mixed seeds

1 handful of seasonal berries

Place the dried apricots in a blender. Pour in the milk, then peel and tear in the bananas. Finely grate in the orange zest, then squeeze in all the juice. Remove the stalk from the bay and finely chop the leaf. Halve the vanilla pod lengthways and scrape out the seeds, then add them to the blender with the bay (pop the vanilla pod in a pot of honey to infuse it with extra flavour, for other meals). Blitz for a few minutes, until super-smooth, then in a bowl mix with the oats and pop into the fridge for at least 2 hours, preferably overnight.

For each portion, add the yoghurt and grate over the apple or pear, mixing it through if you like. Toast your nuts and seeds – I like to mix it up each time; try pistachios, cashews, almonds, chia, poppy, sunflower or linseeds – crush and scatter over, then serve with fresh berries.

> This will keep in the fridge for a good 2 days and is a perfect portable breakfast – simply add the toppings each morning and you're away.

CALORIES	FAT	SAT FAT	PROTEIN	CARBS	SUGAR	FIBRE	5 MINUTES PLUS SOAKING
358kcal	10.6g	2.4g	10.4g	53.2g	23.7g	8.9g	

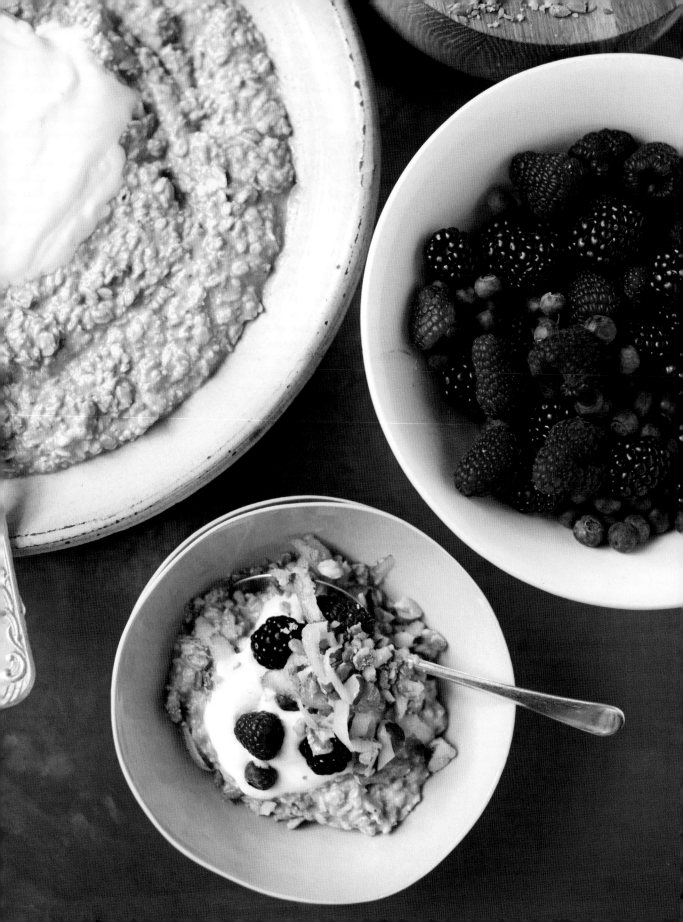

PAN-COOKED MUSHROOMS
TOMATO, PANCETTA, SPINACH & CHEESE

_ This lovely balanced breakfast heroes the humble mushroom, which is a great source of _
copper, one of the essential nutrients our nervous system needs to function efficiently

SERVES 1

6 chestnut mushrooms

1 ripe tomato

olive oil

white wine vinegar

Tabasco chipotle sauce

1 slice of seeded wholemeal
 bread

1 rasher of smoked pancetta

1 handful of baby spinach

1 tablespoon cottage cheese

Trim off the rim and stalk of the mushrooms and place the mushrooms in a bowl (keeping the trimmings for another day). Halve the tomato through the stalk, add to the bowl with 1 teaspoon each of oil and vinegar and a few dashes of Tabasco, then toss together. Place a large non-stick frying pan on a medium heat and put the tomato and mushrooms into the pan, cut side down, along with the slice of bread and the pancetta.

I like to let everything cook and colour for 10 to 15 minutes, turning the tomato and bread halfway. Keep an eye on the pancetta and move it on top of the bread once crispy. Let the mushrooms get really golden on their underside before flipping them. For the last couple of minutes, shake all the ingredients to one side and add the spinach to wilt down. Season to perfection.

Place the toast on your plate, pile the spinach on top, followed by the cottage cheese, tomato and pancetta. Serve with an extra dash of Tabasco, with those lovely golden mushrooms on the side, season to taste and tuck straight in.

CALORIES	FAT	SAT FAT	PROTEIN	CARBS	SUGAR	FIBRE	20 TO 25 MINUTES
247kcal	11.8g	2.8g	10.4g	23.3g	5.9g	4.6g	

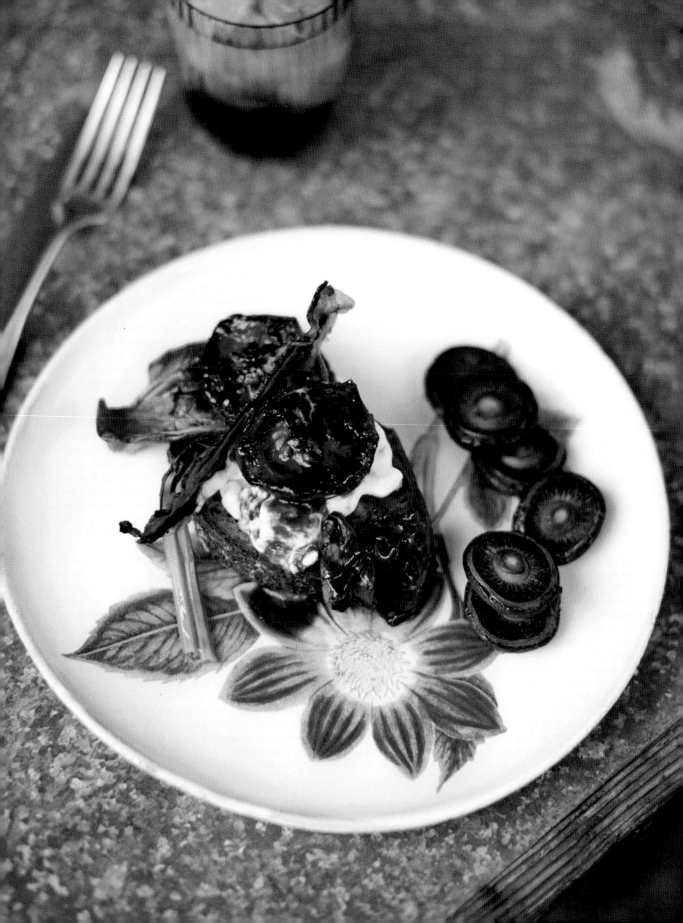

EARL GREY BANANA BREAD
GRIDDLED PEACHES, YOGHURT & NUTS

— Potassium-packed bananas keep our nervous system in good shape, assisting our internal body communication and helping us to maintain healthy blood pressure —

SERVES 8

1 Earl Grey teabag

50g unsweetened dried banana

50g dried dates

50g pecan nuts

150g wholemeal self-raising flour

50g rye flour

1 level teaspoon baking powder

2 large ripe bananas

2 large eggs

50ml maple syrup

4 tablespoons olive oil

FOR EACH PORTION

1 ripe peach or nectarine

balsamic vinegar

1 heaped tablespoon natural
  yoghurt

1 tablespoon whole almonds

Preheat the oven to 180°C/350°F/gas 4. Line a 1.5-litre loaf tin with a scrunched sheet of wet greaseproof paper. Make a cup of Earl Grey tea with 100ml of boiling water, removing the teabag after 3 minutes. In a food processor, blitz the dried banana, destoned dates, pecans, flours, baking powder and a pinch of sea salt until finely chopped. Add the peeled bananas, eggs, syrup, oil and Earl Grey tea, and blitz again until combined.

Tip the mixture into your prepared tin, give it a light tap to flatten the top, pull the paper up at the sides so it's nice and even, then bake for 50 to 55 minutes, or until nicely golden and an inserted skewer comes out clean. Gently lift the bread out of the tin and transfer to a wire rack to cool.

To serve, I like to toast two slices of banana bread per portion, then serve with a halved and destoned peach or nectarine that's been grilled on a hot griddle pan to bring out all that wonderful natural sweetness, then tossed in a drizzle of balsamic vinegar (you could even add a drizzle of manuka honey too). Add a dollop of yoghurt, a sprinkling of crushed, toasted almonds, and tuck on in. A scattering of fresh baby mint leaves would also be delicious. Store any extra portions in an airtight container, where it will keep for 2 to 3 days.

CALORIES	FAT	SAT FAT	PROTEIN	CARBS	SUGAR	FIBRE	1 HOUR 10 MINUTES
389kcal	19.6g	2.8g	9.8g	44.6g	25.6g	4.7g	

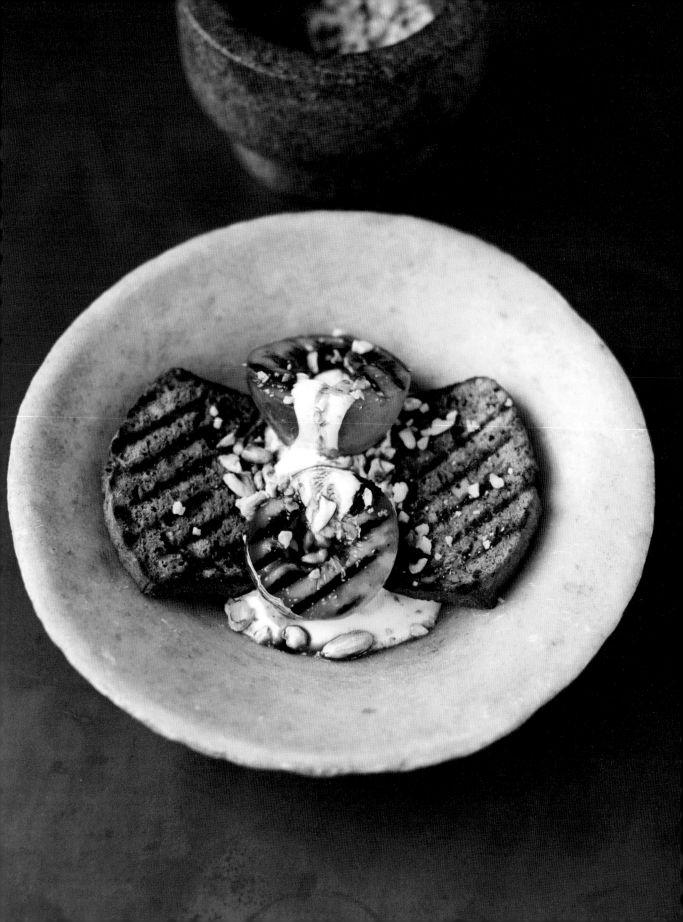

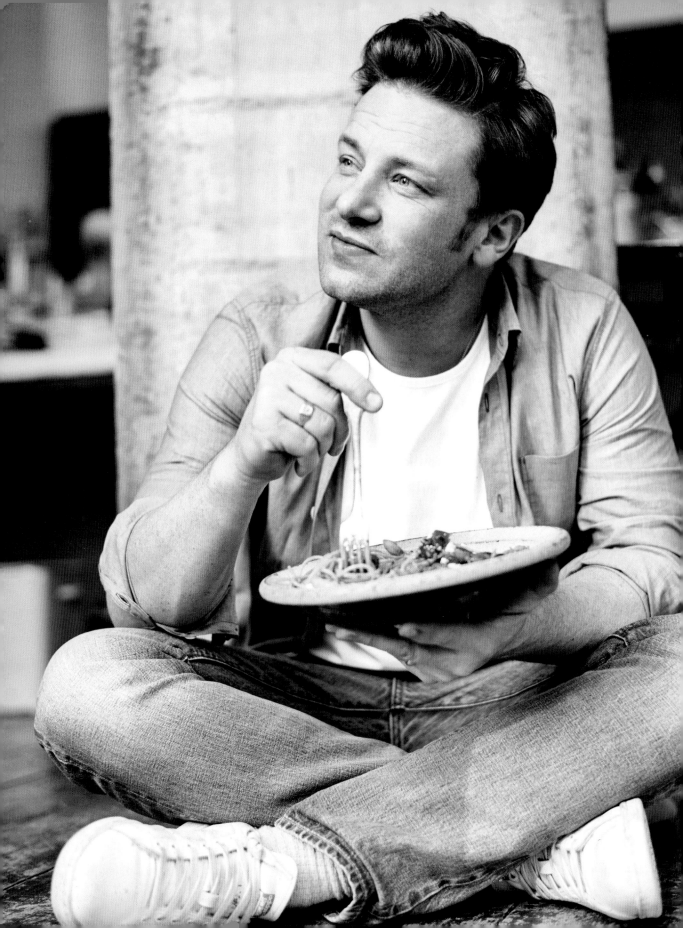

LUNCH

Lunch is a really important meal for me, especially when I'm at work. Essentially it's our opportunity to keep our energy levels up, keeping us focused and helping us get the most out of the rest of the day. You'll find a wide range of tasty meals in this chapter: all of them are straightforward and quick to rustle up, and some can be made ahead, boxed up and taken to work to be enjoyed at your leisure. All the recipes have a nice mix of the food groups and are less than 600 calories per portion – the dinner recipes are the same, meaning you can mix things up between the chapters, if you feel like widening your repertoire.

TASTY FISH TACOS
GAME-CHANGING KIWI, LIME & CHILLI SALSA

_ Just one haddock fillet provides us with a source of seven different essential _
vitamins and minerals, plus this colourful dish gives us three of our 5-a-day

SERVES 2

100g plain wholemeal flour

2 ripe kiwi fruit

4 spring onions

1 fresh jalapeño or green chilli

1 bunch of fresh coriander (30g)

2 limes

Tabasco chipotle sauce

¼ of a small red cabbage (150g)

1 tablespoon red wine vinegar

½ an orange

1 red or yellow pepper

2 x 120g fillets of firm white fish,
   such as haddock, skin on,
   scaled and pin-boned

olive oil

2 tablespoons natural yoghurt

In a bowl, mix the flour and a pinch of sea salt with 60ml of water to form a dough. Knead for a couple of minutes, then put aside. Peel the kiwi fruit, cut in half and put into a large dry non-stick frying pan on a medium heat with the green halves of the spring onions and the deseeded chilli. Lightly scald it all, turning every now and again, then place in a blender with half the coriander, the juice of 1 lime and a few shakes of chipotle Tabasco. Blitz until smooth, then taste and season to perfection. Very finely slice the red cabbage, ideally on a mandolin (use the guard!), scrunch with the remaining coriander leaves and the vinegar and orange juice, then season to perfection.

To make your tacos, divide the dough into four balls and roll out each one thinly. Cook each through in a non-stick pan for just 1 minute on each side until soft, turning when you see bubbles. Cover with a tea towel to keep warm.

Slice up the whites of the spring onions. Deseed the pepper and cut into 1cm dice. Slice the fish into 2cm strips, then toss with the spring onion, pepper and 1 tablespoon of oil. Return the pan you used for your tacos to a high heat and cook the fish mixture for around 4 minutes, or until the fish is cooked through and lightly golden. Divide the yoghurt, fish and veg between your warm tacos. Serve with the dressed red cabbage, that killer salsa and lime wedges for squeezing over, then devour!

CALORIES	FAT	SAT FAT	PROTEIN	CARBS	SUGAR	FIBRE	35 MINUTES
418kcal	10.6g	1.8g	35.2g	48.3g	16.8g	8.4g	

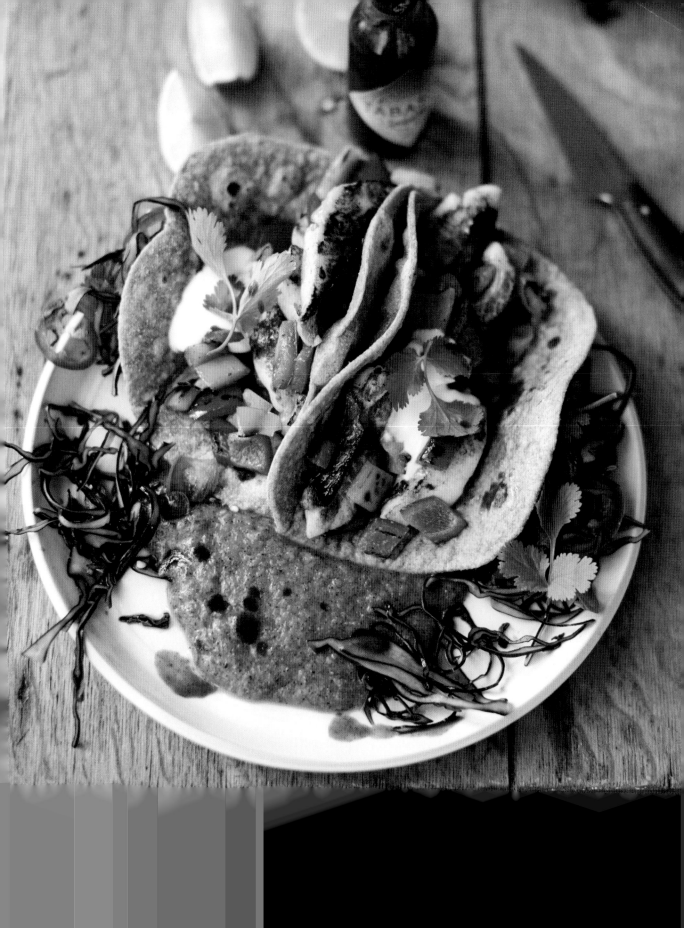

ASIAN CRISPY BEEF
BROWN RICE NOODLES & LOADSA SALAD

— Beef is packed with zinc, which we need in order to make DNA and to metabolize — key vitamins and minerals, enabling us to utilize the best of what we eat

SERVES 2

1 tablespoon unsalted peanuts

2 cloves of garlic

5cm piece of ginger

sesame oil

2 star anise

200g lean beef mince

1 teaspoon runny honey

1 teaspoon fish sauce

1 teaspoon low-salt soy sauce

2 limes

150g brown rice noodles

2 spring onions

1 fresh red chilli

200g fresh mixed salad veg,
    such as round lettuce, carrot,
    radishes, cress, spinach

4 sprigs of fresh coriander

Lightly toast the peanuts in a dry frying pan, then crush in a pestle and mortar and put aside. Peel and finely chop the garlic and ginger. Put 1 tablespoon of sesame oil and the star anise into the frying pan on a medium-high heat. Add the mince, breaking it apart with a wooden spoon, followed by half the garlic and ginger and the honey. Stir-fry for 5 minutes to crisp up and get golden brown. Meanwhile, crush the remaining garlic and ginger into a paste in the pestle and mortar, then muddle in the fish and soy sauces and lime juice to make a dressing. Cook the noodles according to the packet instructions. Trim the spring onions, then finely slice with the chilli (deseed if you like). Prep the salad veg, breaking the lettuce leaves apart and matchsticking or finely slicing any crunchy veg so it's all a pleasure to eat.

Load up your plates with that lovely salad veg, then drain and add the noodles. Spoon over the dressing, sprinkle over the crispy beef, chilli, spring onions and crushed peanuts, pick over the coriander leaves and tuck in.

CALORIES	FAT	SAT FAT	PROTEIN	CARBS	SUGAR	FIBRE	25 MINUTES
440kcal	20.3g	6g	27.5g	37.8g	10.7g	2.8g	

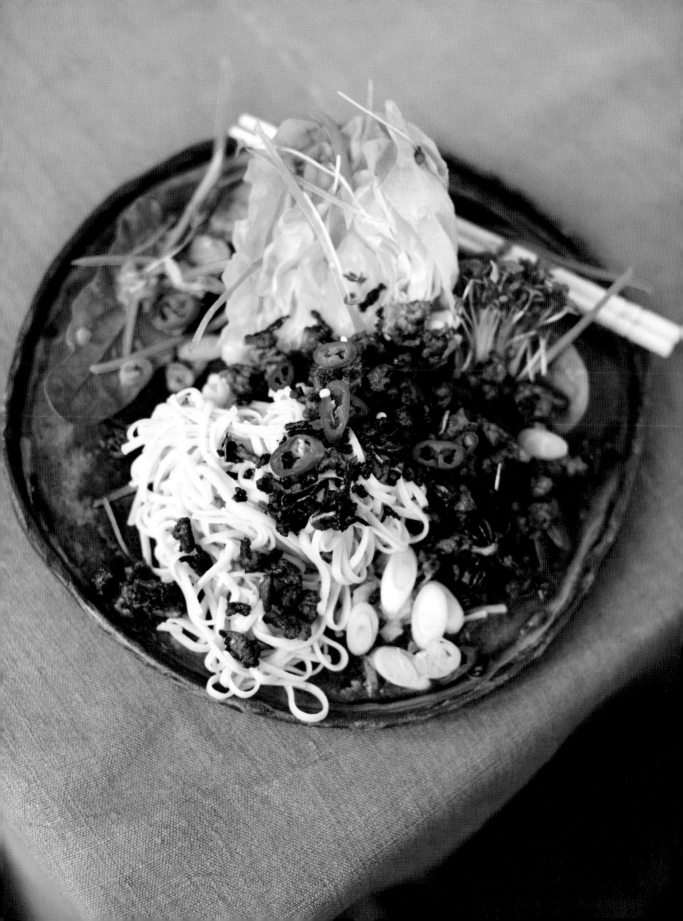

HAPPINESS PASTA
SWEET TOMATO, AUBERGINE & RICOTTA

— As well as being very low in saturated fat compared to most other cheeses, ricotta is also —
high in calcium, a nutrient vital in keeping our teeth and bones nice and strong

SERVES 4

2 aubergines

1–2 fresh red chillies

40g pine nuts

2 cloves of garlic

1 bunch of fresh basil (30g)

olive oil

2 x 400g tins of plum tomatoes

300g dried wholewheat fusilli

200g ricotta cheese

10g Parmesan cheese

Sit a double-layer bamboo steamer over a large pan of boiling salted water. Halve the aubergines lengthways and add to the baskets skin side up, with the whole chillies. Cover and steam for 25 minutes, or until soft and tender, then remove. Transfer the chillies to a small bowl and cover with clingfilm.

Lightly toast the pine nuts in a large casserole pan on a medium heat, then lightly crush in a pestle and mortar. Peel and finely slice the garlic and finely chop the basil stalks, then add to the pan with 1 tablespoon of oil and return to the heat to cook until golden. Tip the tomatoes into the pan through your hands, crushing and scrunching them up as you go. Fill each tin with water, swirl it around, and add to the pan with a good pinch of sea salt and black pepper. Bring to the boil, then simmer gently for 30 minutes, or until reduced by half, roughly chopping and adding the aubergines for the last 10 minutes.

Meanwhile, cook the pasta in the pan of boiling salted water according to the packet instructions, then drain, reserving a mugful of cooking water. Peel and deseed the chillies, then finely chop and stir into the sauce. Tear in most of the basil leaves and season to perfection. Toss the pasta and ricotta through the sauce, loosening with a little reserved water if needed. Serve with the pine nuts and remaining basil leaves scattered over, with a grating of Parmesan.

CALORIES	FAT	SAT FAT	PROTEIN	CARBS	SUGAR	FIBRE	1 HOUR
472kcal	18.9g	5.3g	20.5g	60.2g	12g	10g	

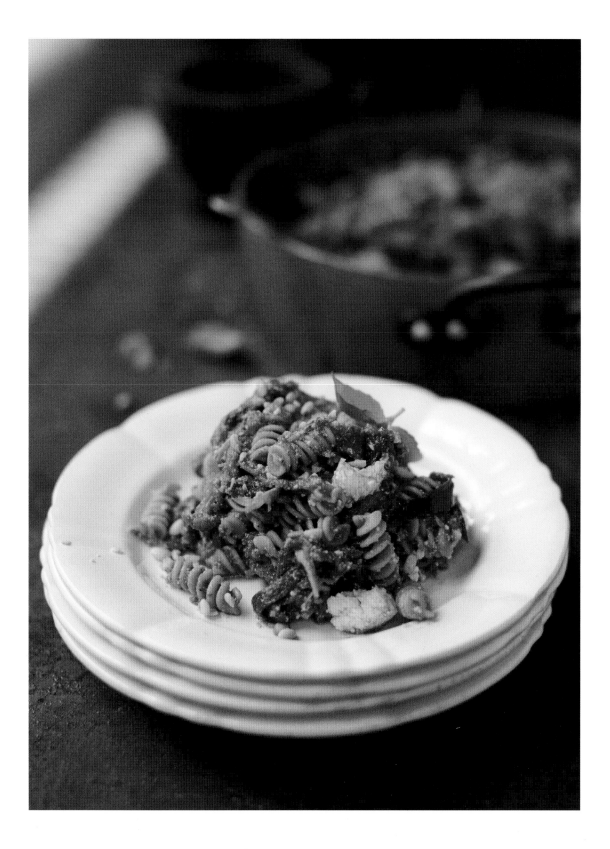

ORANGE GARDEN SALAD
BRESAOLA & GIANT RYE CRISPBREADS

— Hunt down these giant rye crispbreads, they're fantastic – plus, rye is a great source of —
zinc, which is good for cognitive function and helps keep our nails and skin healthy

SERVES 2

1 orange

extra virgin olive oil

red wine vinegar

½ a red onion

1 handful of enoki or chestnut
mushrooms

½ a bunch of fresh flat-leaf
parsley (15g)

1 red chicory

2 large handfuls of mixed
watercress and rocket

1 giant rye crispbread

20g Parmesan cheese

6 thin slices of bresaola

Top and tail the orange, then, standing it on its flat bottom, trim off the peel. Segment the orange into a bowl, squeezing the juice from the centre over the top. Add a pinch of sea salt and black pepper and 1 tablespoon each of oil and vinegar. Peel and very finely slice the red onion, ideally on a mandolin (use the guard!), pick apart or slice the mushrooms, pick and finely chop the parsley leaves, then add it all to the bowl and mix together well.

Finely slice the stalk end of the chicory, going about halfway up, then click apart the more delicate whole leaves and place gently on top of the salad with the watercress and rocket, tossing together only moments before serving.

Using your giant crispbread as a plate (you can use smaller ones and just divide the topping between them, if that's what you've got), arrange the salad on top, then use a speed-peeler to shave over the Parmesan. Arrange the bresaola over the top in waves, then serve. Simple, vibrant, easy and delicious.

CALORIES	FAT	SAT FAT	PROTEIN	CARBS	SUGAR	FIBRE	15 MINUTES
329kcal	10.7g	3.2g	15.8g	45.9g	13g	3.6g	

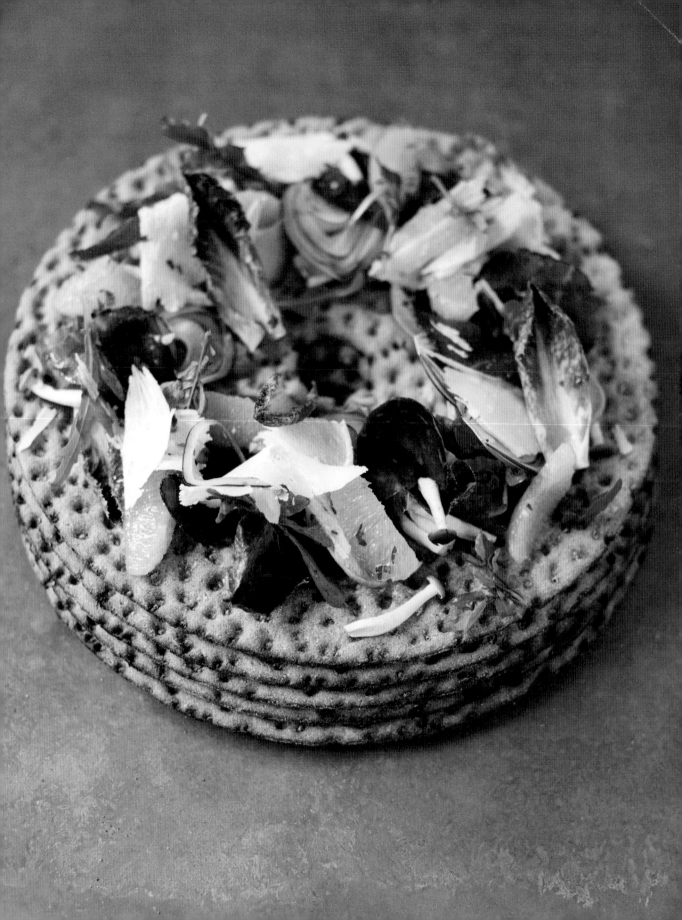

HEALTHY CHICKEN CAESAR
AWESOME SHREDDED SALAD & CROUTONS

— Finely sliced cauliflower isn't just delicious – when it's eaten raw we get twice as much vitamin B6 and three times as much potassium, keeping our nervous systems healthy —

SERVES 2

1 lemon

15g Parmesan cheese

2 anchovy fillets in oil

4 heaped tablespoons natural
    yoghurt

½ teaspoon English mustard

1 teaspoon Worcestershire sauce

white wine vinegar

extra virgin olive oil

1 small red onion

½ a small cauliflower (300g)

1 romaine lettuce

olive oil

1 sprig of fresh rosemary

2 x 120g skinless chicken breasts

1 thick slice of wholemeal bread

Finely grate the lemon zest and Parmesan into a large bowl. Slice and add the anchovies, along with the yoghurt, mustard and Worcestershire sauce. Squeeze in half the lemon juice, add 1 tablespoon of vinegar and 2 tablespoons of extra virgin olive oil and mix to make your dressing.

Now you're going to turn regular salad into a thing of beauty by either taking your time with good knife skills, or ideally, investing in a mandolin for ease, elegance and accuracy (use the guard!). Start by peeling and very finely slicing the red onion, then stir it through the dressing. Click off and discard any tatty outer leaves from the cauliflower, then very finely slice it. Finely slice the lettuce by hand and pile both on top of the dressed onion, tossing together only moments before serving.

Put 1 teaspoon of olive oil in a frying pan on a medium heat. Pick the rosemary leaves over the chicken and lightly season it on both sides, flattening it slightly with the heel of your hand. Cook for 4 minutes on each side, or until golden and cooked through. Cube the bread and toast alongside the chicken, moving regularly until evenly golden and gnarly, removing only when super-crispy. Toss the salad together and season to perfection, slice up the chicken and serve with a sprinkling of croutons and lemon wedges for squeezing over.

CALORIES	FAT	SAT FAT	PROTEIN	CARBS	SUGAR	FIBRE	25 MINUTES
418kcal	17.5g	4.9g	43g	23.3g	12.5g	6.1g	

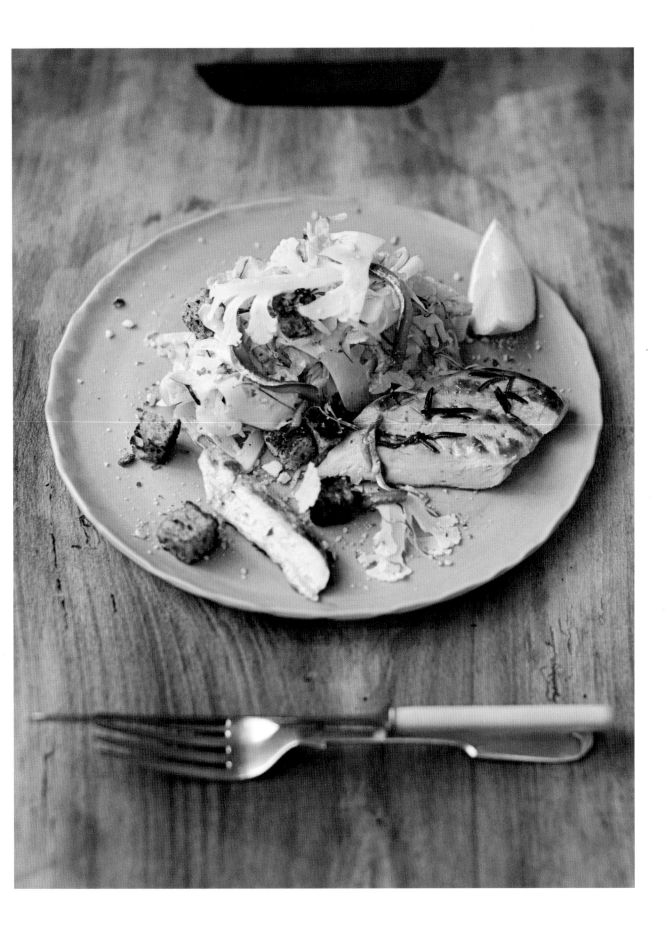

SPROUTING SEED SALAD
SMOKY BACON & BALSAMIC DRESSING

— Look for small sprouting seeds, which contain more health-promoting bioactive compounds —
that are reputed to help protect our cells from cancer and certain cardiovascular diseases

SERVES 2

1–2 slices of rye bread (150g)

1 rasher of smoked streaky bacon

olive oil

2 small cloves of garlic

1 sprig of fresh rosemary

3 tablespoons balsamic vinegar

100g baby spinach

1 large or 2 small roasted peeled
  red peppers in brine

300g mixed sprouts, such as
  alfalfa, lentil, chickpea,
  mung bean

30g feta cheese

Tear the rye bread and whiz into crumbs in a food processor, then toast in a large non-stick dry frying pan on a medium heat until really crisp and gnarly. Once done, decant into a small dish, leaving the pan on the heat.

Finely chop the bacon and place in the pan with 1 tablespoon of oil. While it crisps up, peel and finely slice the garlic, and pick and finely chop the rosemary leaves. Toss into the pan, then, when lightly golden, remove from the heat and add the balsamic and a splash of water to make your dressing.

Pile the spinach leaves into a nice serving bowl. Finely chop the pepper, then in a separate bowl toss with all the sprouts, half the breadcrumbs and the balsamic dressing, then spoon over the spinach. Sprinkle over the remaining breadcrumbs, crumble over the feta and serve.

CALORIES	FAT	SAT FAT	PROTEIN	CARBS	SUGAR	FIBRE	
317kcal	8.6g	3.2g	16g	42.3g	14.2g	10.6g	15 MINUTES

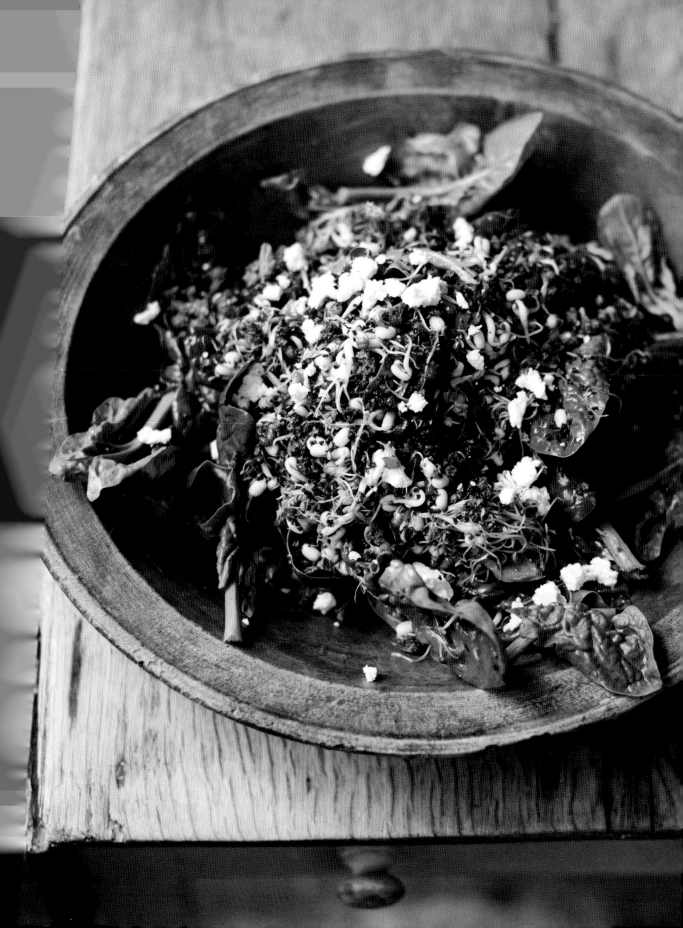

AMAZING MEXICAN TOMATO SOUP
SWEET POTATO CHIPS, FETA & TORTILLA

Sweet potato is a great non-starchy carb, so it counts towards our 5-a-day tally, plus it contains more vitamin C than regular potatoes, which our bodies need and utilize every day

SERVES 2

1 sweet potato (250g)

olive oil

1 teaspoon ground coriander

2 small wholemeal tortillas

4 spring onions

1 fresh red chilli

½ a bunch of fresh coriander (15g)

750g ripe tomatoes

2 cloves of garlic

½ x 660g jar or 1 x 400g tin of chickpeas

30g feta cheese

1 lime

Preheat the oven to 200°C/400°F/gas 6. Wash the sweet potato, trim a 1cm slice off the side to give you a flat edge to rest it on, then carefully cut it all lengthways into 1cm slices, and again into 1cm chips. Toss with 1 teaspoon of oil and the ground coriander, then season lightly with sea salt and black pepper. Roast for 30 to 35 minutes, or until tender and caramelized at the edges. Place the tortillas in the oven for the last 5 minutes to crisp up.

Meanwhile, trim the spring onions and finely slice with the chilli (deseed if you like) and the coriander stalks. Remove the cores from the tomatoes and chop them into quarters. Put half the whites of the spring onions, half the chilli and the coriander leaves aside on a small plate, then place the rest in a large casserole pan on a medium-high heat with 2 teaspoons of oil. Crush in the garlic, fry for 2 minutes, then add the tomatoes. Tip in the chickpeas and their juice, top up with 600ml of boiling water and put the lid on. Simmer for 20 minutes, then season to perfection. Mash up the tomatoes, then keep warm over the lowest heat until the sweet potato chips are done.

To serve, smash the crispy tortillas into the soup, add the sweet potato chips and half the coriander leaves and gently mix together – the tortillas will suck up the lovely juices, giving that perfectly soggy texture. Season to perfection, then coarsely grate over the feta, sprinkle with the reserved spring onions and chilli and the rest of the coriander leaves, and serve with wedges of lime.

CALORIES	FAT	SAT FAT	PROTEIN	CARBS	SUGAR	FIBRE	
596kcal	15.6g	4.8g	24.4g	91g	23.3g	20.3g	45 MINUTES

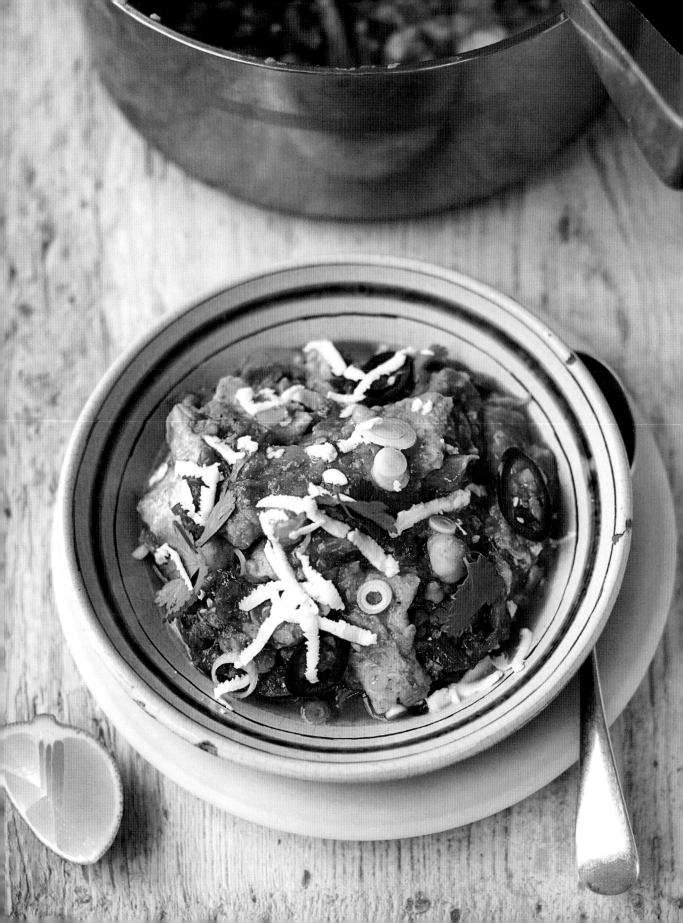

TOMATO & OLIVE SPAGHETTI
GARLIC BREAD & SARDINE SPRINKLES

Protein-rich sardines are high in omega 3, and are packed with vitamins and minerals such as chloride, which helps us to digest our food super-efficiently

SERVES 2

4 large ripe mixed-colour tomatoes

8 black olives (stone in)

extra virgin olive oil

½ a lemon

150g dried wholewheat spaghetti

40g tinned sardines in oil

1 clove of garlic

dried red chilli flakes

1 slice of seeded wholemeal bread

20g feta or ricotta cheese

2 sprigs of fresh basil

Prick the tomatoes and plunge into a pan of boiling salted water for 30 seconds, then scoop out onto a plate, saving the pan of water for your pasta. Destone the olives and tear into quarters in a large bowl, then place a sieve on top. As soon as the tomatoes are cool enough to handle, peel away and discard the skin, then cut them into quarters. Deseed, placing the seedy cores in the sieve and chopping the flesh into 1cm chunks. Push the seedy cores through the sieve so the juice dresses the olives (discard the sieve contents), then toss with the chopped tomatoes, 1 tablespoon of oil and a squeeze of lemon juice. Taste, season to perfection and put aside. Cook the spaghetti in the pan of boiling salted water according to the packet instructions.

Pick away the spine bones from the sardines – don't worry about the smaller bones as they'll get smashed up and you won't notice them. Place in a food processor, along with the peeled garlic and a good pinch of chilli flakes. Tear in the bread and blitz to fine crumbs, then tip into a dry frying pan on a medium heat. Toast the sprinkles until golden, tossing regularly.

Drain the spaghetti and toss straight into the bowl of dressing. Divide between your plates, drizzle with a little oil and scatter over some hot sprinkles, serving the rest in a bowl on the side to add as you eat. Crumble over the feta or ricotta, pick over the basil leaves and serve right away.

CALORIES	FAT	SAT FAT	PROTEIN	CARBS	SUGAR	FIBRE	25 MINUTES
449kcal	14.5g	3.5g	19.7g	64.3g	9g	9.6g	

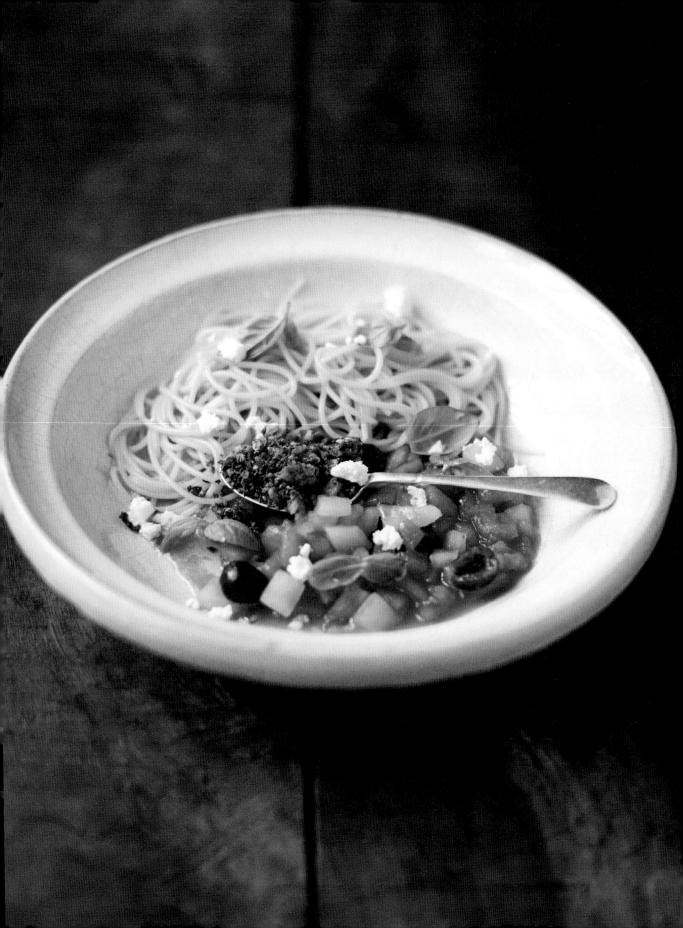

EASY SCANDI CRISPBREADS
PICKLED HERRINGS, RAINBOW VEG

— Protein-rich jarred herrings and fibre-packed spelt and rye flours for the Scandi crispbreads are all brilliant store-cupboard staples that enable you to rustle up a quick and easy lunch —

SERVES 2

1 x 7g sachet of yeast

olive oil

200g mixed flour (equal parts spelt, rye, wholemeal, bran), plus extra for dusting

1 tablespoon porridge oats

½ teaspoon fennel seeds

2 x 80g jarred pickled herring fillets with pickling liquor

1 small red onion

1 handful of raw crunchy veg, such as mixed-colour beets, carrots, radishes

4 sprigs of fresh dill

2 tablespoons white wine vinegar

2 tablespoons natural yoghurt

1 punnet of cress

cayenne pepper

Preheat the oven to 220°C/425°F/gas 7. Fill a jug with 130ml of tepid water, add the yeast and 1 tablespoon of oil, then mix with a fork until combined and leave for 5 minutes. Place all the flour and a good pinch of sea salt in a large mixing bowl. Make a well in the middle, pour in the yeast mixture and mix into dough. Knead on a flour-dusted surface for a few minutes until smooth, then return to the bowl, cover and leave for 15 minutes.

Divide the dough into two equal balls. Tear off two large squares of greaseproof paper and dust with flour, then roll out a dough ball between the sheets until 25cm in diameter. Peel back the top sheet and from a height sprinkle over half the oats and fennel seeds, then replace the paper and roll again to press them in. Remove the top sheet, then transfer the dough and base paper onto a baking tray. Repeat the process, then bake both breads for 15 minutes, or until golden at the edges and crisp, turning for the last 2 minutes.

Meanwhile, for the topping, drain 50ml of liquor from the herring jar into a large shallow platter. Peel the red onion and very finely slice with the crunchy veg, ideally on a mandolin (use the guard!). Finely chop the dill leaves, then slice the herring fillets 1cm thick. Add all this to the platter of liquor, along with the vinegar. Gently mix together, then leave for a few minutes.

Serve the crispbreads with the pickled herring and veg (leave the salty pickling liquor behind), spooning over some yoghurt and adding small pinches of cress and cayenne pepper to garnish.

CALORIES	FAT	SAT FAT	PROTEIN	CARBS	SUGAR	FIBRE	35 MINUTES
595kcal	20.8g	4.4g	32.2g	75g	11.4g	19.9g	

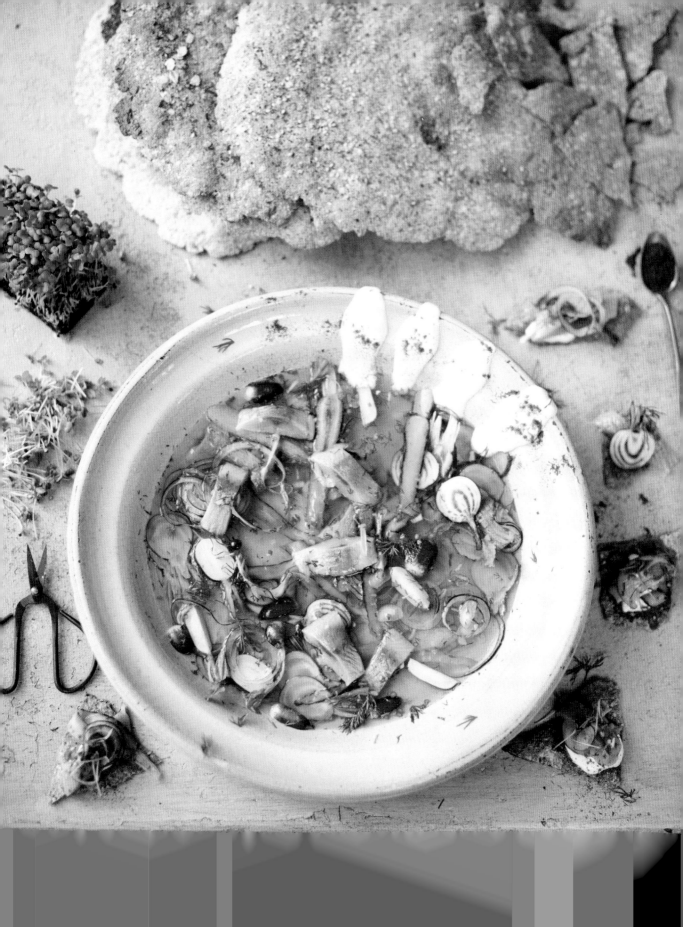

PORTABLE JAM JAR SALADS - PART ONE

These delicious, colourful lunches will cause massive office envy. Make balanced jars by layering up carb, protein, veg and a little dairy. Keep in the fridge and mix before serving

BOTH SERVE 1

BRITISH SALAD

Spoon **150g of cooked pearl barley** (75g if cooking from scratch) into the base of a 1-litre jam jar. Add **1 peeled, coarsely grated raw beetroot.** Grate **1 small eating apple,** mix with **2 heaped tablespoons of fat-free natural yoghurt, 1 tablespoon of extra virgin olive oil** and **1 heaped teaspoon of jarred grated horseradish,** then season to taste and spoon over the beetroot. Make up the rest of your jar with **1 handful each of watercress and baby spinach,** a few ripe cherry tomatoes, **100g of cooked thinly sliced lean roast beef,** the leaves from **2 sprigs of fresh tarragon** and **4 smashed walnuts,** then lid on.

CALORIES	FAT	SAT FAT	PROTEIN	CARBS	SUGAR	FIBRE	
539kcal	54.4g	5.1g	39.1g	40.7g	20.1g	5.4g	20 MINUTES

ITALIAN SALAD

Spoon **150g of cooked wholewheat pasta** (75g if cooking from scratch) into the base of a 1-litre jam jar. Halve and deseed **2 large ripe tomatoes,** then whiz up in a blender with **½ a fresh red chilli,** the leaves from **1 sprig of fresh basil,** the **juice of ½ a lemon** and **1 tablespoon of extra virgin olive oil,** season to taste and spoon over the pasta. Make up the rest of your jar with **2 more chopped ripe tomatoes, 2 handfuls of rocket, 75g of drained jarred tuna,** the leaves from **2 more sprigs of fresh basil** and **15g of shaved Parmesan cheese.** Top with **1 wedge of lemon** for squeezing over later, then lid on.

CALORIES	FAT	SAT FAT	PROTEIN	CARBS	SUGAR	FIBRE	
565kcal	19.6g	4.4g	38.8g	61.7g	13.9g	10.3g	20 MINUTES

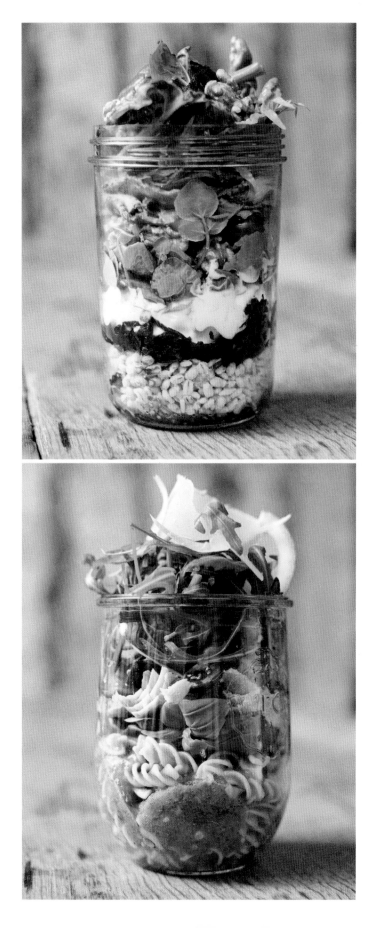

PORTABLE JAM JAR SALADS - PART TWO

— Once you've got the hang of this principle, go to town mixing up your combos to —
embrace seasonal produce, use up any leftovers and keep your veg drawer clean

BOTH SERVE 1

GREEK SALAD

Spoon **150g of cooked bulgur wheat** (75g if cooking from scratch) into the base of a 1-litre jam jar, then finely chop and sprinkle over the leaves from **2 sprigs of fresh dill**. Mix **2 heaped tablespoons of fat-free natural yoghurt** and **1 tablespoon of extra virgin olive oil** together, then season to taste and spoon over the bulgur. Make up the rest of your jar with **½ a shredded little gem lettuce, 4 olives** (destoned and torn into quarters), **1 sliced ripe tomato, 5cm of sliced cucumber, 100g of shredded cooked chicken**, the roughly chopped leaves from **2 sprigs of fresh flat-leaf parsley, 15g of feta cheese** and **1 teaspoon of toasted sesame seeds**. Top with **1 wedge of lemon** for squeezing over later, then lid on.

CALORIES	FAT	SAT FAT	PROTEIN	CARBS	SUGAR	FIBRE	20 MINUTES
413kcal	20.3g	4.9g	31.9g	25.9g	8.6g	4.8g	

MOROCCAN SALAD

Spoon **150g of cooked wholewheat couscous** (75g if cooking from scratch) into the base of a 1-litre jam jar. Add the seeds from **½ a pomegranate**. Mix **2 heaped tablespoons of fat-free natural yoghurt** with **1 tablespoon of extra virgin olive oil** and **1 teaspoon of finely chopped preserved lemon**, then season to taste and spoon over the couscous. Make up the rest of your jar with **5cm of sliced cucumber, ¼ of a shredded round lettuce, ½ a coarsely grated carrot, 1 peeled and sliced blood orange, 60g of drained chickpeas**, the torn leaves from **2 sprigs of fresh mint and 2 sprigs of fresh coriander, 15g of feta cheese, 1 good pinch each of toasted sesame seeds, chopped pistachios and cumin seeds**, then lid on.

CALORIES	FAT	SAT FAT	PROTEIN	CARBS	SUGAR	FIBRE	20 MINUTES
598kcal	20.1g	4.6g	22g	86.3g	24.7g	14.1g	

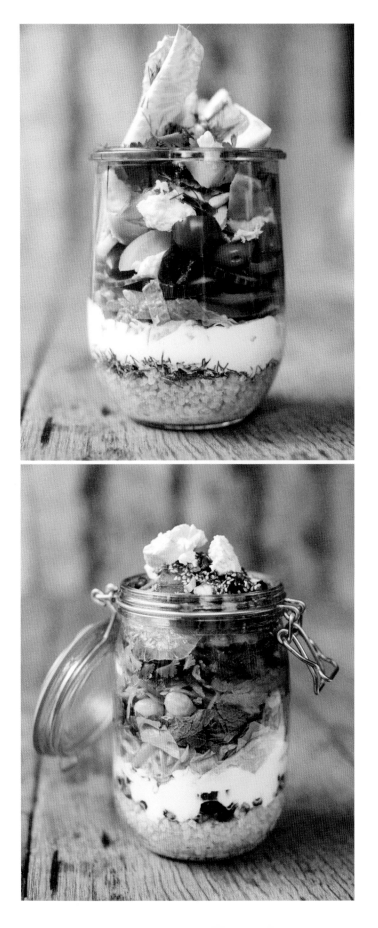

SKINNY CARBONARA
SMOKY BACON, PEAS, ALMONDS & BASIL

— Humble little peas are a source of nine different micronutrients, and are especially high in thiamin, a B vitamin that helps our hearts to function properly —

SERVES 2

200g freshly podded or
 frozen peas

1 tablespoon flaked almonds

1 small clove of garlic

½ a bunch of fresh basil (15g)

15g Parmesan cheese

1 lemon

150g wholewheat spaghetti

1 rasher of smoked streaky bacon

olive oil

1 large egg

100g fat-free natural yoghurt

Put a pan of boiling salted water on the heat for your pasta, dunk a sieve containing the peas into the water for just 30 seconds, then put aside, leaving the pan on the heat. Very lightly toast the almonds in a dry non-stick frying pan on a medium heat, then blitz until fine in a food processor. With the processor still running, peel and drop in the garlic, a pinch of sea salt, the basil leaves, the finely grated Parmesan and the lemon juice. Blitz until it comes together, then pulse in the peas, to try and keep a bit of texture.

Cook the pasta in the boiling salted water according to the packet instructions. Meanwhile, very finely slice the bacon and fry slowly in the frying pan with 1 teaspoon of oil on a medium-low heat until golden and crispy, then use a slotted spoon to transfer to kitchen paper, so the flavoursome fat stays in the pan. Scoop in three-quarters of your pea mixture to heat through.

Whisk the egg and yoghurt together well. When the pasta's done, reserving a mugful of cooking water, drain the pasta and toss straight into the pea pan, mixing well, then take the pan off the heat (this is very important, otherwise the egg will scramble when you add it, and we don't want that). Pour in the egg mixture and toss until evenly coated, silky and creamy, loosening with cooking water if needed. Taste and season to perfection, and serve topped with the remaining pea mixture and the crispy bacon. It might be skinny, but it's beautifully light and delicious. Enjoy!

CALORIES	FAT	SAT FAT	PROTEIN	CARBS	SUGAR	FIBRE	20 MINUTES
493kcal	16.4g	5.2g	27g	63.6g	9.2g	11.5g	

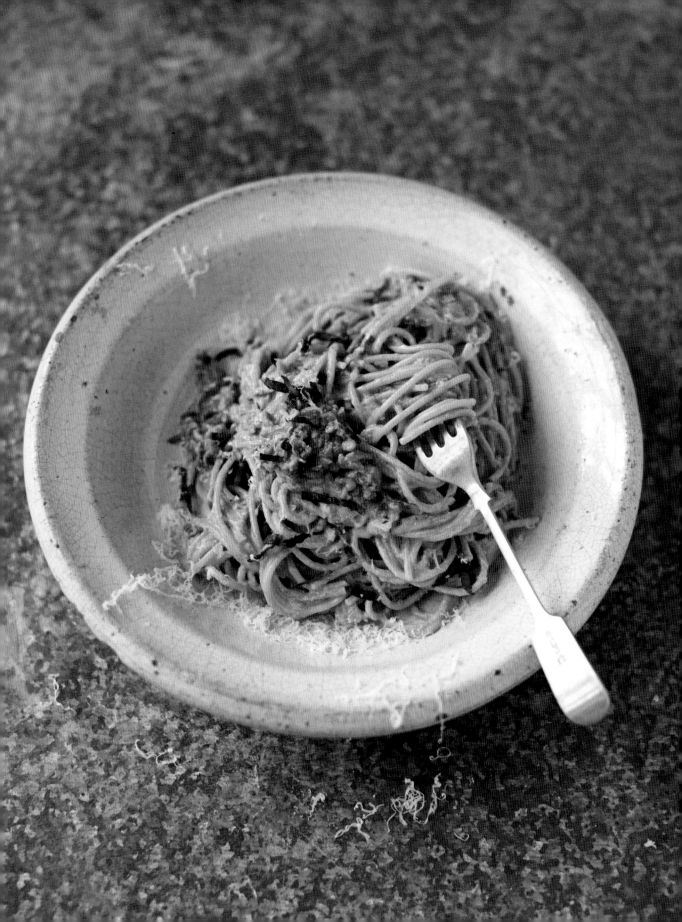

ROASTED SWEET POTATOES
BLACK BEANS & JALAPEÑO TOMATO SALSA

— Jam-packed with flavour, not only does this dish give us three of our 5-a-day, the black beans —
are a great source of protein, and actually contain more protein than any other beans

SERVES 2

2 x 200g sweet potatoes

100g brown rice

250g ripe mixed-colour tomatoes

2 spring onions

1 x 200g jar of jalapeños

½ a bunch of fresh coriander
(15g)

1 red onion

olive oil

1 level teaspoon cumin seeds

1 x 400g tin of black beans

2 heaped teaspoons cottage
cheese

Preheat the oven to 180°C/350°F/gas 4. Wash the sweet potatoes, then season and roast for 1 hour, or until cooked through. After 30 minutes, cook the rice according to the packet instructions, then drain. Roughly chop the tomatoes, trim and finely slice the spring onions and place both in a bowl. Tip the jalapeños and their liquor into a blender and rip in most of the coriander, reserving a few pretty leaves. Blitz until super-smooth, then return to the jar, using 2 tablespoons worth to dress the tomatoes and spring onions (keep the rest of the dressing in the fridge for other meals).

Peel and finely chop the onion. Put a pan on a medium heat with 1 teaspoon of oil and the cumin seeds. Fry for 30 seconds then stir in the onion and a splash of water. Cook and stir for 8 minutes, or until softened, then add the beans and all their juice. Reduce the heat and cook for a further 5 minutes until thick and oozy, stirring occasionally. Taste and season to perfection, loosening with a splash or two of boiling water before serving, if needed.

Divide the beans, rice and tomato salsa between your plates. Split open the sweet potatoes and add one to each plate. Spoon over the cottage cheese, season with black pepper and finish with your reserved coriander leaves.

CALORIES	FAT	SAT FAT	PROTEIN	CARBS	SUGAR	FIBRE	
600kcal	6.8g	1.7g	23.4g	109.5g	20.8g	28.6g	1 HOUR

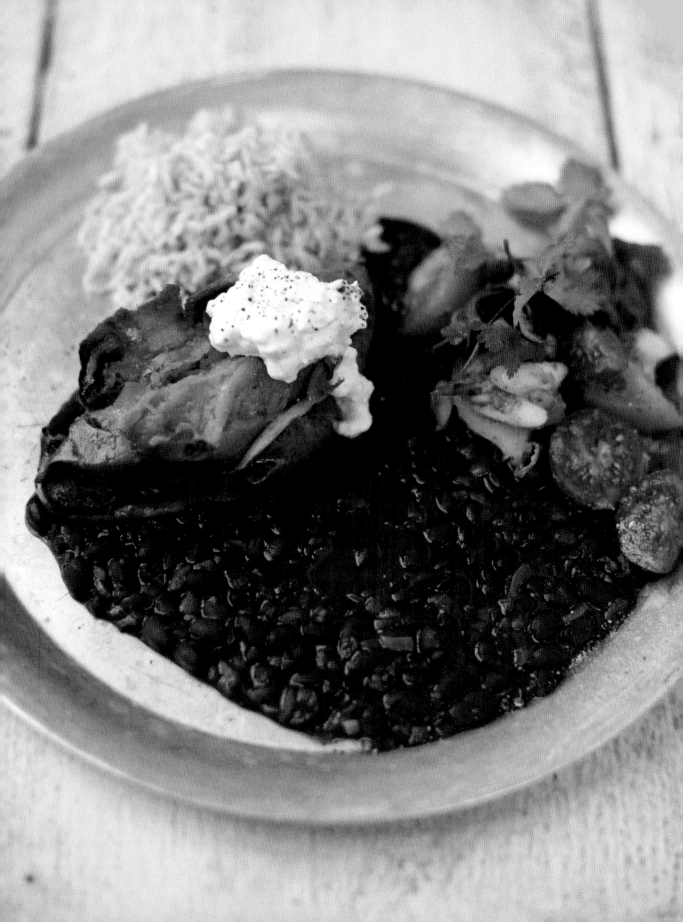

BEETS & SARDINES
HORSERADISH, YOGHURT & RYE BREAD

Sardines are packed with omega-3 fatty acids, which help keep our cholesterol levels healthy and our hearts happy. They're also a great vitamin D and calcium source for healthy bones

SERVES 2

300g mixed-colour raw
  baby beets

1 tablespoon balsamic vinegar

2 teaspoons jarred grated
  horseradish

4 heaped tablespoons fat-free
  natural yoghurt

8 fresh sardine fillets, skin on
  and scaled

extra virgin olive oil

1 lemon

4 sprigs of fresh dill

4 small slices of seeded rye bread

Trim off and reserve any nice beetroot leaves, then scrub the beets clean. Cook in a pan of boiling water for around 35 minutes, or until tender, depending on their size, steaming any reserved leaves in a colander over the pan for the last couple of minutes (you could use vac-packed beets here instead, for convenience, in which case skip straight to the blending stage). Drain the beets, reserving a little cooking water, then put half of them (preferably purple ones) into a blender with the vinegar and horseradish. Blitz until super-smooth, loosening with a splash of cooking water, if needed, then taste and season to perfection. Divide the yoghurt between two plates, spread it out, and marble the blitzed beetroot through it – get creative!

Place a dry non-stick frying pan on a medium heat and add the sardine fillets, skin side down. Cook on the skin side only for around 4 minutes, to ensure you get mega crispy skin and soft juicy flesh – don't move them!

Meanwhile, quarter the remaining beets and toss in 1 teaspoon of oil and a squeeze of lemon juice with any steamed leaves. Divide between your plates, followed by the crispy sardines. Pick the dill leaves and sprinkle over, then serve with rye bread and a wedge of lemon on the side for squeezing over. I like it both ways, but toasted rye bread gives you an even nicer, nuttier flavour.

CALORIES	FAT	SAT FAT	PROTEIN	CARBS	SUGAR	FIBRE	45 MINUTES
543kcal	21.4g	6g	51.8g	35.7g	17.8g	7.4g	

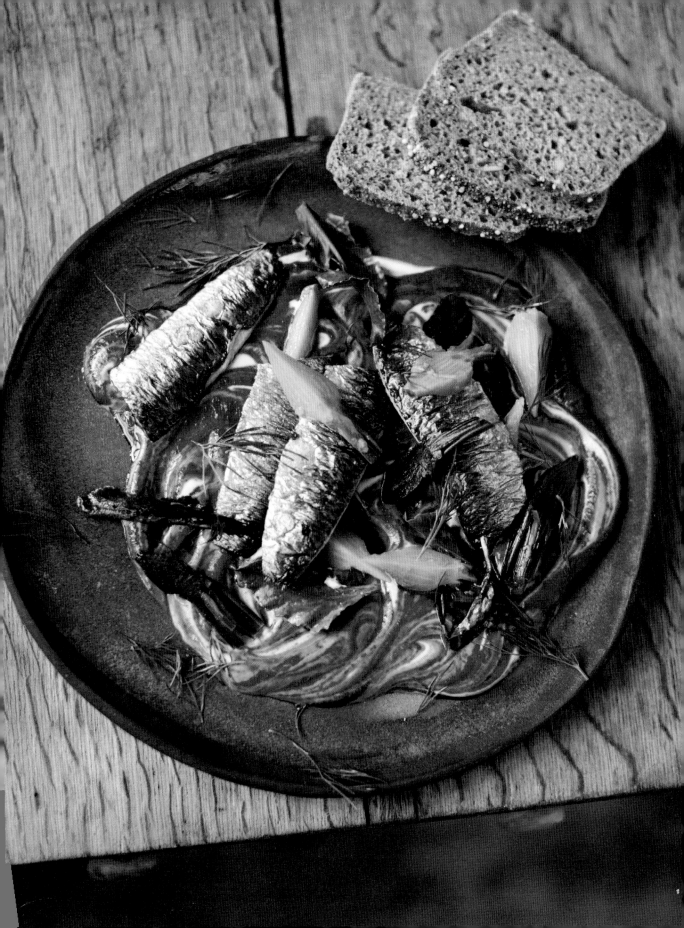

SUPER GREEN SOUP
CHICKPEAS, VEG & SMOKY CHORIZO

_ When nutrient-rich kale is boiled, protective antioxidant 'polyphenols' escape into the _
water, so using it for your soup adds extra goodness, plus we get two of our 5-a-day

SERVES 4

1 onion

2 cloves of garlic

olive oil

500g potatoes

1 x 400g tin of chickpeas

1 sprig of fresh rosemary

2 sprigs of fresh thyme

1 fresh bay leaf

1 litre really good chicken stock

150g kale and/or cavolo nero

80g quality chorizo

Peel and finely slice the onion and garlic, then put into a casserole pan on a medium heat with 1 tablespoon of oil and a splash of water. Cook for about 10 minutes, or until softened, stirring regularly.

Meanwhile, chop the potatoes into 2cm dice (leave the skin on for extra nutrients and fibre). Drain the chickpeas. Tie the rosemary, thyme and bay together, then stir into the pan with the chopped potatoes and chickpeas. Cover with the stock, bring to the boil, then reduce to a simmer for 30 minutes, or until the potatoes are cooked through.

Strip the kale and/or cavolo nero off the stalks, then roughly chop. Remove the herb bunch from the pan, then add the greens and submerge for 10 minutes. Finely slice the chorizo and gently fry in a pan on a medium heat until golden, then add to the soup with any drips of spicy flavoursome fat. The kale tends to suck up a lot of the lovely stock, so top up by stirring in a good splash of boiling water just before serving, if needed.

CALORIES	FAT	SAT FAT	PROTEIN	CARBS	SUGAR	FIBRE	
356kcal	11.9g	3.1g	21g	42.6g	4.9g	8.3g	50 MINUTES

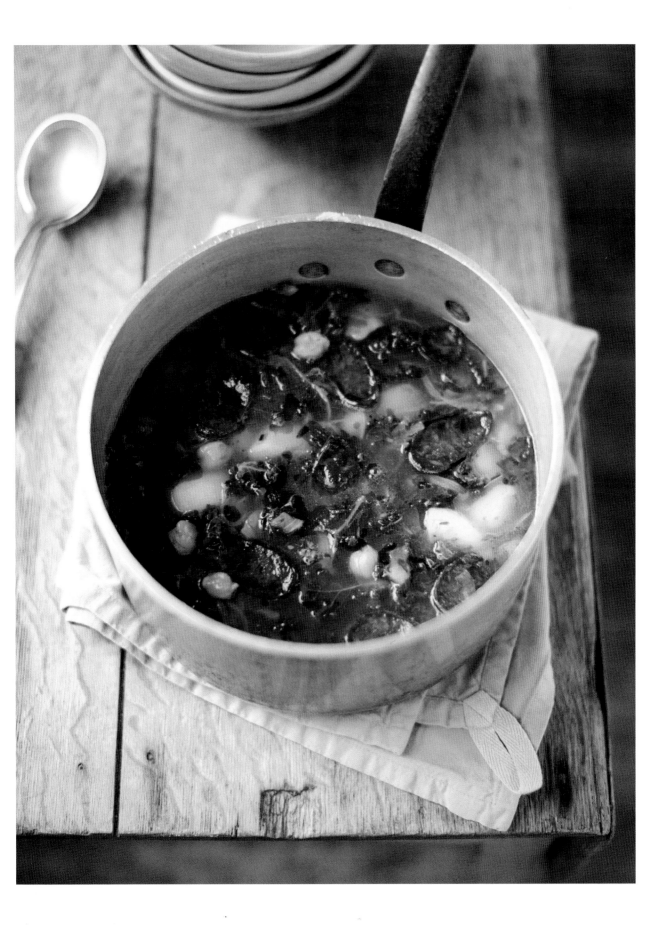

HERBY PASTA SALAD
RADISHES, APPLES, FETA & BRESAOLA

— The beauty of this simple dish is that all the wonderful veg gives us two of our 5-a-day, —
as well as a massive boost of vitamin C, providing us with more than our daily need

SERVES 4

300g fregola or giant
   wholewheat couscous

1 lemon

1 orange

extra virgin olive oil

4 spring onions

4 spears of asparagus

2 sticks of celery

1 courgette

1 red pepper

1 fresh red chilli

2 tablespoons sun-dried tomatoes

1 bunch of fresh mint (30g)

1 eating apple

1 handful of radishes

120g thinly sliced bresaola

30g feta cheese

1 pomegranate

Cook the fregola or giant couscous according to the packet instructions, then drain. Squeeze all the lemon and orange juice into a large bowl and mix with 2 tablespoons of oil. Trim and finely slice the spring onions and stir through the dressing. Trim the asparagus, celery and courgette, deseed the pepper, then take pride in finely dicing it all by hand with the chilli and sun-dried tomatoes (I think it's nice taking the time to do jobs like this – it improves your knife skills and is strangely satisfying).

Pick and finely chop the mint leaves, then add to the dressing with all the chopped veg and the drained fregola or giant couscous. Mix well, then taste and season to perfection. On a mandolin (use the guard!), very finely slice the apple and radishes. Plate up the herby pasta salad, arranging the slices of apple, radish and bresaola around the plates. Crumble over the feta, then halve the pomegranate and, holding each half cut side down in your fingers, bash the back with a spoon so that all the jewels tumble over the salad.

CALORIES	FAT	SAT FAT	PROTEIN	CARBS	SUGAR	FIBRE	30 MINUTES
474kcal	14.5g	3g	21.7g	67.3g	15.6g	5.5g	

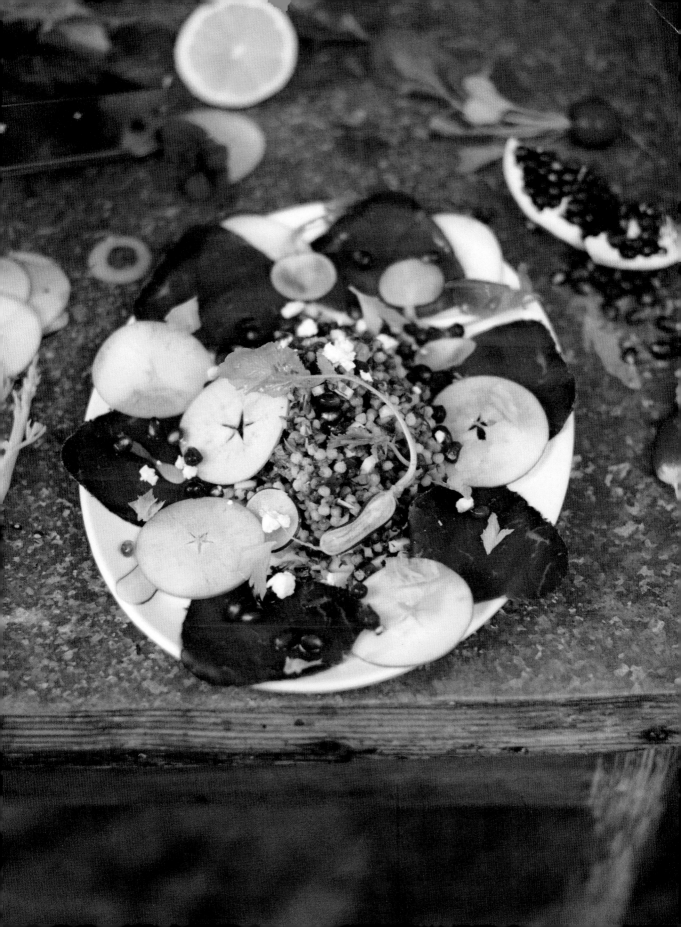

HOT-SMOKED TROUT
GREEN LENTILS, FRESH TOMATO SAUCE

— Hot-smoked trout is delicious and a great get-ahead ingredient. It's very low in saturated — fat and is a good source of protein, helping our muscles to grow and repair

SERVES 2

2 large handfuls of mixed
  seasonal greens, such as
  chard, spinach, kale

150g green lentils

extra virgin olive oil

red wine vinegar

Tabasco sauce

2 x 350g whole hot-smoked
  trout or 200g skinless
  hot-smoked trout fillets

1 teaspoon jarred grated
  horseradish

1 tablespoon natural yoghurt

100g ripe cherry tomatoes

Preheat the oven to 180°C/350°F/gas 4. Tear any tough stalks off the greens. Cook the lentils according to the packet instructions, steaming the greens above the pan for the last 5 minutes. Remove the greens to a board and finely chop them. Drain the lentils, toss with the chopped greens and dress with 1 tablespoon each of oil and vinegar and a shake of Tabasco, then season to perfection. You can serve these hot or at room temperature, which is my preference. Divide between plates when you're ready to serve your fish.

Place the trout on a baking tray and pop into the oven to warm through for 15 minutes, slightly less if using fillets. Meanwhile, stir the horseradish through the yoghurt, then divide and spoon over the lentils. Pick the cherry tomatoes into a blender, add a splash of vinegar and blitz until super-smooth, then season to taste and spoon over the yoghurt. Serve with the trout. Nice with some fresh wholemeal bread on the side to complete your balanced meal.

CALORIES	FAT	SAT FAT	PROTEIN	CARBS	SUGAR	FIBRE	35 MINUTES
274kcal	12.1g	2.4g	27.5g	13.3g	3.9g	6.1g	

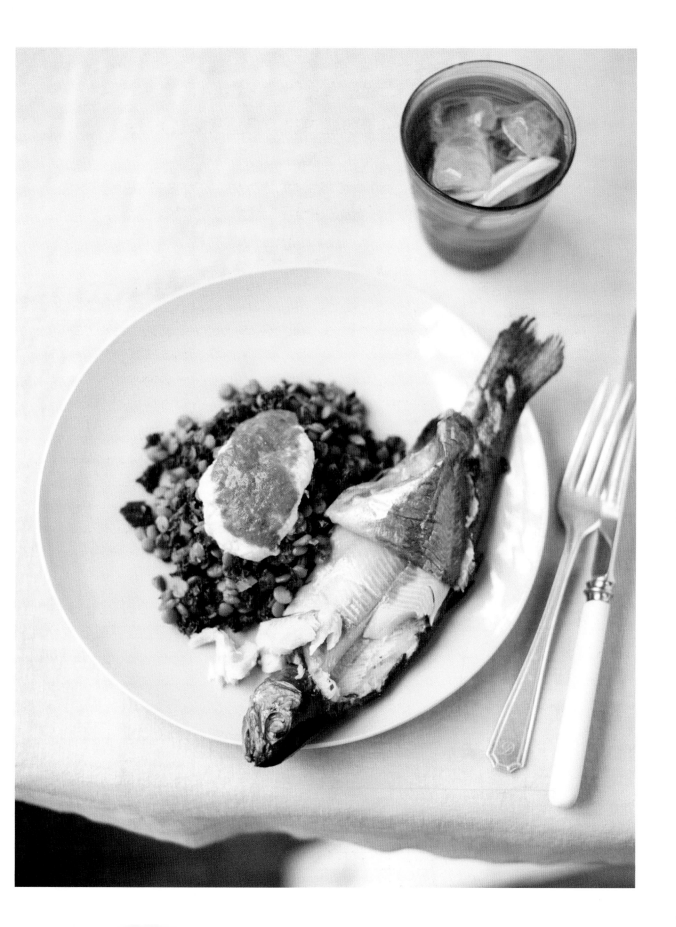

TASTY VEG OMELETTE
RAW TOMATO & CHILLI SALSA

— Eggs are the most brilliant source of protein – eating two gives us over a day's worth of
vitamin B$_{12}$, helping us produce red blood cells. Plus, we get three of our 5-a-day here —

SERVES 2

150g potatoes

olive oil

1 red onion

1 red pepper

1 yellow pepper

4 large eggs

1 handful of frozen peas

2 large ripe tomatoes

½–1 fresh red chilli

1 lemon

2 handfuls of rocket

15g Parmesan cheese

optional: Tabasco chipotle sauce

Wash the potatoes and chop into 1cm dice, then put into a 25cm non-stick frying pan on a medium heat with 1 tablespoon of oil and a good splash of water and toss well. Peel the onion, deseed the peppers, chop both into 1cm dice as well, then toss into the pan. Cook gently for 15 minutes on a medium-low heat, or until softened and lightly golden, adding splashes of water if needed, and tossing regularly. Meanwhile, beat the eggs with a pinch of sea salt and black pepper for 2 minutes so they're light and fluffy.

Toss the peas into the pan, then pour in the egg mixture. Use a rubber spatula to thoroughly mix it all together and begin to cook the eggs, then push it out flat, cover with a lid and leave to cook through for 5 minutes, or until set on the top and golden on the bottom. While that cooks, halve the tomatoes and remove the cores, deseed the chilli, place both in a blender with half the lemon juice and blitz until smooth, then taste and season to perfection.

Loosen around the edge of the omelette with the spatula, then place a large plate or board over the pan and in one bold, careful movement, flip it over onto the plate or board. Dress the rocket with the remaining lemon juice, pile in the centre, and finely grate over the Parmesan. Serve the omelette warm with the salsa, and a shake of Tabasco chipotle sauce is nice too.

CALORIES	FAT	SAT FAT	PROTEIN	CARBS	SUGAR	FIBRE	40 MINUTES
406kcal	22.3g	5.5g	22.9g	31.3g	15.7g	6.5g	

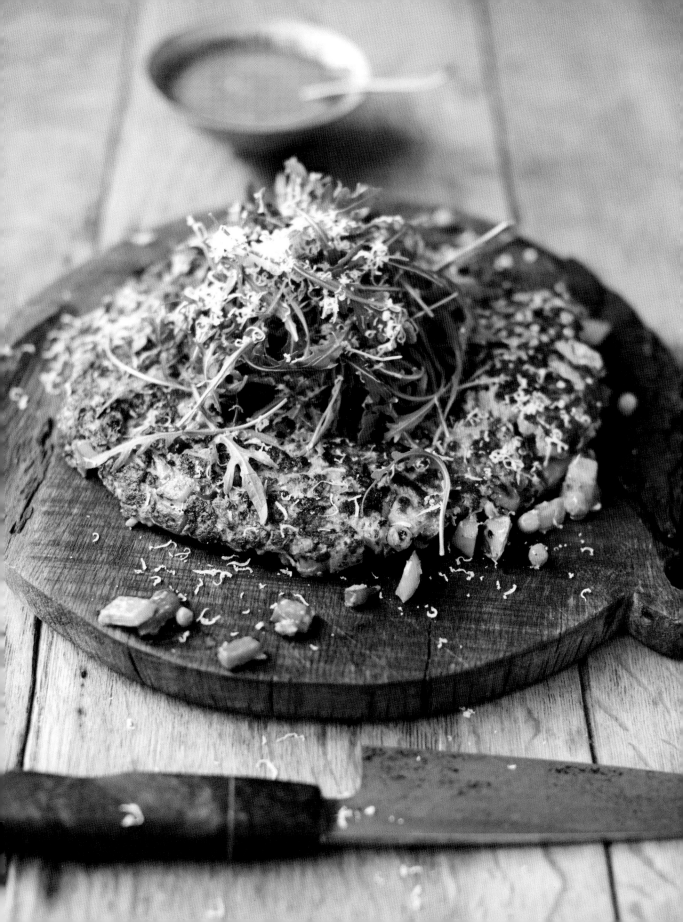

COSY SQUASH SOUP
CHICKPEA SALAD FLATBREADS

— You've gotta love butternut squash, it's such an all-rounder on the nutrition front, including being nice and high in vitamin A, keeping our skin healthy and helping us to see properly —

SERVES 6

1 large butternut squash (1.5kg)

½ a bunch of fresh thyme (15g)

2 heaped teaspoons harissa

olive oil

2 onions

1 fresh red chilli

3 oranges

2 litres really good veg stock

1 x 660g jar of quality chickpeas

1 large red onion

red wine vinegar

extra virgin olive oil

1 big bunch of fresh flat-leaf parsley (60g)

3 tablespoons whole almonds

6 small wholewheat flatbreads

80g feta cheese

Preheat the oven to 180°C/350°F/gas 4. Halve the squash lengthways, scoop out the seeds and chop into 2cm chunks. Place in a large roasting tray, strip over the thyme leaves and toss with half the harissa and 1 teaspoon of olive oil. Roast for 1 hour, or until golden and cooked through.

While the squash cooks, peel the onions and slice with the chilli (deseed if you like). Cook very gently in a casserole pan on the lowest heat with 1 teaspoon of olive oil and a splash of water, stirring regularly and adding more water as needed. When the squash is done, add it to the pan, finely grate in the zest of 1 orange, cover with the stock, then bring to the boil and simmer for 15 minutes. Blitz with a hand blender until smooth, loosening with water if needed, then have a taste and season carefully to perfection.

Meanwhile, drain the chickpeas and toss with the remaining harissa in a large non-stick frying pan on a high heat. Toast until crispy and on the edge of catching, then remove. Peel and very finely slice the red onion, ideally on a mandolin (use the guard!). Place in a bowl, then top, tail, peel and segment the oranges, adding them to the bowl and squeezing any juice from the centre over the top. Add 1 tablespoon each of vinegar and extra virgin olive oil, then pick in the parsley leaves, toss together and season to perfection.

Return the frying pan to the heat and toast the almonds, then remove and finely chop while you quickly toast the flatbreads. Fold them in half, pile in the salad and chickpeas, crumble in the feta, then roll up and squash ready for dunking. Divide the soup between bowls and scatter over the almonds.

CALORIES	FAT	SAT FAT	PROTEIN	CARBS	SUGAR	FIBRE	1 HOUR 20 MINUTES
414kcal	11g	1.5g	16.9g	63g	17g	13.2g	

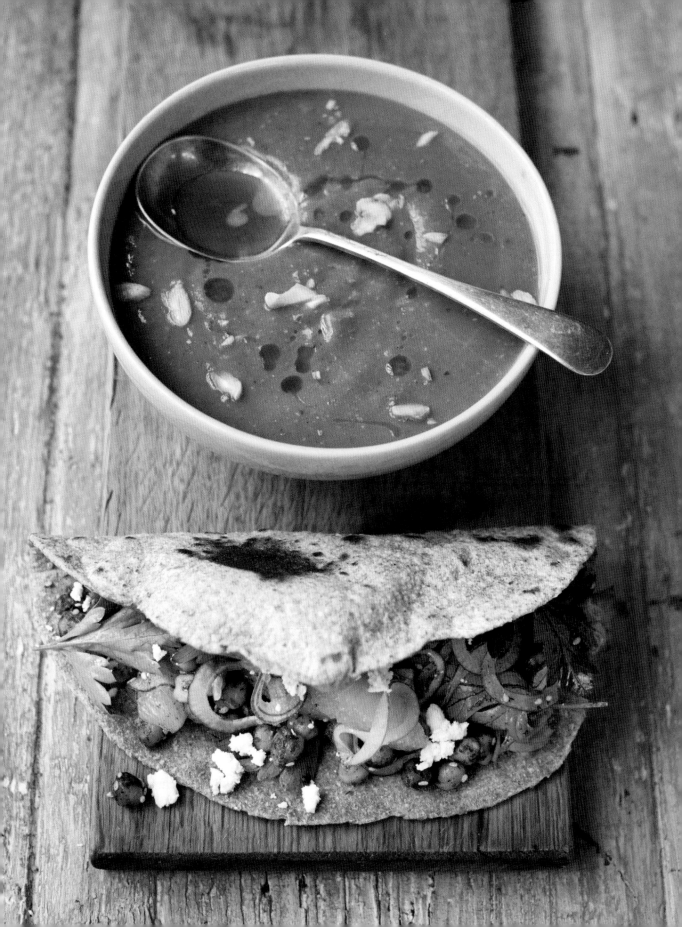

SEARED TUNA
SICILIAN COUSCOUS & GREENS

— I love having fresh sustainably sourced tuna once in a while – it's easy to cook and
high in selenium, which helps keep our nails and hair super-strong and healthy —

SERVES 2

4 ripe mixed-colour tomatoes

1½–2 fresh red chillies

2 sprigs of fresh basil

2 lemons

150g wholewheat couscous

2 cloves of garlic

1 x 225g piece of tuna

1 whole nutmeg, for grating

1 teaspoon dried oregano

olive oil

1 teaspoon baby capers

4 spring onions

1 bunch of asparagus (300g)

1 large handful of Swiss chard

30g feta cheese

First up, a cool method to make a really flavoursome couscous – we're going to feed it with cold liquid, rather than heating it. Simply quarter the tomatoes, deseed 1 chilli, and place in a food processor with the basil leaves, the zest and juice from 1 lemon, a pinch of sea salt and black pepper, plus 150ml of cold water. Blitz until smooth, tip the mixture into a bowl, stir in the couscous, then cover and leave aside for 1 hour to do its thing.

When the couscous has sucked up all the flavour, taste and season to perfection. Peel the garlic and finely slice with the remaining chilli. Season the tuna with pepper and a few scrapings of nutmeg, then pat with the oregano and 1 teaspoon of oil. Sear in a non-stick frying pan on a high heat for 1 to 2 minutes on each side, adding the chilli, garlic and capers when you flip it, and gently jiggling it about to sear it all nicely.

Transfer the contents of the pan to a board, returning the pan to a medium heat. Trim the spring onions and asparagus, then halve lengthways, halve the chard stalks and put it all into the hot pan with a good splash of water. Cover with a lid and steam for 4 minutes, or until just cooked through. Fluff up the couscous, crumble over the feta, pop the veg on top, slice up the tuna and serve with lemon wedges for squeezing over.

CALORIES	FAT	SAT FAT	PROTEIN	CARBS	SUGAR	FIBRE	15 MINUTES
543kcal	13g	4.5g	45.2g	64.7g	10.4g	10.3g	PLUS SOAKING

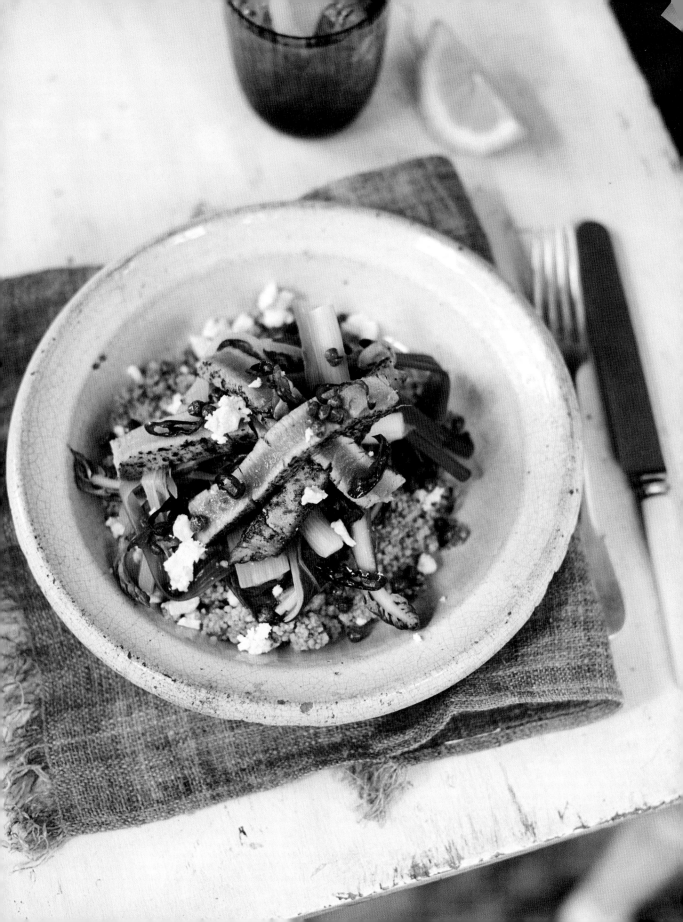

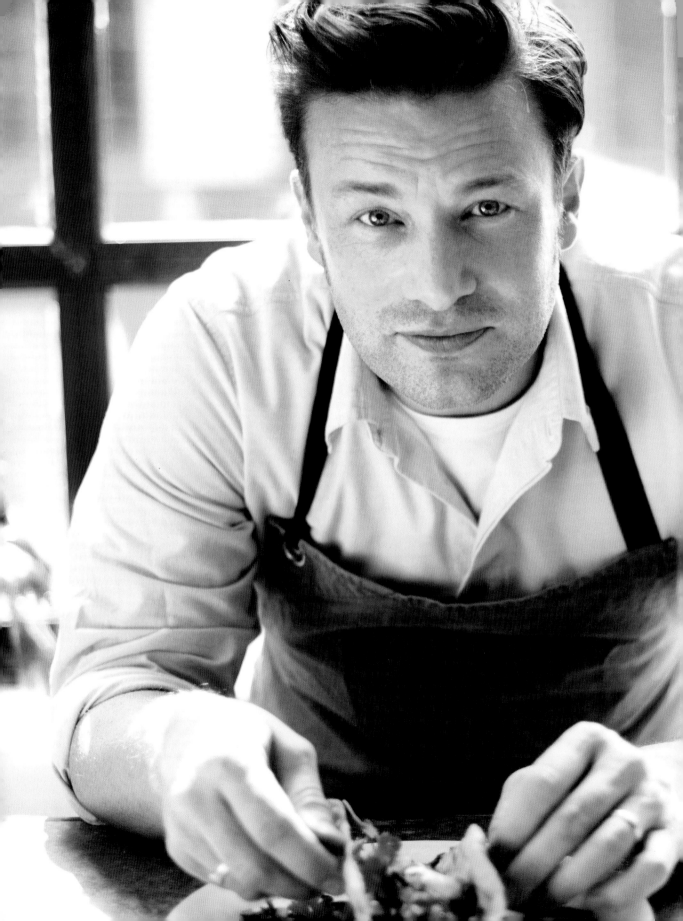

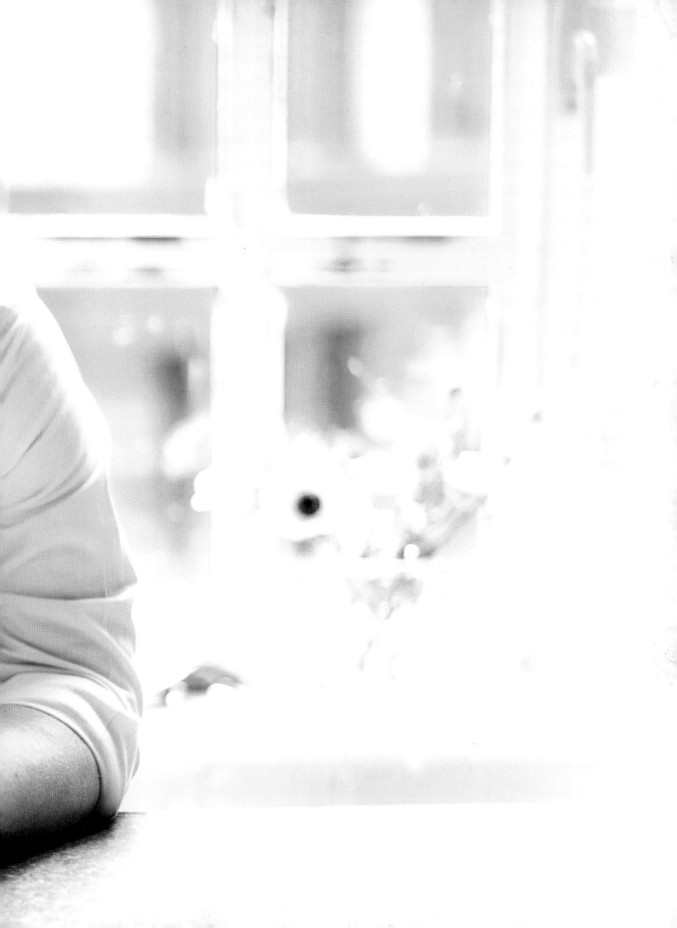

HEALTHY CHICKEN CLUB
TOMATO, LETTUCE, PEAR & TARRAGON

___ Chicken is a lean protein source that's packed with B vitamins and the mineral phosphorus, ___
which – along with calcium – makes up the matrix of our bones and teeth

SERVES 2

3cm piece of cucumber

1 small ripe pear

2 spring onions

½ a little gem lettuce

2 sprigs of fresh tarragon

2 tablespoons natural yoghurt

1 teaspoon English mustard

1 tablespoon cider vinegar

cayenne pepper

150g leftover cooked skinless
    chicken breast

2 super-thick slices of wholemeal
    bread

1 ripe beef tomato

2 small handfuls of watercress

½ a lemon

Halve the cucumber and remove the watery core, then in long strokes coarsely grate the cucumber and pear on a box grater. Scrunch them in your hands to remove some of the excess juice, then place in a bowl. Trim and finely slice the spring onions, shred the little gem, pick and finely chop the tarragon (you could also use mint or basil leaves), and place it all in the bowl with the yoghurt, mustard and vinegar. Mix well, then taste and season to perfection, using a little cayenne to spice things up. Slice up the chicken.

Toast the bread in a dry frying pan until golden on both sides – placing a little weight on top will help it to colour evenly and give you a great contrast between crispy outside and soft centre. I like to use two super-thick slices, and once toasted, place a bread knife in between the two edges and slice the bread horizontally in half, but you could use four thinner slices, if you prefer.

Finely slice the tomato and divide between two pieces of toast. Sprinkle with a little sea salt, then spoon over some dressed salad. Add the chicken and the rest of the dressed salad, toss the watercress in lemon juice and pile on top, then top with the other toasts. Skewer up some cornichons, radishes, cherry tomatoes, whatever you've got, and use them to hold the sandwiches together.

CALORIES	FAT	SAT FAT	PROTEIN	CARBS	SUGAR	FIBRE	20 MINUTES
271kcal	4.8g	1.4g	24.6g	34.2g	14.2g	6.8g	

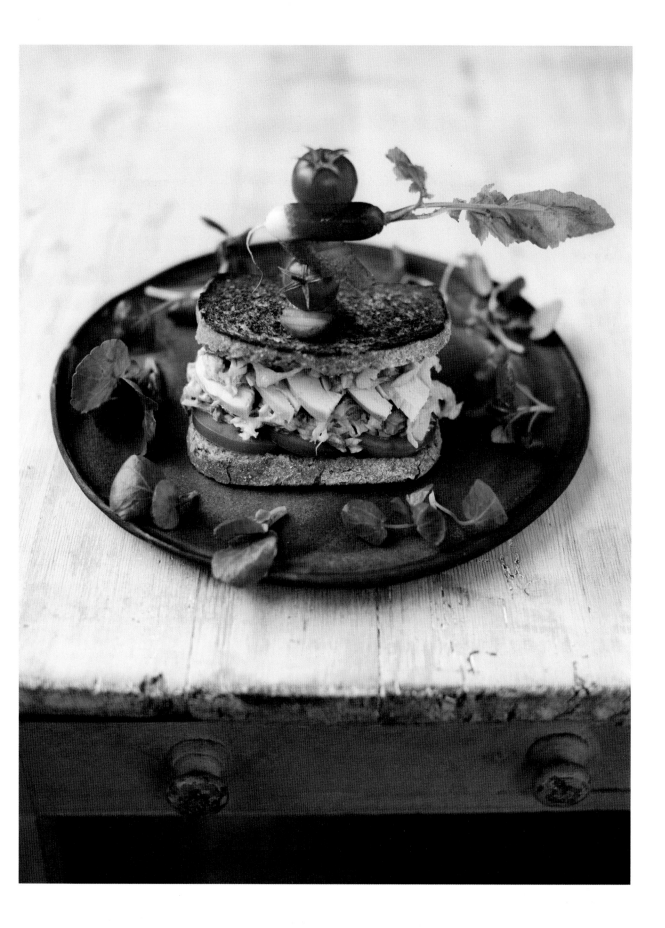

CHICKEN & GARLIC BREAD KEBABS
BLOOD ORANGE, SPINACH & FETA

__ Bursting with vitamin C, the blood orange's vibrant colour comes from anthocyanin, __
an antioxidant reputed to help in the prevention of many degenerative diseases

SERVES 2

2 sprigs of fresh rosemary

2 cloves of garlic

extra virgin olive oil

1 tablespoon white wine vinegar

cayenne pepper

2 x 120g skinless chicken breasts

2 thick slices of wholemeal bread

8 fresh bay leaves

2 blood oranges (use regular
    oranges if out of season)

100g baby spinach

1 lemon

1 tablespoon balsamic vinegar

20g feta cheese

Pick the rosemary leaves and smash up in a pestle and mortar with a pinch of sea salt. Peel and crush in the garlic, then muddle in 1 tablespoon of oil, the vinegar and a generous pinch of cayenne. Chop the chicken and bread into 2cm chunks and, in a bowl, toss and mix well with the marinade until evenly coated. Take a little care in skewering up the chicken and bread chunks, randomly interspersing them with the bay leaves on four short skewers and using hardy rosemary stalks, wooden or metal skewers as appropriate. Of course, check that the skewers will fit inside your largest non-stick frying pan.

Place the frying pan on a medium-high heat. Lay the skewers in the pan and cook for 4 to 5 minutes on each side, or until cooked through and golden. I like to place a lid and weight on top so that the chicken makes really nice contact with the pan and gets super-crispy.

Meanwhile, top and tail the blood oranges, trim off the peel, then slice into rounds. Dress the spinach with a squeeze of lemon juice and a drizzle of oil, arrange on your plates with the blood oranges and drizzle with the balsamic. Top with the kebabs, crumble over the feta and serve with lemon wedges.

CALORIES	FAT	SAT FAT	PROTEIN	CARBS	SUGAR	FIBRE	30 MINUTES
444kcal	12.8g	3.3g	39.2g	45g	22.3g	8.2g	

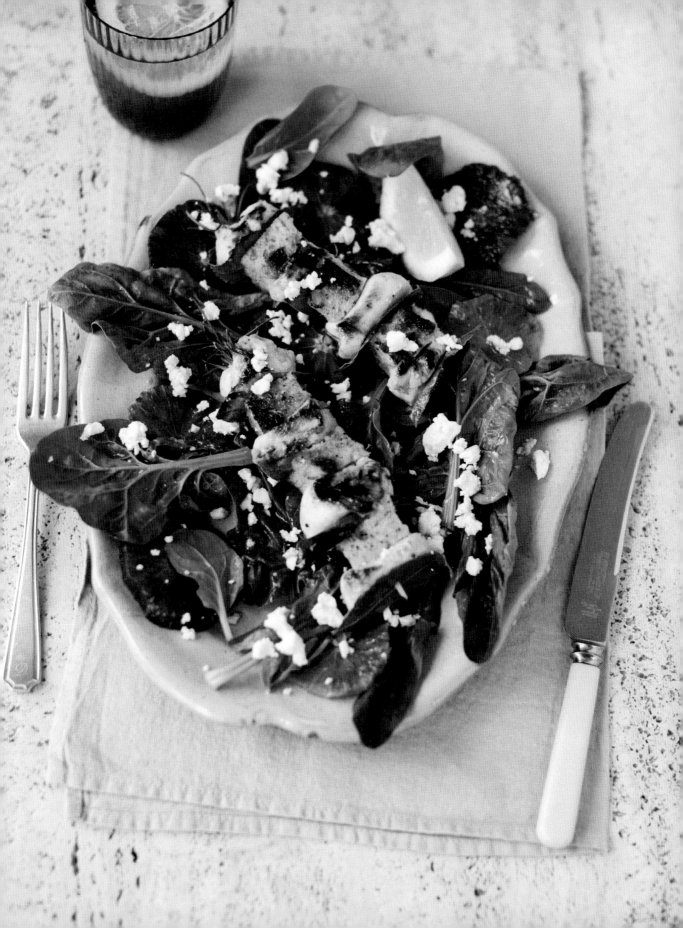

WHOLEWHEAT SPAGHETTI
SPROUTING BROCCOLI, CHILLI & LEMON

— Broccoli is a brilliant source of vitamin C, which we need for lots of things, one of which
is keeping our immune systems in tip-top condition to help us fight illness —

SERVES 2

150g dried wholewheat spaghetti

2 cloves of garlic

olive oil

1 lemon

1 pinch of dried red chilli flakes

4 anchovy fillets in oil

200g sprouting broccoli

2 heaped tablespoons
   cottage cheese

Cook the spaghetti in a pan of boiling salted water according to the packet instructions. Meanwhile, peel and finely slice the garlic and put it into a large non-stick frying pan on a medium heat with 2 tablespoons of oil. Finely grate in half the lemon zest and add the chilli flakes and anchovies. Fry for a couple of minutes, while you trim the broccoli and split any larger stalks in half lengthways. Add the broccoli to the frying pan with a spoonful of pasta water, then cover and leave to steam for 5 minutes, or until tender.

Use tongs to transfer the spaghetti straight from the water into the frying pan and toss together, along with the cottage cheese. Squeeze in half the lemon juice, loosen with a splash of cooking water if needed, then divide between your plates. Finish with a grating of lemon zest and a pinch of black pepper.

CALORIES	FAT	SAT FAT	PROTEIN	CARBS	SUGAR	FIBRE	15 MINUTES
438kcal	17.9g	3.2g	17.9g	54.9g	5.7g	10.1g	

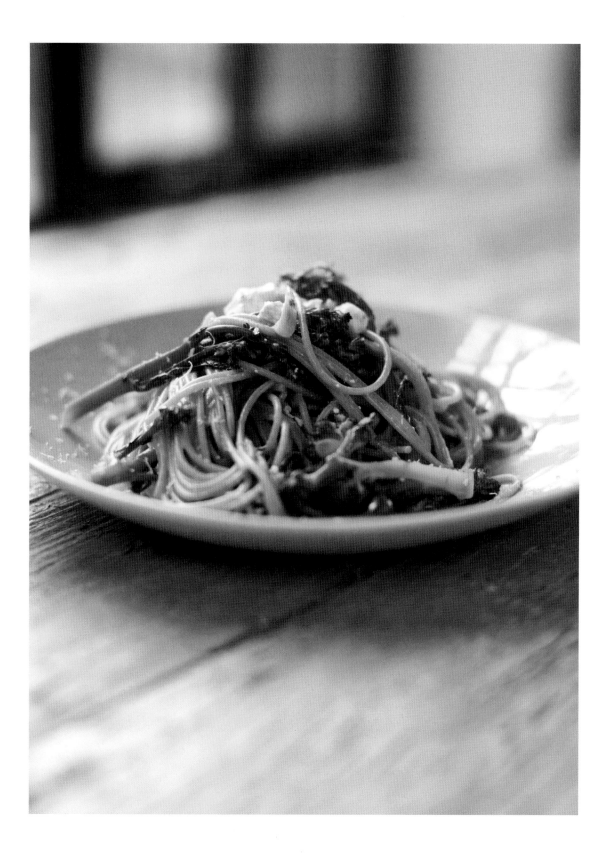

MEXICAN GAZPACHO
FLATBREADS & GARNISHES

— This super-refreshing dish packs in a massive four of our 5-a-day and has a very —
high water content, so aids hydration, something we can all benefit from

SERVES 2

1 large egg

1 corn on the cob

2 sticks of celery

200g chunk of watermelon

½ a cucumber

200g ripe tomatoes

2 spring onions

½ a bunch of fresh coriander
   (15g)

½ a clove of garlic

120g roasted peeled red peppers
   in brine

1 tablespoon jarred jalapeños
   in pickling liquor

2 limes

1 large wholemeal tortilla

1 handful of ice cubes

For your garnishes, boil the egg in a small pan of boiling salted water for 8 minutes, then drain and peel under cold water. Grill the corn on a hot griddle pan, turning regularly until nicely charred all over.

Meanwhile, trim the celery (reserving any yellow leaves) and peel the watermelon, then roughly chop with the cucumber and tomatoes and place in a blender. Rip in the green half of the spring onions and most of the coriander (reserving a few leaves). Peel and add the garlic, then add the peppers and the jalapeños with 1 tablespoon of their liquor. Finely grate in the lime zest, squeeze in all the juice and put aside while you finish your garnishes.

Trim and finely slice the whites of the spring onions and pop on a plate with your reserved celery and coriander leaves. Slice the egg (preferably with an old-school egg slicer!) and cut the kernels off the corn. Toast and tear up the tortilla. Add it all to your garnishes plate.

Blitz the gazpacho until super-smooth, then season to absolute perfection. Add the ice cubes and blitz again, then divide between bowls, cups or glasses. Serve with your plate of garnishes for dipping, dunking and topping.

CALORIES	FAT	SAT FAT	PROTEIN	CARBS	SUGAR	FIBRE	20 MINUTES
252kcal	6.5g	1.8g	11.5g	37g	14.8g	6.8g	

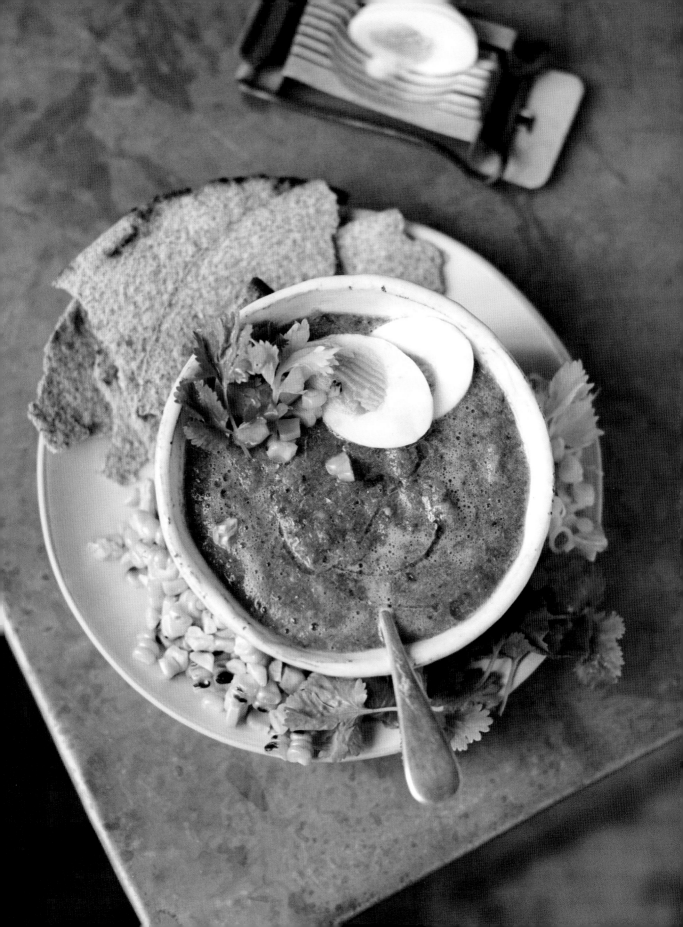

SUPER SUMMER SALAD
WATERMELON, RADISHES, QUINOA & FETA

— Quinoa is an awesome grain packed with many essential vitamins and minerals, —
as well as protein. This refreshing salad gives us four of our 5-a-day

SERVES 4

250g regular, black or red quinoa

4 spring onions

120g roasted peeled red peppers
   in brine

1 slice of wholemeal bread

1 tablespoon Tabasco chipotle
   sauce

extra virgin olive oil

1 large orange

40g blanched hazelnuts

1 small red onion

100g radishes

1 fresh red chilli

2 limes

½ a bunch of fresh mint (15g)

2 small red or green chicory

750g chunk of watermelon

80g feta cheese

Cook the quinoa according to the packet instructions, removing from the heat 2 minutes early (this is to give you a beautiful texture when you dress it later). While it cooks, cut off the green parts of the spring onions and place in a blender with the peppers, bread, chipotle Tabasco, 1 tablespoon of oil and the orange juice. Blitz until super-smooth, then season to perfection to make a dressing. Once the quinoa is ready, drain it well, then, while still steaming hot, toss with the dressing. Toast the hazelnuts in a dry frying pan, tossing for 4 minutes, or until golden, then smash up in a pestle and mortar and, in a large serving bowl or on a big beautiful platter, fold through the quinoa.

Peel the onion, then very finely slice with the radishes and chilli, ideally on a mandolin (use the guard!). Finely grate all the lime zest over the veg and squeeze over the juice, then mix together with your hands. Pick and tear over the mint leaves, reserving the pretty baby leaves for garnish.

Trim and finely slice the chicory and the whites of the spring onions and scatter over the quinoa. Peel and finely slice the watermelon and arrange on top of the salad. Sprinkle over the lime-dressed veg and reserved mint, then grate over the feta in long strokes. Keep it pretty or toss together before tucking in. Also nice served with a little cured meat, such as prosciutto.

CALORIES	FAT	SAT FAT	PROTEIN	CARBS	SUGAR	FIBRE	45 MINUTES
474kcal	19.9g	4.6g	16.7g	61.7g	24.1g	3.4g	

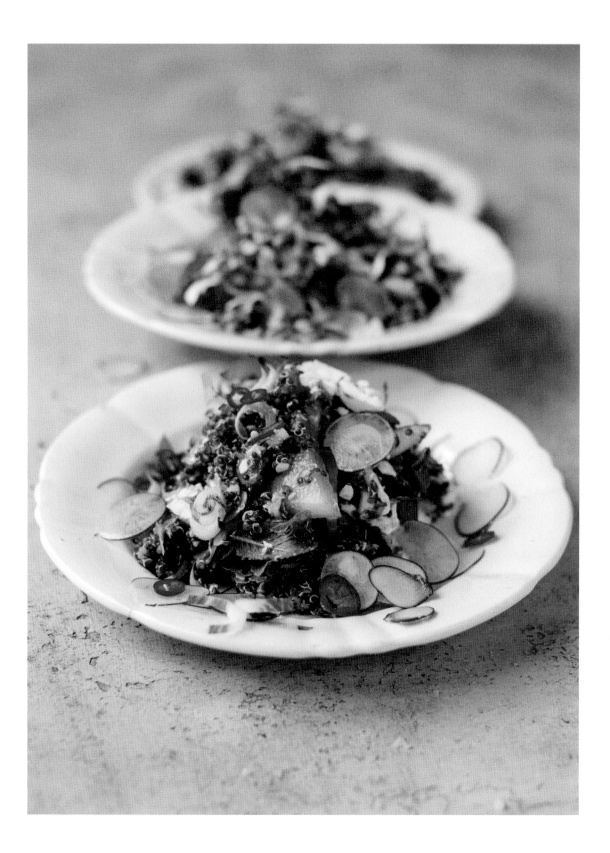

ASIAN GREEN SALAD
TOFU, NOODLES & SESAME SPRINKLE

__ Silken tofu is a delight to eat, a wonderful carrier of flavours, and is packed with both __
protein and calcium. This busload of nutritious greens contains two of our 5-a-day

SERVES 2

1 bunch of asparagus (300g)

½ a head of broccoli

100g sugar snap peas

200g silken tofu

150g brown rice noodles

2cm piece of ginger

1 clove of garlic

2 limes

2 tablespoons low-salt soy sauce

2 tablespoons sesame oil

1 tablespoon balsamic vinegar

1 sheet of nori

1 heaped tablespoon sesame
    seeds

1 teaspoon dried red chilli flakes

Sit a double-layer bamboo steamer over a large pan of boiling salted water. Trim the woody ends off the asparagus, then halve the spears at an angle. Cut the broccoli into small florets, peeling and slicing the stalk. Arrange both asparagus and broccoli in the top steamer layer with the sugar snaps. Chop the tofu into bite-sized chunks and place in the bottom layer. Pop the noodles into the boiling water under the steamer. Boil and steam everything hard for 4 minutes, or until the veg are only just cooked, but still green and full of life.

Meanwhile, peel the ginger and garlic and finely grate into a bowl, adding the zest and juice of 1 lime. Mix in the soy, sesame oil and vinegar to make a dressing. For your sprinkle, finely tear the sheet of nori into a blender, add a small pinch of sea salt and black pepper and blitz until fine. Toast the sesame seeds and chilli flakes in a dry pan until lightly golden, then tip into the blender and whiz to combine.

Reserving some cooking water, drain the noodles and toss with the veg, tofu and dressing, loosening with a splash of reserved water, if needed. Scatter over a little sesame sprinkle, keeping the rest for another day, and serve with lime wedges for squeezing over, to taste.

CALORIES	FAT	SAT FAT	PROTEIN	CARBS	SUGAR	FIBRE	
459kcal	22.4g	3.9g	22.5g	41.4g	11.8g	7.7g	15 MINUTES

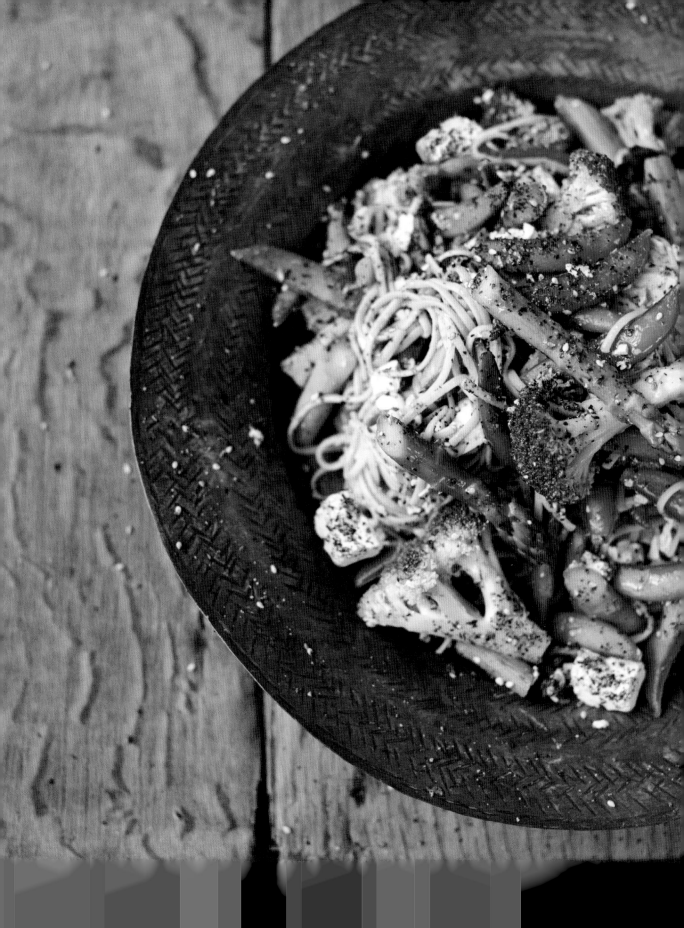

SEARED TURMERIC CHICKEN
HOUMOUS, PEPPERS, COUSCOUS & GREENS

_____ Turmeric is super-high in iron – allowing our blood to transport oxygen efficiently so we feel less tired – and contains manganese, keeping our bones strong and healthy _____

SERVES 2

2 sprigs of fresh oregano

1 level teaspoon ground turmeric

olive oil

2 x 120g skinless chicken breasts

200g seasonal greens, such as
   baby spinach, Swiss chard

150g wholewheat couscous

½ a bunch of fresh mint (15g)

1 lemon

1 tablespoon blanched hazelnuts

2 large or 4 small roasted peeled
   red peppers in brine

¼ x skinny houmous (see page
   230) or 2 tablespoons natural
   yoghurt

optional: hot chilli sauce

Pick and finely chop the oregano leaves, then place in a bowl with the turmeric, a pinch each of sea salt and black pepper and 2 tablespoons of oil to make a marinade. Toss the chicken in the marinade and leave aside.

Blanch the greens in a large pan of boiling water until just tender enough to eat but still vibrant in colour, then drain, reserving the water. In a bowl, just cover the couscous with boiling greens water, season, pop a plate on top and leave for 10 minutes. Pick and finely chop the mint leaves and stir into the fluffy couscous with the juice of half a lemon, then season to perfection. Toast the hazelnuts in a large dry non-stick frying pan on a medium-high heat, removing and crushing in a pestle and mortar once lightly golden. Return the frying pan to a high heat and cook the chicken for 4 minutes on each side, or until cooked through, turning halfway and adding the peppers when you flip the chicken. Reheat the greens, if needed.

Meanwhile, you can either make a quick houmous (put three-quarters into the fridge for another day if making a full batch) or simply use yoghurt – both options are delicious. Serve the chicken with the couscous, peppers, greens and houmous or yoghurt, scattered with the hazelnuts and with a lemon wedge on the side. Nice with a drizzle of hot chilli sauce too.

CALORIES	FAT	SAT FAT	PROTEIN	CARBS	SUGAR	FIBRE	30 MINUTES
579kcal	20.6g	3.2g	41.4g	58.5g	4.2g	7.6g	

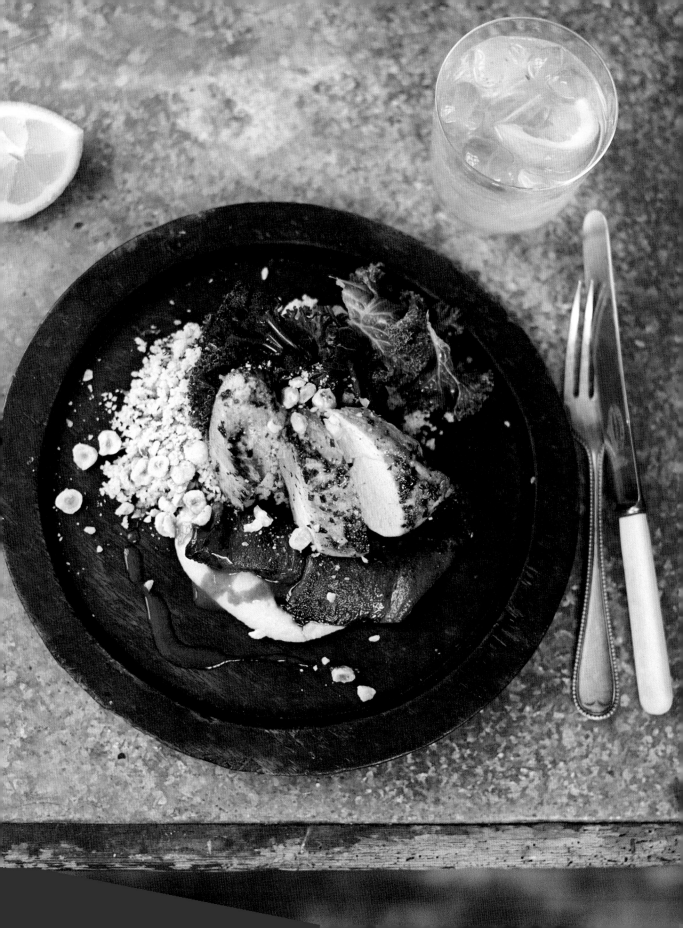

SALMON CEVICHE
CHOPPED SALAD, BLACK RICE BALLS

— Salmon is a fantastic source of vitamin D, which helps keep our bones, teeth and muscles healthy – we get it naturally from sunlight, but it's useful to top up from food too —

SERVES 2

150g black rice

1 red onion

2 large lemons

1 lime

1 pomegranate

1 clove of garlic

1 fresh red chilli

½ a cucumber

½ a ripe avocado

1 handful of ripe mixed-colour
tomatoes

½ a bunch of fresh coriander
(15g)

2 x 120g fillets of super-fresh
salmon, skin off and pin-boned

Cook the rice according to the packet instructions, then drain and leave to cool. Meanwhile, peel and very finely slice the red onion, ideally on a mandolin (use the guard!). Place in a large bowl with 2 really good pinches of sea salt and squeeze over the lemon and lime juice (don't worry about the salt – the liquid is to cure the fish, not for drinking). Halve the pomegranate and squeeze the juice from one half through a sieve into the bowl. Hold the other half cut side down in your fingers and bash the back of it with a spoon so that all the jewels tumble out into the liquor.

Peel the garlic, then finely slice with the chilli and add to the bowl. Peel the cucumber, halve lengthways and use a teaspoon to remove the watery core, then slice 2cm thick and add to the bowl. Peel and destone the avocado and chop the same size, along with the tomatoes, then roughly chop most of the coriander leaves and stir it all into the bowl. Chop the salmon into 1cm x 2cm chunks and gently mix them into the bowl, being sure to submerge everything in the ceviche liquid. Leave for 10 minutes, to cure the salmon.

Meanwhile, use a spoon to mix and mash the rice for a couple of minutes, until it gets sticky. Wet your clean hands and roll little portions of rice into balls. Drain away most of the ceviche liquid, then sprinkle over the remaining coriander leaves and serve right away with the rice balls.

CALORIES	FAT	SAT FAT	PROTEIN	CARBS	SUGAR	FIBRE	40 MINUTES
452kcal	24.2g	4.6g	30.5g	27.1g	9.7g	7.2g	

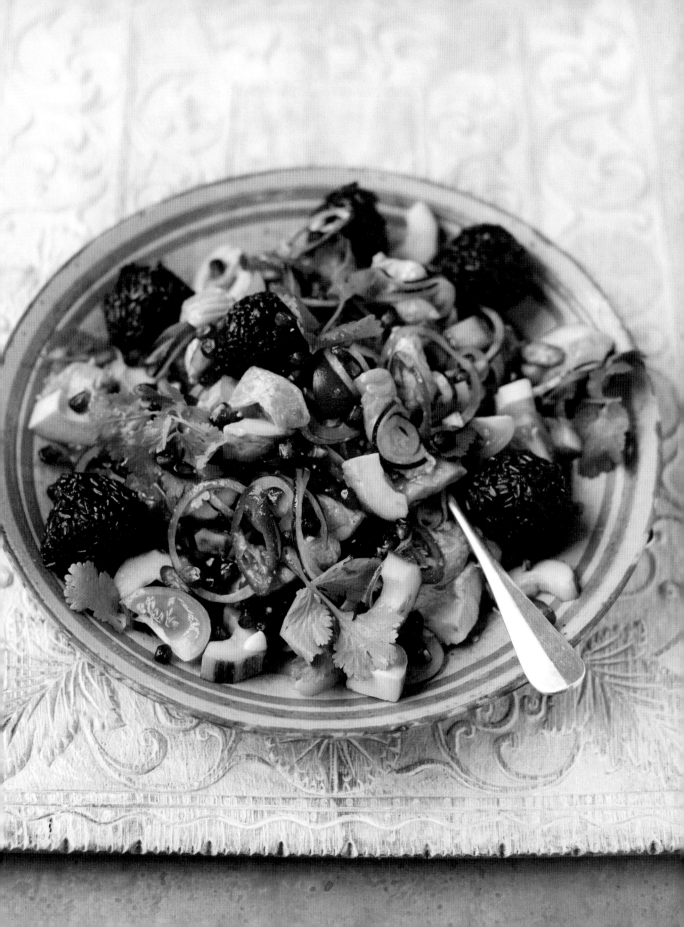

ASIAN STIR-FRIED VEG
CRISPY SESAME NOODLE OMELETTE

— This is an easy, delicious, balanced way to pack in a portion of your 5-a-day.
Eggs are our protein of choice, helping to keep us feeling full until dinner time —

SERVES 1

75g brown rice noodles

2 large mixed handfuls of
asparagus, baby corn,
carrots, beansprouts

3cm piece of ginger

1 clove of garlic

½ a fresh red chilli

sesame oil

1 teaspoon sesame seeds

2 large eggs

1 spring onion

3 sprigs of fresh coriander

1 lime

low-salt soy sauce

Cook the noodles according to the packet instructions, then drain. Trim the woody ends off the asparagus and chop up the stalks, halving the tips lengthways to help them cook. Halve the baby corn lengthways and matchstick the carrot. Peel and finely chop the ginger and garlic, finely slice the chilli (deseed if you like), and put into a 30cm non-stick frying pan on a medium-high heat with 1 teaspoon of sesame oil. Toss for 1 minute, then add the asparagus, corn, carrot, beansprouts and a pinch of sesame seeds. Toss and stir-fry for 5 minutes, then tip on to a plate, returning the pan to the heat.

Drizzle 1 teaspoon of sesame oil into the pan, randomly scatter in the noodles in a fairly even layer, then sprinkle over the remaining sesame seeds and leave to nicely crisp up while you beat the eggs with a splash of water. Pour the eggs over the crispy noodles, swirling them around the pan, then cover and reduce the heat to low. Leave to cook through for a couple of minutes while you trim and finely slice the spring onion and pick the coriander leaves.

Loosen the edges of the omelette with a rubber spatula and slide onto a plate. Pile the stir-fried veg in the centre, then scatter over the spring onions and coriander leaves. Serve with a squeeze of lime juice and a drizzle of soy sauce.

CALORIES	FAT	SAT FAT	PROTEIN	CARBS	SUGAR	FIBRE	15 MINUTES
392kcal	19.1g	4.5g	19.5g	36.6g	5g	2.5g	

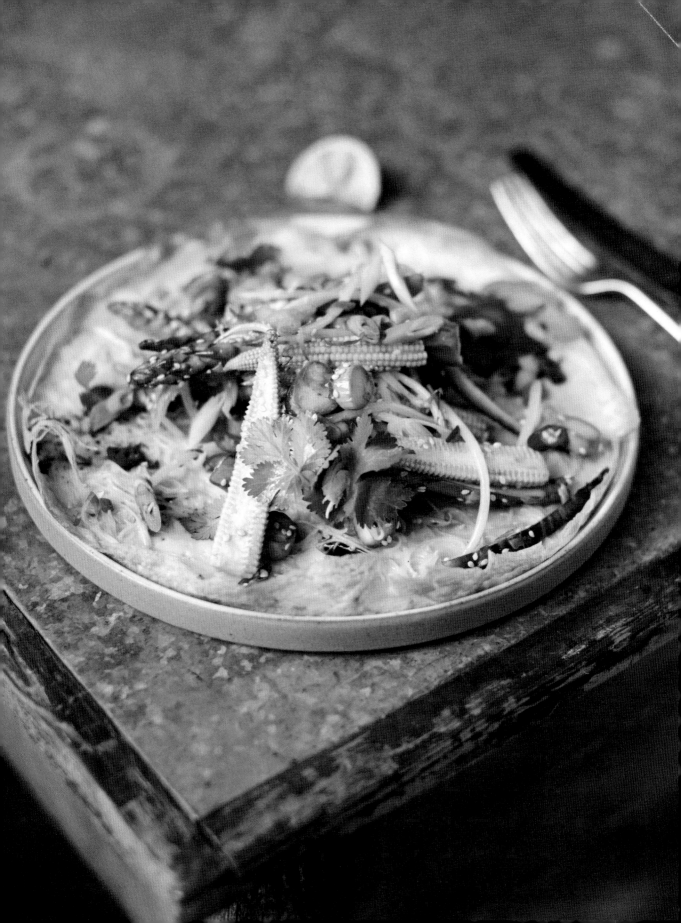

SQUASH IT VEG SANDWICH
HOUMOUS, AVOCADO & COTTAGE CHEESE

—   This delicious hand-held veg-packed beauty gives us two of our 5-a-day, while sunflower   —
seeds and cottage cheese balance the mix with some all-important protein

SERVES 2

2 seeded wholemeal rolls

200g crunchy mixed seasonal
veg, such as baby carrots, raw
baby beets, cauliflower, peppers,
radishes, cucumber, freshly
podded peas, asparagus

1 eating apple

1 tablespoon sunflower seeds

½ a bunch of fresh dill or
mint (15g)

1 tablespoon balsamic vinegar

extra virgin olive oil

2 tablespoons skinny houmous
(page 230)

2 tablespoons cottage cheese

½ a ripe avocado

I like to pop the rolls into the oven and turn it on to a low temperature so they can warm through while I prep everything else.

Lay out a clean tea towel. Wash and trim all your veg, deseeding any peppers and the apple, then pile in the middle of the tea towel with the sunflower seeds. Tear over the dill or mint leaves, then pull up the edges of the tea towel to make a bundle. Holding it firmly, bash and squash it with a rolling pin to crush up all the veg. Simply stop when you think everything is an agreeable size to eat. As crazy as it might seem, by squashing up the veg you create more surface area for the dressing to stick to, you start to break down hard vegetables, and in turn they start to release their natural juices and flavours, which makes it all taste and eat even better.

Tip the veg into a bowl and dress with the vinegar and 1 tablespoon of oil, then season to perfection. Halve your warm rolls and spread the bases with houmous and the lids with cottage cheese. Peel, destone and finely slice the avocado and layer on top of the houmous. Pile as much of the dressed squashed veg on to the bases of the rolls as you can, pop the lids on and squeeze together. Serve any remaining veg on the side, and get stuck in!

CALORIES	FAT	SAT FAT	PROTEIN	CARBS	SUGAR	FIBRE	20 MINUTES
397kcal	17.7g	3.7g	14.1g	47.7g	15.2g	8.8g	

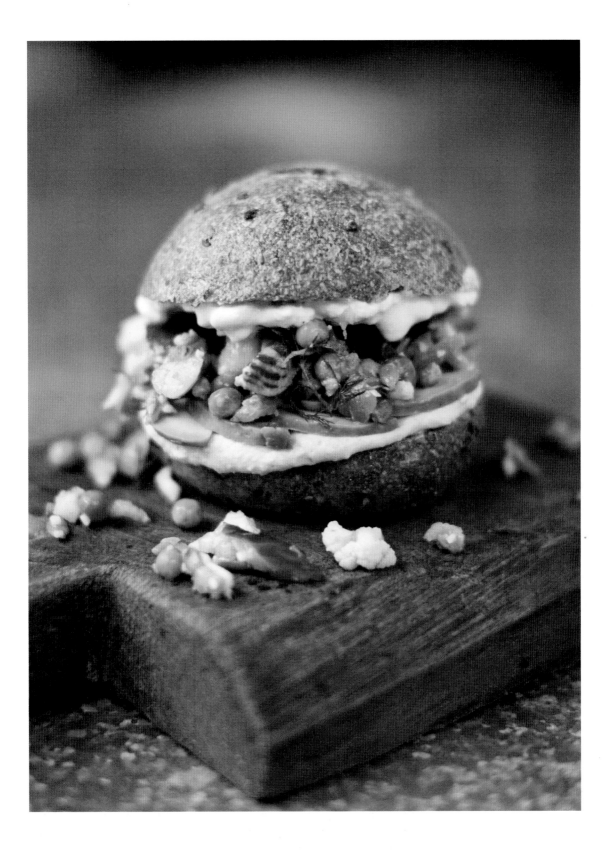

MY RUSSIAN SALAD
GOLDEN PAPRIKA CHICKEN

Inspired by the popular classic and celebrating loads of veg, including two of our 5-a-day, I've re-worked the traditional mayo-based dressing to make it super-healthy here

SERVES 4

400g mixed-colour raw baby beets and small carrots

400g potatoes

1 bunch of asparagus (300g)

100g freshly podded peas

2 x 180g skinless chicken breasts

olive oil

smoked paprika

3 tablespoons natural yoghurt

2 tablespoons cottage cheese

1 heaped teaspoon Dijon mustard

1 tablespoon white wine vinegar

2 anchovy fillets in oil

2 cornichons

1 teaspoon baby capers

¼ of a bunch of fresh dill (5g)

Cook the beets in a small pan of boiling water for around 10 minutes, or until tender. Trim the carrots, halving any larger ones lengthways and cut the potatoes into 2cm dice, then cook in a separate pan of boiling salted water for 8 minutes, or until tender. Trim the woody ends off the asparagus and slice the stalks 1cm thick, leaving the tips whole. Add to the potato pan with the peas for 2 more minutes, then drain it all in a colander and leave to steam dry.

Rub the chicken breasts with 1 tablespoon of oil, a generous pinch of paprika and a little seasoning, then cook for 10 minutes in a non-stick frying pan on a medium-high heat, or until golden and cooked through, turning halfway.

Meanwhile, put the yoghurt, cottage cheese, mustard, vinegar and a pinch of black pepper into a large serving bowl. Very finely chop the anchovies, cornichons, capers and dill, add to the bowl and mix well. Stir in the potatoes, carrots, asparagus and peas, then taste and season to perfection. Peel and slice the beets, then fold through gently to maintain all the beautiful colours. Slice up and pile on the chicken, dust with a little extra paprika and tuck in.

CALORIES	FAT	SAT FAT	PROTEIN	CARBS	SUGAR	FIBRE	25 MINUTES
315kcal	7.9g	2g	31.3g	31.2g	11.1g	5.8g	

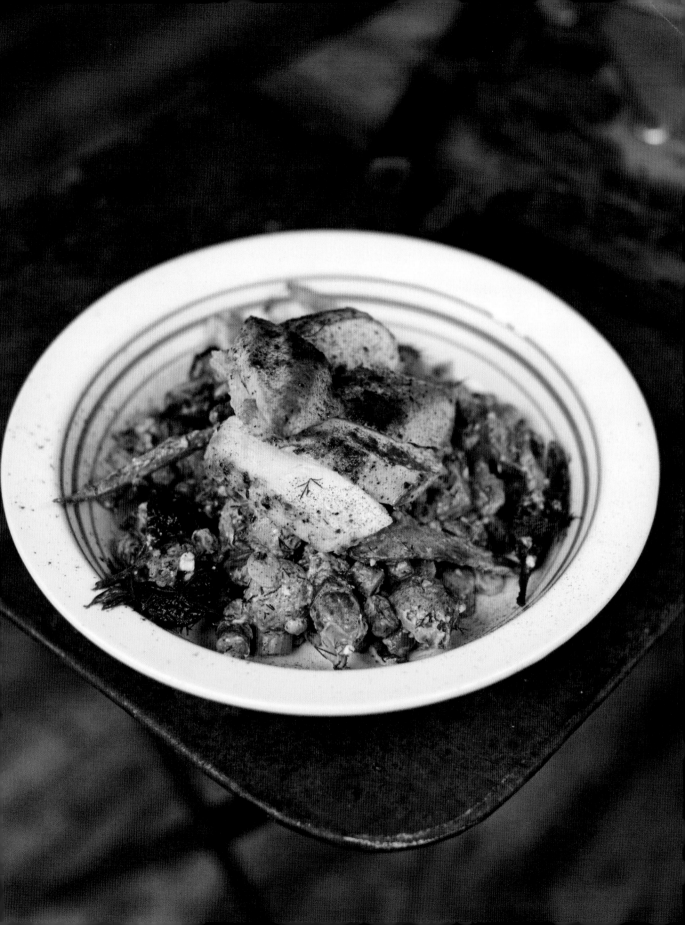

SESAME SEARED SALMON
TAHINI AVOCADO & SHRED SALAD

— As well as this delicious dish giving us three of our 5-a-day, salmon is full of vitamin D, —
which our bodies need for absorbing calcium, keeping our bones and teeth healthy

SERVES 2

150g brown rice noodles

2 limes

2 x 100g fillets of salmon, skin
on, scaled and pin-boned

4 teaspoons sesame seeds

1 clove of garlic

4 teaspoons tahini

8cm piece of cucumber

2 small carrots

2 raw baby beets

1 punnet of cress

1 ripe avocado

extra virgin olive oil

½–1 fresh red chilli

2 sprigs of fresh coriander

Cook the noodles according to the packet instructions, then drain and toss in a little squeeze of lime juice. Carefully slice each of the salmon fillets lengthways into three. Scatter the sesame seeds over a board and press one side of the salmon slices into the seeds to form a crust. Place a large dry non-stick frying pan over a medium heat, and once hot, add the salmon sesame side down. Leave for 2 to 3 minutes, or until golden, flip over to cook for just 1 more minute, then remove from the heat.

Peel the garlic and pound into a paste with a pinch of sea salt in a pestle and mortar, then muddle in the tahini, the remaining lime juice and a splash of water to make a wicked dressing. Use a box grater to coarsely grate the cucumber, carrots and beets, keeping them in separate piles and dividing between two plates. Snip and divide up the cress, then divide up the noodles.

Halve, peel and destone the avocado and add one half to each plate, then pour the dressing into the wells and add a few drips of oil. Lay the salmon alongside, then finely slice the chilli and scatter over with the coriander leaves. Toss everything together at the table and enjoy.

CALORIES	FAT	SAT FAT	PROTEIN	CARBS	SUGAR	FIBRE	20 MINUTES
552kcal	33.1g	6g	28.4g	35.1g	8g	6.2g	

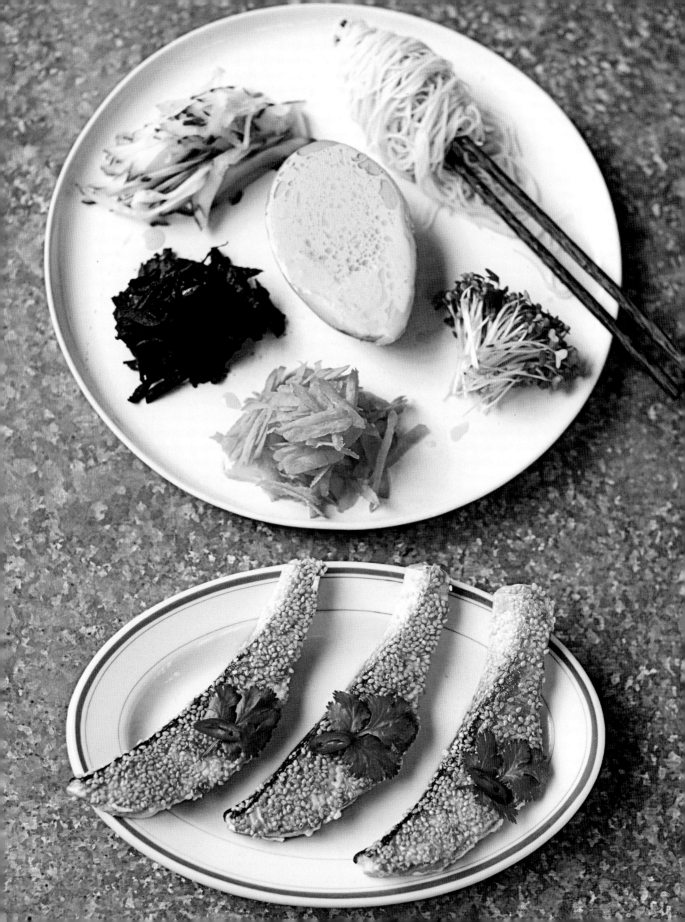

GRILLED CORN & QUINOA SALAD
MANGO, TOMATOES, HERBS, AVO, FETA

_ Giving us two of our 5-a-day, this colourful salad also uses quinoa – it's a brilliant, _
tasty grain packed with both protein and fibre, and is also gluten-free

SERVES 4

250g regular, black or red quinoa

1 small ripe mango

1 ripe avocado

300g ripe mixed-colour tomatoes

2 limes

extra virgin olive oil

2 corn on the cob

2 cloves of garlic

4 rashers of smoked streaky
   bacon

1 fresh red chilli

olive oil

20g feta cheese

½ a bunch of fresh coriander
   or mint (15g)

Cook the quinoa according to the packet instructions, then drain. Peel and destone the mango and avocado, then roughly chop or slice the flesh, along with the tomatoes. In a large bowl, toss them with the lime zest and juice, 2 tablespoons of extra virgin olive oil and a pinch of sea salt and black pepper. Leave to macerate while you grill the corn cobs on a hot griddle pan until nicely charred, then carefully slice off the kernels.

Peel the garlic and finely slice with the bacon and chilli (deseed if you like). Put it all into a small frying pan on a medium heat with 1 teaspoon of olive oil. Stir and cook until lightly golden, tossing regularly. Tip into the bowl of macerated veg, add the quinoa and corn and toss it all together, then taste and season to perfection. Divide between your plates, crumble over the feta, pick over the herb leaves and serve.

CALORIES	FAT	SAT FAT	PROTEIN	CARBS	SUGAR	FIBRE	25 MINUTES
438kcal	20.6g	4.4g	15.3g	51.2g	9.4g	3.3g	

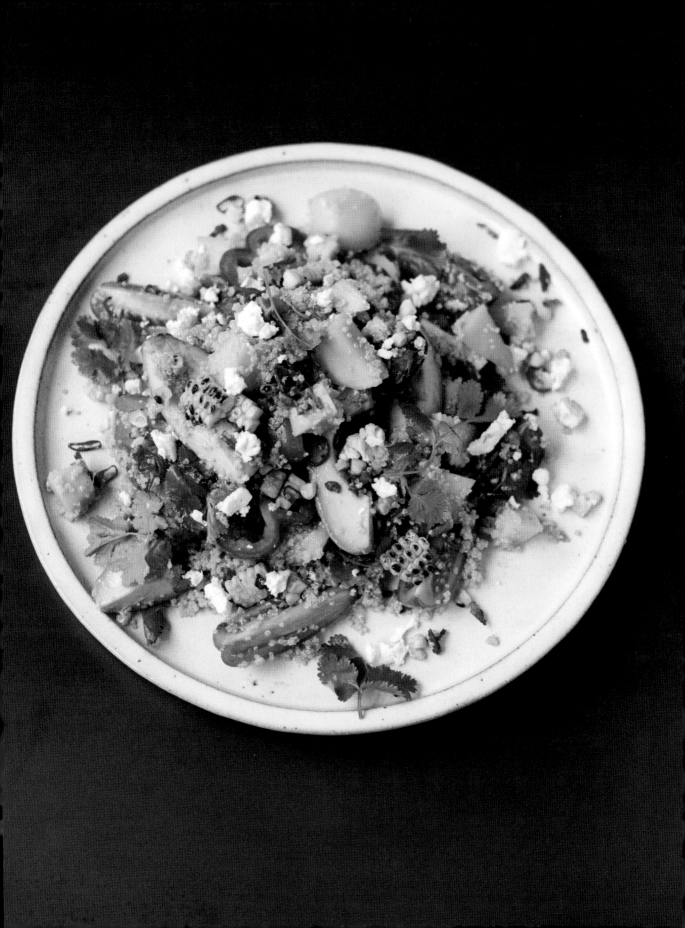

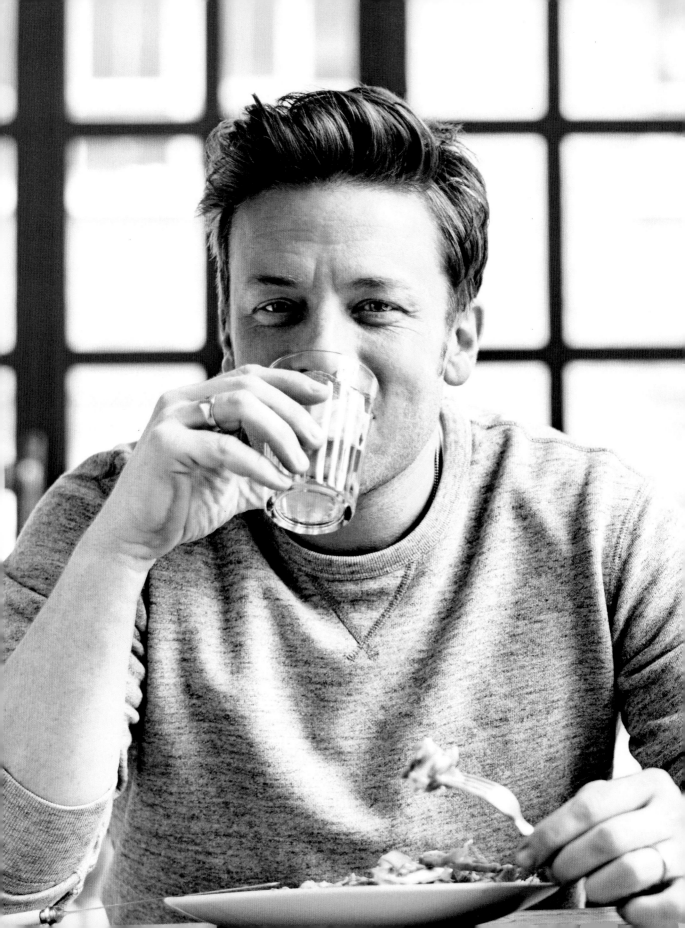

DINNER

What I've set out to achieve in this chapter is the perfect balance between super-fast, get-it-out pronto recipes, and medium-length recipes, for those evenings when you've got a little more time on your hands. And there's a whole host of inspiration from around the world in these dishes to really get your taste buds going. All the recipes have a nice mix of the food groups and are less than 600 calories per portion, so they can be enjoyed at lunchtime too, if that works for you. Whenever you can, take the time to sit at the table and really enjoy your meal, sharing it with loved ones if they're about.

BOMBAY CHICKEN & CAULI
POPPADOMS, RICE & SPINACH

Cumin and turmeric are great sources of iron, and teaming them with lemon juice like I've done here means our bodies can absorb that all-important iron really efficiently

SERVES 2

100g brown rice

½ a small cauliflower (400g)

½ a bunch of fresh mint (15g)

6 tablespoons natural yoghurt

1 lemon

1 heaped teaspoon each of ground turmeric, medium curry powder

1 tablespoon balsamic vinegar

2 cloves of garlic

3cm piece of ginger

2 x 120g skinless chicken breasts

1 level teaspoon each of cumin seeds, black mustard seeds

4 uncooked poppadoms

60g baby spinach

1 fresh red chilli

Preheat the oven to 220°C/425°F/gas 7. Cook the rice in a pan of boiling salted water according to the packet instructions. Chop the cauliflower into thin wedges and place in a sieve above the rice, then cover and steam for 15 minutes. Pick the mint leaves into a blender (reserving a few baby leaves). Add 3 tablespoons of yoghurt, half the lemon juice and a splash of water to the blender, then blitz for 1 minute until super-smooth and green. Decant into a nice dish and pop into the fridge for later.

Without washing the blender, add the remaining yoghurt and lemon juice, the turmeric, curry powder and balsamic. Crush in the garlic, then peel, finely chop and add the ginger. Blitz until super-smooth to make a marinade, then pour into a large baking tray. Lightly score the chicken breasts to increase the surface area and toss in the marinade. When the time's up on the cauliflower, tip it into the chicken tray, quickly toss together, sprinkle over the cumin and black mustard seeds, then place in the oven for 15 minutes, or until the chicken is cooked through and the cauli is gnarly.

When the rice is done, drain it, catching some of the water in the pan, then sit the sieve of rice back over the pan, cover, and place on the lowest heat to keep warm. One-by-one, puff up your dry poppadoms in the microwave for around 30 seconds each. Slice and divide up the chicken, with the cauli, rice, spinach and poppadoms. Drizzle with the dressing, then finely slice and scatter over the chilli. Finish with the baby mint leaves and tuck on in.

CALORIES	FAT	SAT FAT	PROTEIN	CARBS	SUGAR	FIBRE	
546kcal	13.1g	3.5g	48g	63.6g	13.8g	7.6g	40 MINUTES

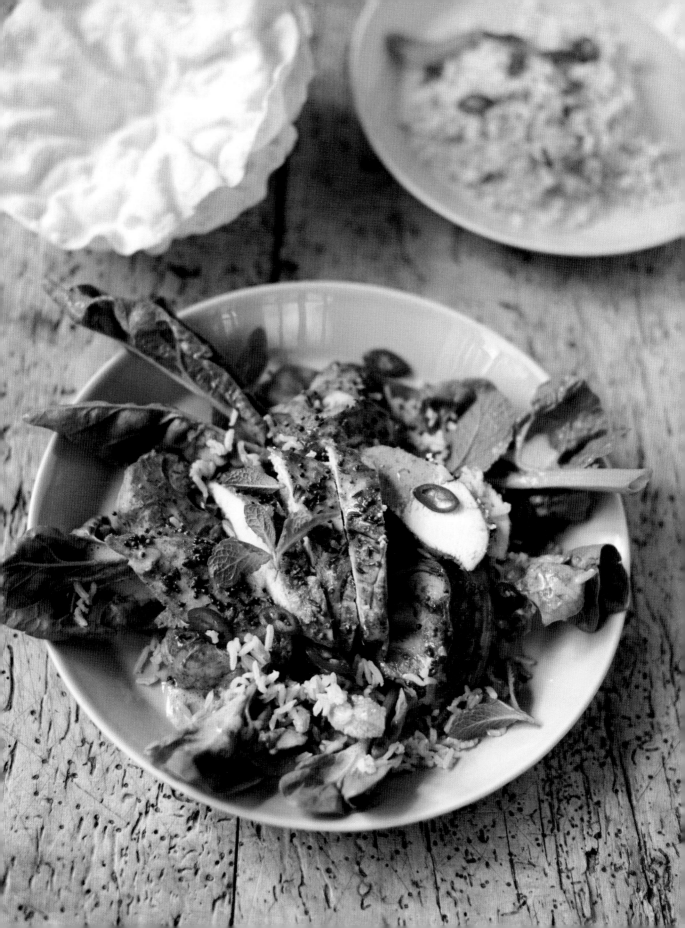

MEGA VEGGIE BURGERS
GARDEN SALAD & BASIL DRESSING

— Tofu is a brilliant carrier of flavours, plus it's high in protein, low in saturated fat and a great source of calcium and phosphorus, both of which make for strong and healthy bones —

SERVES 4

350g firm silken tofu

1 large egg

75g wholemeal breadcrumbs

2 heaped teaspoons Marmite

8 ripe tomatoes

1 tablespoon red wine vinegar

2 sprigs of fresh basil

4 soft wholemeal buns

400g mixed seasonal salad veg,
 such as cucumber, red cabbage,
 apples, cress, baby spinach

½ x creamy basil dressing
 (see page 226)

olive oil

2 sprigs of fresh rosemary

50g Cheddar cheese

50g gherkins

Wrap the tofu in a clean tea towel, then squeeze and wring it out to remove the excess liquid (about 4 tablespoons should come out – it's messy, but really important to do this for great burger texture later). Place the tofu in a bowl, scraping it off the tea towel. Crack in the egg, then add the breadcrumbs and Marmite. Mix and scrunch together really well with clean hands, then shape into 4 even-sized patties that'll fit nicely in your buns once cooked.

Roughly chop the tomatoes and put into a dry non-stick frying pan on a high heat with a pinch of black pepper, a splash of water and the vinegar. Squash the tomatoes with a potato masher, cook for 10 to 15 minutes, or until thick and delicious, then tear in half the basil leaves and season to perfection (I sometimes add a pinch of dried red chilli flakes too, for a kick). If you want to plump up your buns, pop them into a warm oven for a few minutes.

Meanwhile, finely slice or prep all the salad veg, and make the creamy basil dressing. Place 2 teaspoons of oil in a large non-stick frying pan on a medium heat. Pick the rosemary leaves into the pan in four piles, place the patties on top and cook for 3 minutes on each side, or until golden. Slice or grate the cheese, place on the patties, reduce the heat to low, then cover and leave to melt for 3 to 4 minutes. Spread the tomato sauce into the buns, then sandwich the cheesy burgers and sliced gherkins inside. Toss the salad with the dressing, serve alongside the burgers and enjoy – totally awesome.

CALORIES	FAT	SAT FAT	PROTEIN·	CARBS	SUGAR	FIBRE	45 MINUTES
424kcal	15.7g	4.6g	24.9g	44.8g	12.1g	9.3g	

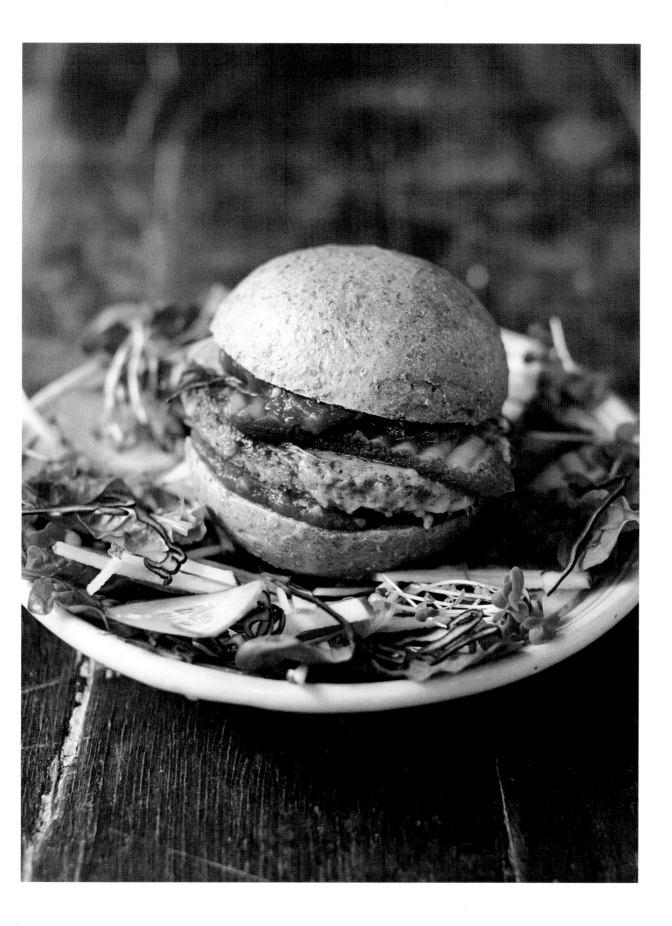

SPELT SPAGHETTI
VINE TOMATOES & BAKED RICOTTA

— Spelt spaghetti has an incredible nutty taste and is a great alternative to regular spaghetti as —
it's high in wheat bran fibre, or beta-glucans, which help keep our cholesterol levels in check

SERVES 4

olive oil

½ a bunch of fresh thyme (15g)

4 cloves of garlic

½–1 fresh red chilli

1 lemon

500g ripe mixed-colour cherry
  tomatoes, on the vine

250g best-quality ricotta cheese

320g dried spelt spaghetti

4 handfuls of rocket

optional: balsamic vinegar

Preheat the oven to 180°C/350°F/gas 4. Pour 3 tablespoons of oil into a small bowl. Run the bunch of thyme under a hot tap for 3 seconds to reawaken it, then shake dry and strip the leaves into the oil. Peel the garlic, then finely slice it with the chilli and add to the bowl. Finely grate in the lemon zest, add a pinch of sea salt and black pepper and mix together. Lay the cherry tomatoes in a 30cm x 40cm baking tray. Rub the flavoured oil all over the ricotta and place in the centre of the tray, then gently rub the remaining oil over the tomatoes. Add a splash of water to the tray, place in the oven and roast for 45 minutes, then remove. With 10 minutes to go, cook the spaghetti in a pan of boiling salted water according to the packet instructions.

Lift the ricotta out of the tray, then shake the tomatoes off the vines, discarding the stalks. Add half a mug of pasta water to the tray and gently shake to loosen all the sticky goodness from the base. Drain the spaghetti and toss straight into the tray with a squeeze of lemon juice, season to perfection, then break that beautiful ricotta over the top. Sprinkle over the rocket, toss together well, then serve. My missus likes this with a little drizzle of balsamic, too.

CALORIES	FAT	SAT FAT	PROTEIN	CARBS	SUGAR	FIBRE	1 HOUR
492kcal	18.9g	5.8g	16.3g	61.7g	9.2g	7g	

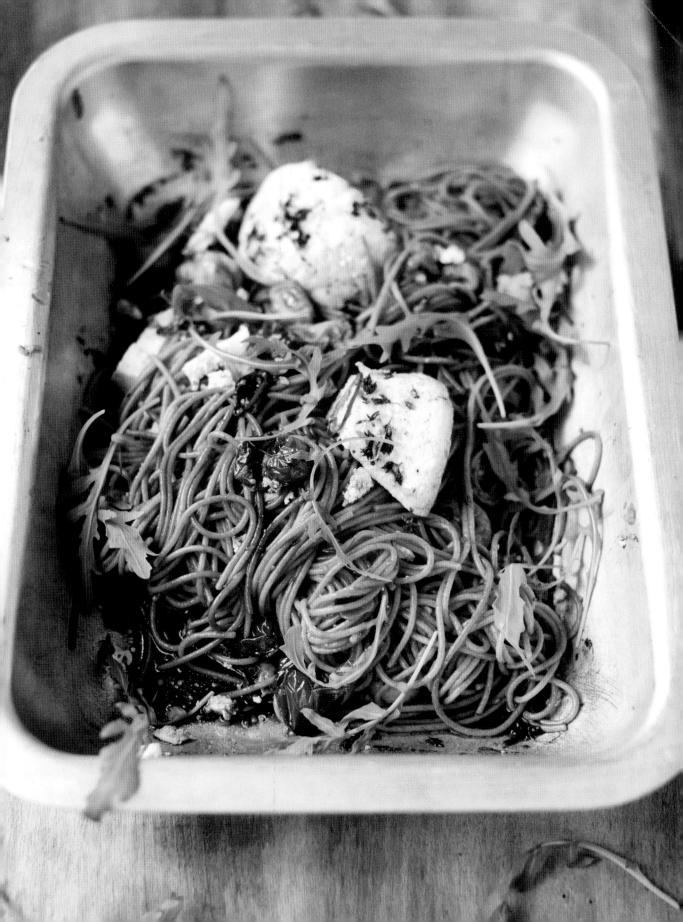

SEARED GOLDEN CHICKEN
MINT SAUCE & SPRING VEG FEST

All the super-fresh spring veg in this dish give us two of our 5-a-day and ensure it's a really nutritious meal packed with vitamin C, which our bodies need for pretty much everything!

SERVES 2

olive oil

white wine vinegar

dried red chilli flakes

2 x 120g skinless chicken breasts

1 bunch of asparagus (300g)

100g freshly podded or
    frozen broad beans

100g freshly podded or
    frozen peas

1 bunch of fresh mint (30g)

20g feta cheese

2 slices of seeded wholemeal
    bread

Place 1 tablespoon each of oil and vinegar in a bowl with a pinch of chilli flakes. Add the chicken breasts and massage them with all that flavour, then transfer to a medium non-stick frying pan on a medium-high heat to cook for around 8 minutes, or until golden and cooked through, turning regularly.

Meanwhile, put a large pan on a high heat and half-fill with boiling water. Trim the woody ends off the asparagus, then slice the stalks 1cm thick, leaving the tips whole. Quickly cook in the water with the broad beans and peas for just 3 minutes. Remove one large ladleful of veg and water to a blender, then drain the rest of the veg and divide between your serving bowls. Quickly rip the top leafy tender-stalked half of the mint into the blender, then pick in the rest of the larger leaves. Add 2 tablespoons of vinegar, a drizzle of oil and a pinch of sea salt and blitz until super-smooth.

Place the seared golden chicken on top of the veg, spoon over the mint sauce and crumble over the feta, then serve with a slice of bread on the side to mop up all the delicious juices. What a beautifully simple, seasonal recipe.

CALORIES	FAT	SAT FAT	PROTEIN	CARBS	SUGAR	FIBRE	15 MINUTES
468kcal	18g	4.2g	45.5g	32.3g	6.1g	11g	

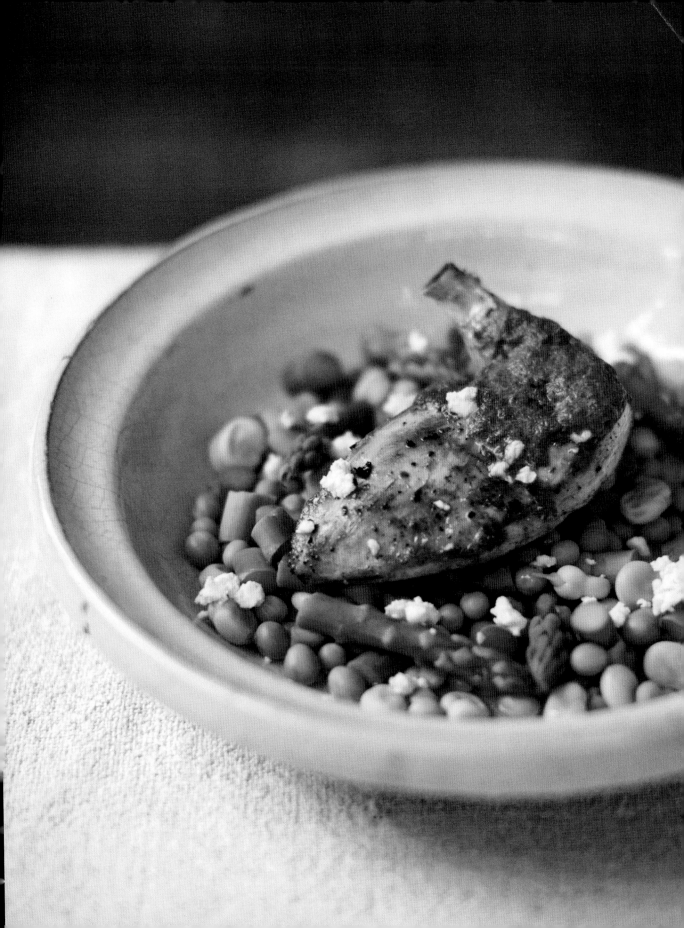

EASY CURRIED FISH STEW
PRAWNS, WHITE FISH & SWEET TOMATOES

_ Prawns are super-high in vitamin B12, which our metabolic and nervous systems
need to function properly, plus it helps to prevent us from feeling tired _

SERVES 6

6 spring onions

1 fresh red chilli

5cm piece of ginger

olive oil

1 handful of curry leaves

1 teaspoon black mustard seeds

1 level teaspoon ground turmeric

½ teaspoon each of chilli powder,
    cumin seeds, fennel seeds

12 large raw shell-on king prawns

300g brown rice

250g ripe mixed-colour cherry
    tomatoes

1 x 400g tin of light coconut milk

6 x 100g white fish fillets, such as
    bream or haddock, skin on,
    scaled and pin-boned

1 lemon

12 uncooked poppadoms

Trim the spring onions and finely slice with the chilli, then peel and matchstick the ginger. Put a 25cm shallow casserole pan on a medium heat with 1 tablespoon of oil, the spring onions, chilli, ginger, curry leaves and all the spices. Stir and fry for 5 minutes, or until lightly golden.

Meanwhile, remove the prawn heads and stir them into the pan as you go for serious added flavour, then add the rice and 1.2 litres of boiling water. Simmer for 10 minutes while you peel the rest of the prawns (I leave the tails on), then use a small sharp knife to lightly score down the backs and devein them, which will mean they butterfly as they cook. Keep in the fridge until needed.

Halve and add the tomatoes to the pan, then cover with the coconut milk. Simmer for 20 minutes, then cut the fish in half across the middle and place in the pan for a further 10 minutes, or until the fish and rice are cooked through, adding the prawns for the last 5 minutes. Pick out the prawn heads, squeeze out all the lovely juices, then discard, and loosen the stew with a little boiling water, if needed. Have a taste, and season to perfection with sea salt, black pepper and lemon juice. One-by-one, puff up your dry poppadoms in the microwave for around 30 seconds each and serve with the stew.

CALORIES	FAT	SAT FAT	PROTEIN	CARBS	SUGAR	FIBRE	50 MINUTES
454kcal	15.1g	4.6g	30.9g	51.7g	4.3g	3.6g	

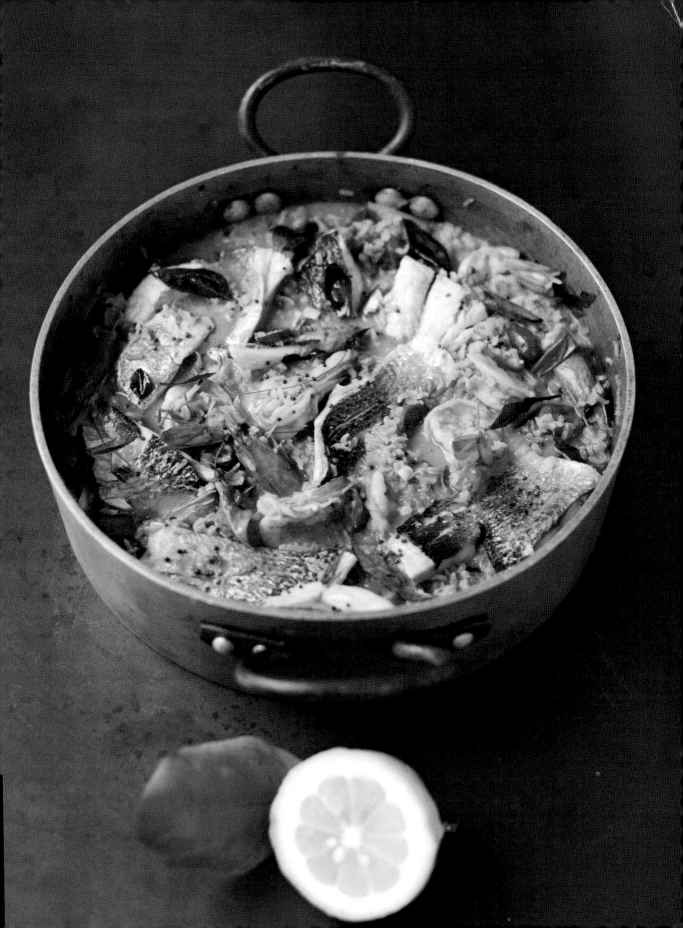

GOLDEN SALMON STEAKS
SWEET PEAS & SMASHED VEG

— Salmon is full of omega-3 fatty acids and is packed with vitamin D, which our bodies need in order to absorb and utilize calcium efficiently, keeping our bones strong and healthy —

SERVES 2

400g mixture of carrots, potatoes and swede

½ a bunch of fresh chives (15g)

2 heaped tablespoons natural yoghurt

olive oil

2 x 180g darnes of salmon, skin on, scaled and bone in

1 teaspoon fennel seeds

300g frozen peas

1 lemon

Wash the carrots and potatoes, peel the swede, then chop it all into 2cm chunks. Cook the swede in a pan of boiling salted water for 10 minutes, then add the carrots and potatoes. Cook for another 15 minutes, or until just soft. Drain and steam dry for 1 minute, then mash. Finely chop and stir in half of the chives, along with the yoghurt, and season to perfection.

Meanwhile, rub a non-stick frying pan on a medium heat with 1 teaspoon of oil, then add the salmon (you could use 2 x 120g fillets, if you prefer). Sprinkle over the fennel seeds and cook for 6 minutes, or until golden and cooked through, turning halfway. You don't need much oil, as the natural fat in the salmon will help it crisp up, while cooking the salmon on the bone ensures it stays juicy – it's cooked when you can easily remove the bone.

Cook the peas in a small pan of boiling water, then drain and add to the salmon pan for 30 seconds, quickly shaking them around to take on some of that lovely flavour. Squeeze half the lemon juice over the salmon, and serve with the smashed veg, sprinkled with the rest of the chives, and extra wedges of lemon for squeezing over.

CALORIES	FAT	SAT FAT	PROTEIN	CARBS	SUGAR	FIBRE	
482kcal	21.2g	4g	42.4g	32.9g	14g	11.9g	30 MINUTES

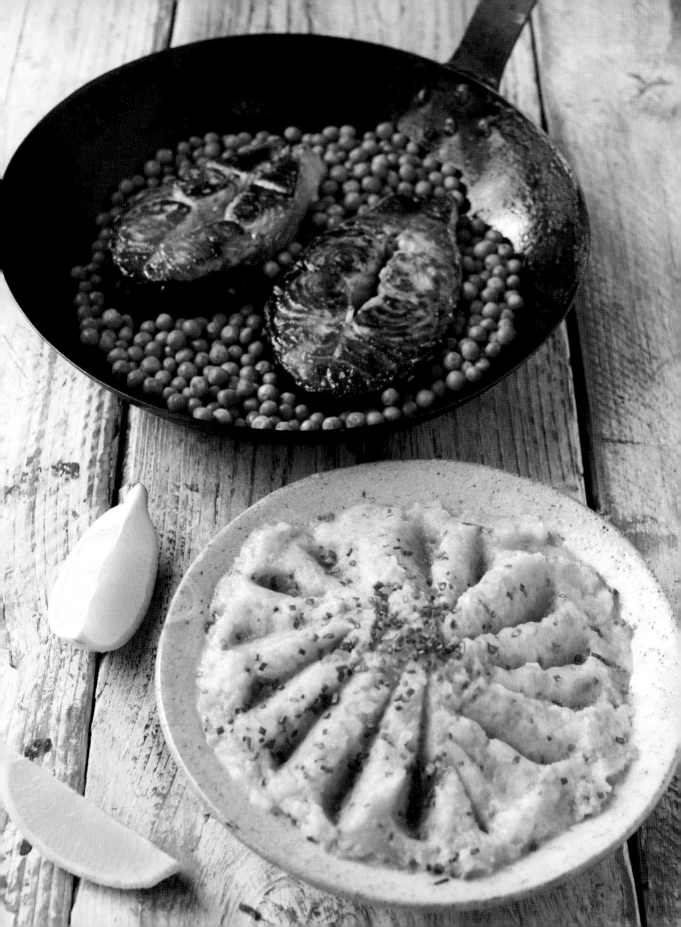

DELICIOUS SQUASH DAAL
SPECIAL FRIED EGGS & POPPADOMS

— Red split lentils are a brilliant source of nutrients, including iron, which we need for making blood cells to transport oxygen around the body, helping to prevent us from getting tired —

SERVES 2
+ 6 LEFTOVER DAAL PORTIONS

8 cloves of garlic

2 fresh red chillies

olive oil

3 teaspoons black mustard seeds

1 heaped teaspoon cumin seeds

1 handful of curry leaves

2 onions

5cm piece of ginger

1 bunch of fresh coriander (30g)

½ a butternut squash (600g)

500g red split lentils

3 tablespoons natural yoghurt

1 lime

2 large eggs

4 uncooked poppadoms

2 handfuls of baby spinach

Start by making a temper. Peel the garlic, then finely slice with the chillies, ideally 1mm thick on a mandolin (use the guard!). Pour 2 tablespoons of oil into a large wide pan on a medium heat and add the mustard seeds, cumin seeds and curry leaves for 1 minute, then the garlic and chillies. Stir so everything's flat, moving regularly until crisp and lightly golden. With a slotted spoon, remove half the temper to a plate, taking the pan off the heat.

Peel the onions and ginger and finely chop with the coriander stalks, then chop the squash into 2cm cubes, leaving the skin on but discarding any seeds. Stir it all into the pan and return to a medium heat for 15 minutes to soften. Stir in the lentils, then 1.5 litres of boiling water. Bring to the boil, then reduce to a gentle simmer and cover for 35 minutes, stirring occasionally. Mash the squash into the daal, taste and season to perfection. Remove 6 portions, bag them up and, once completely cool, freeze for a rainy day when you'll be really grateful it's there, leaving the rest on a low heat to keep warm.

To serve, blitz the coriander leaves, yoghurt, a pinch of sea salt and half the lime juice in a blender until smooth, then decant into a small bowl. Reheat the reserved temper in a non-stick frying pan on a medium-low heat with 1 teaspoon of oil, then divide into two piles and crack an egg over each. Cover and leave to slowly fry on the bottom for 2 or 3 minutes, while they coddle on top. One-by-one, puff up your dry poppadoms in the microwave for around 30 seconds each. Top each portion of daal with a fried egg, and pop some spinach, dressing, poppadoms and a lime wedge on the side.

CALORIES	FAT	SAT FAT	PROTEIN	CARBS	SUGAR	FIBRE	
239kcal	11.6g	2.5g	14.6g	22.3g	7.3g	3.4g	1 HOUR

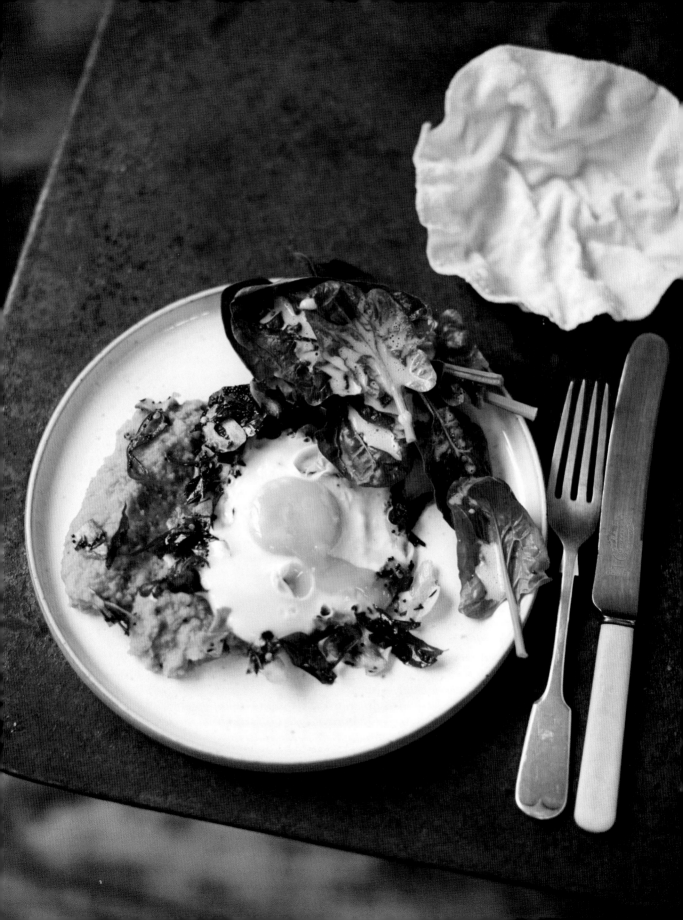

ROASTED SQUASH LAKSA BAKE
CHICKEN, LEMONGRASS, PEANUTS & RICE

Squash is packed with vitamin A, which – and here's a brilliant fact – helps us see in the dark! We also use vitamin A to metabolize iron properly from the food that we eat

SERVES 2

3 sticks of lemongrass

3 cloves of garlic

10cm piece of ginger

2 fresh red chillies

3 spring onions

1 big bunch of fresh coriander (60g)

80ml coconut cream

white wine vinegar

fish sauce

1 really good chicken stock cube

150g mixed brown and wild or brown rice

1 butternut squash (1.2kg)

2 chicken thighs, bone in

sesame oil

1 tablespoon unsalted peanuts

1 lime

Preheat the oven to 180°C/350°F/gas 4. Bash the lemongrass and remove the outer layers, peel the garlic and ginger, trim the chillies and spring onions. Roughly chop it all and place in a blender. Reserving a few nice leaves for garnish, add the bunch of coriander, along with the coconut cream and a good splash each of vinegar and fish sauce. Blitz until smooth, adding splashes of water until you have a nice spoonable consistency, to make a laksa paste.

Crumble the stock cube into a 30cm shallow ovenproof casserole pan and stir in 700ml of boiling water to dissolve it, then add the rice. Carefully slice two 4cm-thick rounds off the bulbous seedy end of the squash and spoon out the seeds (roast them up with a little oil and sea salt to enjoy as a snack, if you like). Remove and discard the chicken skin. On a plate, massage one third of the laksa paste (simply bag up the rest and freeze so you can enjoy big flavour – quickly – on other days) into the squash and chicken, then place them in among the rice. Drizzle with 1 teaspoon of sesame oil, then bake for 1 hour 30 minutes until golden.

Just before serving, lightly toast the peanuts, then bash up in a pestle and mortar. Serve the laksa bake sprinkled with peanuts and the reserved coriander leaves, with lime wedges for squeezing over. Nice with a fresh side salad.

CALORIES	FAT	SAT FAT	PROTEIN	CARBS	SUGAR	FIBRE	
597kcal	17.9g	6g	25.8g	89.1g	16.6g	6.5g	1 HOUR 40 MINUTES

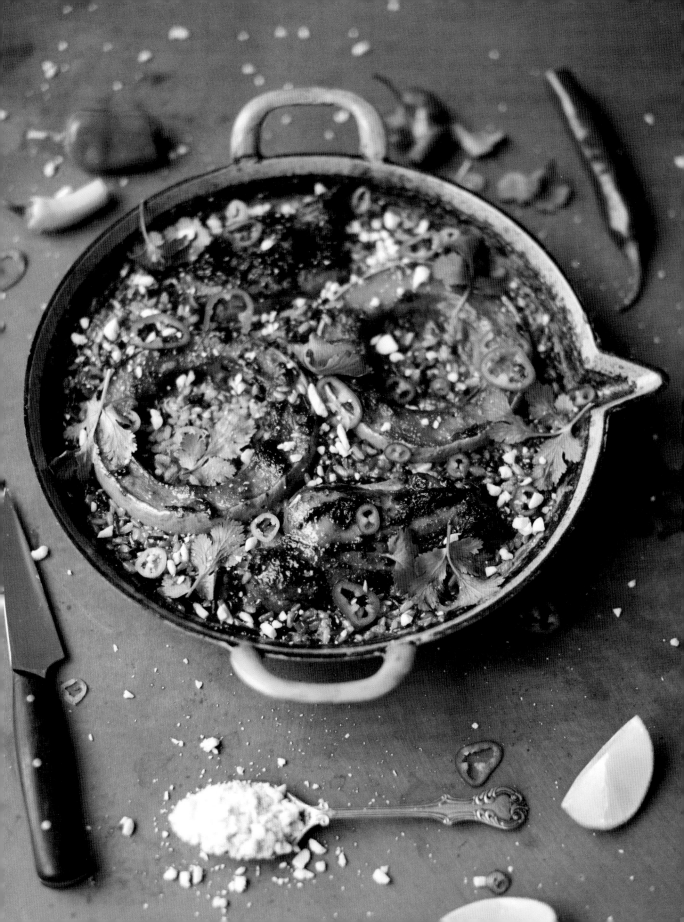

GOLDEN CHICKEN SKEWERS
YELLOW PEPPER SAUCE, BLACK QUINOA

— Black quinoa contains all the goodness of regular quinoa, with the addition of vitamin E, helping protect our cells from damage by stress cells known as free radicals —

SERVES 2

150g regular, black or red quinoa

1 fresh yellow or green chilli

2 yellow peppers

4 spring onions

1 clove of garlic

2 tablespoons cider vinegar

olive oil

2 x 120g skinless chicken breasts

4 sprigs of fresh thyme

½ a ripe avocado

2 sprigs of fresh coriander

optional: natural yoghurt

Cook the quinoa according to the packet instructions, then drain. Deseed the chilli and peppers, quarter the peppers, and put both into a shallow 25cm pan on a medium heat. Trim the spring onions and add the whites to the pan (reserving the green tops). Peel, slice and add the garlic, along with the vinegar, 1 tablespoon of oil and a good splash of water. Cover and simmer for 20 minutes, or until soft and sweet, stirring occasionally. Decant the contents of the pan into a blender, blitz until smooth, then season to perfection.

You can cook your skewers in a hot non-stick frying pan, griddle pan or even under the grill at full whack. Slice the chicken lengthways into 2cm strips, and chop the greens of the spring onions into 2cm chunks. Checking that your skewers will fit inside your frying, griddle or grill pan, divide up the chicken and spring onions, weaving the chicken around the onions. Strip the thyme leaves over the skewers, lightly season, drizzle with 1 teaspoon of oil and rub all over, then cook for around 8 minutes, or until the chicken is golden, charred and cooked through. Meanwhile, peel and slice the avocado.

Pack half the quinoa into a small oil-rubbed bowl or cup, then turn out onto a plate and repeat. Divide the yellow pepper sauce, sliced avocado, coriander leaves and chicken skewers between your plates, then tuck in. This is delicious with a little dollop of yoghurt on the side too, if you like.

CALORIES	FAT	SAT FAT	PROTEIN	CARBS	SUGAR	FIBRE	40 MINUTES
549kcal	19.8g	3.3g	42.4g	53.5g	14.6g	4.3g	

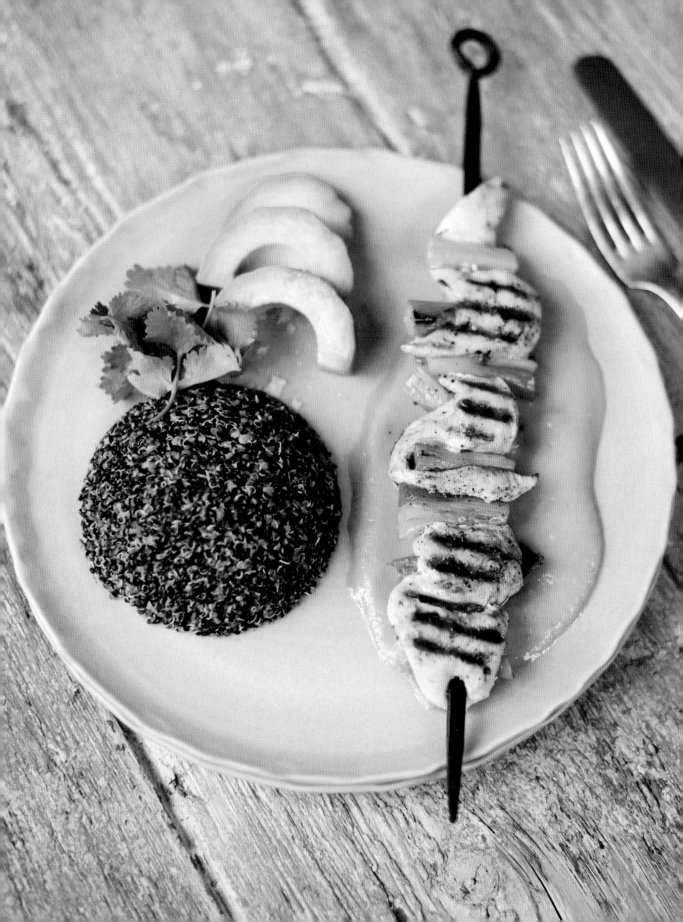

ROASTED MUSTARD MACKEREL
RAINBOW BEETS & BULGUR WHEAT

— Mackerel is a great source of omega-3 fatty acids, is super-rich in protein and packed with iodine, which, through our thyroid gland, helps our metabolism to function efficiently —

SERVES 2

300g raw mixed-colour beets

150g bulgur wheat

olive oil

4 x 75g mackerel or trout fillets, scaled and pin-boned

2 teaspoons Dijon mustard

white wine vinegar

1 tablespoon porridge oats

½ a bunch of fresh thyme (15g)

2 large handfuls of rocket

½ a lemon

2 teaspoons jarred grated horseradish

2 tablespoons natural yoghurt

Preheat the oven to 200°C/400°F/gas 6. Wash the beets, cook in boiling salted water for 30 minutes, or until just tender (depending on their size), then drain and leave until cool enough to handle. Meanwhile, cook the bulgur wheat according to the packet instructions, and drain.

Lay a sheet of wet greaseproof paper in a 25cm x 30cm baking tray and rub it lightly with oil. Evenly spread the bulgur over the tray and place the fish fillets randomly on top. Loosen the mustard with a splash of vinegar, then brush over the skin side of the fish, and sprinkle over the oats. Remove the skin from the beets and finely slice them, ideally on a mandolin (use the guard!), then arrange them around the fish, overlapping the slices and tucking them up to and under the fillets in a nice even layer.

Mix 1 tablespoon of vinegar with 1 teaspoon of oil and a pinch of sea salt and black pepper to make a dressing. Holding the thyme like a brush, use it to dab the dressing all over the beets, then strip over the leaves. Cook at the top of the oven for 15 to 20 minutes, or until the fish is lightly golden and cooked through. Toss the rocket with a squeeze of lemon juice and sprinkle over the top. Stir the horseradish through the yoghurt, season to perfection, then spoon over the fish and tuck in.

CALORIES	FAT	SAT FAT	PROTEIN	CARBS	SUGAR	FIBRE	50 MINUTES
378kcal	9.4g	1g	37.4g	35.9g	13g	6.7g	

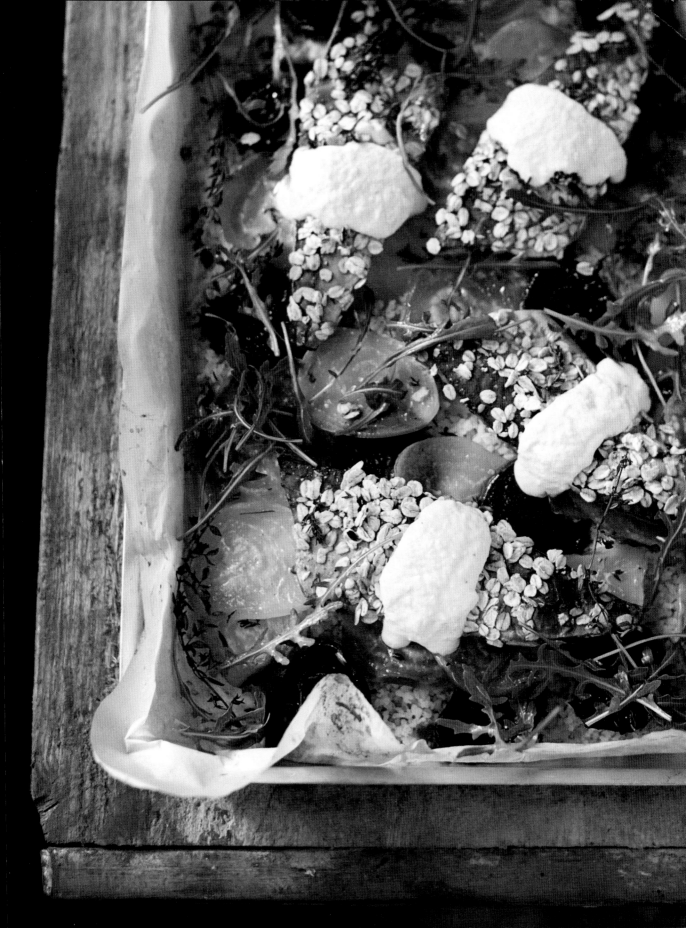

SUPER SQUASH LASAGNE
SPINACH, COTTAGE CHEESE & SEEDS

Using wholewheat lasagne instead of white means we get double the fibre, plus the vitamin A
we get from the squash here helps us to metabolize the iron from the spinach

SERVES 6

olive oil

1 large butternut squash (1.5kg)

1 level teaspoon ground coriander

4 cloves of garlic

1 fresh red chilli

2 tablespoons balsamic vinegar

2 x 400g tins of plum tomatoes

200g baby spinach

60g Parmesan cheese

250g dried wholewheat lasagne
    sheets

400g fat-free cottage cheese

100ml semi-skimmed milk

1 tablespoon sunflower seeds

1 sprig of fresh rosemary

Preheat the oven to 180°C/350°F/gas 4 and rub two large roasting trays with a little oil. Carefully halve and deseed the squash, leaving the skin on, then slice into 1cm half-moon shapes. Lay in a single layer across the trays. Sprinkle over the ground coriander and a pinch of sea salt and black pepper, then roast for 50 minutes, or until soft and lightly golden.

Meanwhile, peel the garlic, deseed the chilli, then finely slice both and place in a large pan on a medium-high heat with 1 tablespoon of oil. Cook for 3 minutes, or until lightly golden, then add the balsamic and tinned tomatoes, breaking them up as you go, and 1 tin's worth of water. Simmer on a medium heat for 15 to 20 minutes, or until slightly thickened, then season to perfection.

To layer up, spread a third of the tomato sauce across the base of a 25cm x 30cm baking dish. Cover with a layer of raw spinach leaves, a layer of roasted squash, a fine grating of Parmesan and a layer of lasagne sheets. Repeat the layers twice more, finishing with lasagne sheets. Loosen the cottage cheese with the milk, mashing the curds a little, then lightly season and spoon over the top. Finely grate over the remaining Parmesan and scatter over the sunflower seeds. Rub the rosemary sprig with oil, then strip the leaves over the top. Bake at the bottom of the oven for 45 minutes, or until golden and bubbling, then serve. Great with a lemon-dressed green salad.

CALORIES	FAT	SAT FAT	PROTEIN	CARBS	SUGAR	FIBRE	1 HOUR 45 MINUTES
438kcal	13.2g	5.4g	21.2g	59g	21.6g	9.4g	

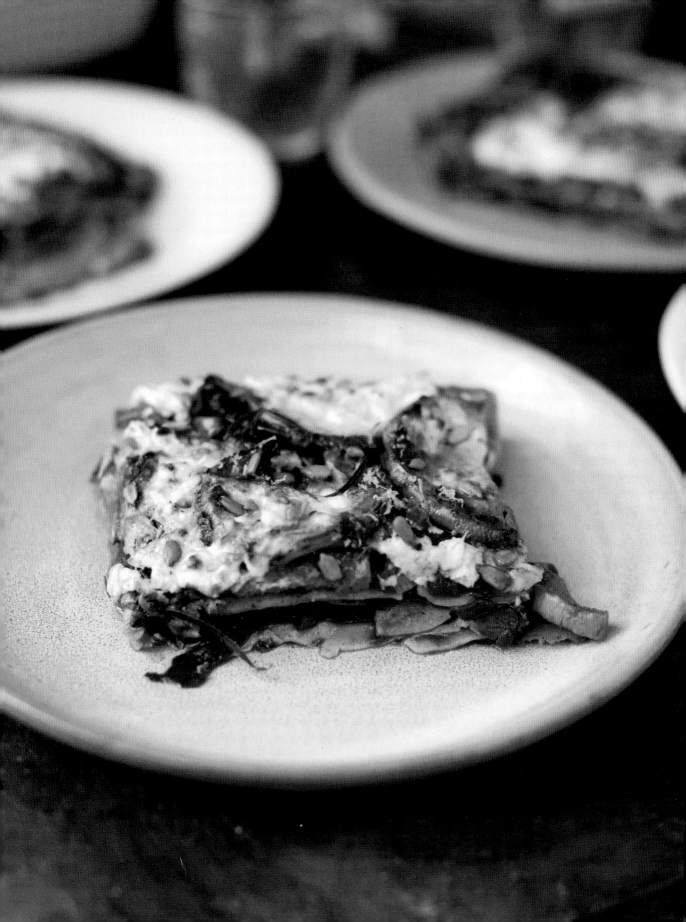

SIZZLING MOROCCAN PRAWNS
FLUFFY COUSCOUS & RAINBOW SALSA

—   Adding a pop of sweetness to this dish, pomegranates are a great source of vitamin B6,
keeping our nervous system healthy so our cells can send signals to each other   —

SERVES 2

2 sprigs of fresh rosemary

2 cloves of garlic

olive oil

1 level teaspoon smoked paprika

1 good pinch of saffron

6 large raw shell-on king prawns

2 oranges

150g wholewheat couscous

400g colourful mixed seasonal
  veg, such as peas, asparagus,
  fennel, courgettes, celery, spring
  onions, red or yellow peppers

1 fresh red chilli

½ a bunch of fresh mint (15g)

1 lemon

2 tablespoons natural yoghurt

1 pomegranate

Strip the rosemary leaves into a pestle and mortar, then peel and add the garlic and pound into a paste with a pinch of sea salt. Muddle in 1 tablespoon of oil, the paprika, saffron and a swig of boiling water to make a marinade. Use little scissors to cut down the back of each prawn shell and remove the vein. Cut 1 orange into wedges, toss with the prawns and the marinade and leave aside for 10 minutes.

Put the couscous into a bowl and just cover with boiling water, then pop a plate on top and leave to fluff up. Take a bit of pride in finely chopping all your colourful seasonal veg and chilli, and put them into a nice serving bowl. Pick a few pretty mint leaves and put to one side, then pick and finely chop the rest and add to the bowl with the juice of the lemon and the remaining orange. Add the couscous, toss together and season to perfection.

Put a large non-stick frying pan on a high heat. Add the prawns, marinade and orange wedges and cook for 4 to 5 minutes, or until the prawns are gnarly and crisp, then arrange on top of the couscous. Dollop with yoghurt, then halve the pomegranate and, holding it cut side down in your fingers, bash the back so the sweet jewels tumble over everything. Sprinkle with the reserved mint leaves and serve.

CALORIES	FAT	SAT FAT	PROTEIN	CARBS	SUGAR	FIBRE	20 MINUTES
572kcal	11.3g	2.4g	30g	91.7g	28.4g	15.9g	

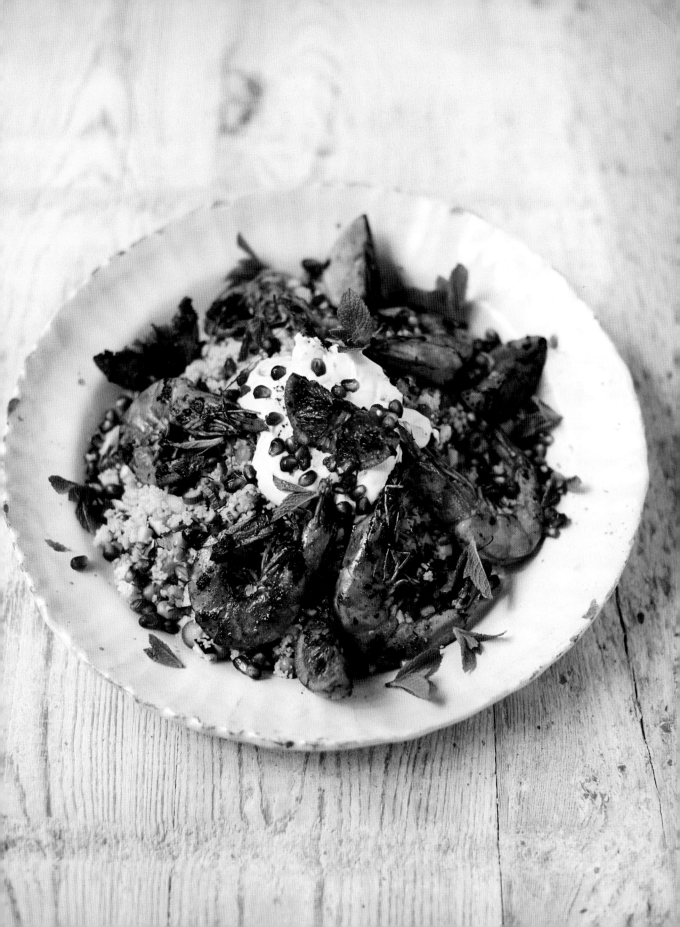

ASIAN STEAMED FISH
BLACK RICE, GREENS & CHILLI SAUCE

— Fresh haddock is a wonderful flaky fish that's low in both fat and saturated fat, as well as being super-high in both selenium and iodine, which help control our metabolism —

SERVES 2

150g black or brown rice

1 lime

2 x 120g fillets of haddock or white fish, skin on, scaled, scored and pin-boned

2cm piece of ginger

1 clove of garlic

1 fresh red chilli

2 spring onions

1 tablespoon low-salt soy sauce

1 tablespoon white wine vinegar

3 ripe cherry tomatoes

2 small bok choi

150g mixed greens, such as sprouting broccoli, asparagus, chard, kale, sugar snap peas

Cook the rice according to the packet instructions, then drain. Get a pan of water on to boil that you can sit a double-layered steamer basket over later. Finely grate the lime zest over the fish fillets and place them in the base layer of the steamer, off the heat.

Squeeze the lime juice into a blender (I like to chuck the squeezed lime halves into the pan of boiling water for added steam aroma). Peel the ginger and garlic, roughly chop and add to the blender. Deseed and add the chilli, trim, roughly chop and add the spring onions, along with the soy, vinegar and tomatoes, then blitz until super-smooth. Season to perfection, then decant into a small cup or bowl and snuggle up alongside the fish.

Trim your bok choi and prep your greens, halving or quartering them lengthways, if needed, to help them cook, and put them into the top steamer basket, above the fish and sauce. Put the lid on and carefully place the stack above the boiling water to steam for 6 minutes, or until the fish is cooked through and the greens are just done but still vibrant in colour. Serve the fish, rice and greens drizzled with your chilli sauce.

CALORIES	FAT	SAT FAT	PROTEIN	CARBS	SUGAR	FIBRE	
416kcal	4g	0.8g	32g	66.8g	6g	4.8g	40 MINUTES

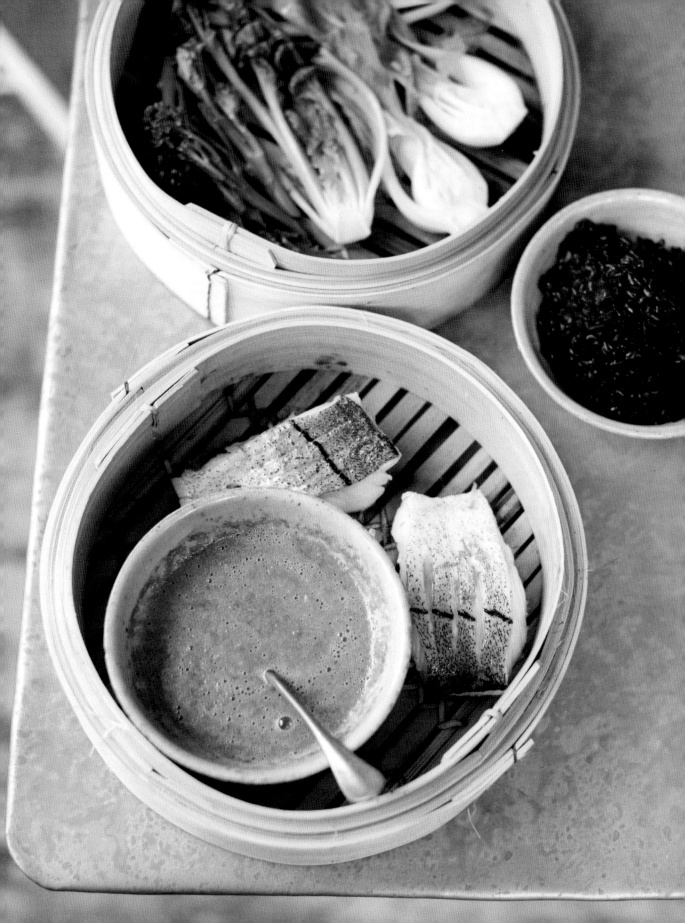

SMOKY VEGGIE FEIJOADA
BLACK BEANS, SQUASH, PEPPERS & OKRA

— Super-protein-packed black beans are a great base to this veggie version of the classic
Brazilian dish, and with all the veg we get loads of fibre and four of our 5-a-day too! —

SERVES 2
+ 4 LEFTOVER FEIJOADA PORTIONS

½ a butternut squash (600g)

olive oil

1 heaped teaspoon each of
   ground coriander, smoked
   paprika

3 mixed-colour peppers

2 red onions

4 cloves of garlic

4 fresh bay leaves

2 x 400g tins of black beans

100g okra

150g brown rice

2 ripe mixed-colour tomatoes

½–1 fresh red chilli

1 bunch of fresh coriander (30g)

1 lime

2 tablespoons natural yoghurt

Preheat the oven to 200°C/400°F/gas 6. Halve and deseed the squash, then carefully chop into 3cm chunks. In a large roasting tray, toss and massage it with 1 teaspoon of oil, the ground coriander and a pinch of sea salt and black pepper. Deseed the peppers and cut into 3cm chunks, then, in a separate tray, toss and massage them with 1 teaspoon of oil and the smoked paprika. Place both trays in the oven for 35 minutes, or until softened.

Meanwhile, peel and finely chop ¼ of an onion and put aside, then roughly chop the rest and place in a large casserole pan on a low heat with 1 tablespoon of oil. Crush in the garlic, add the bay leaves and a good splash of water and cook for 20 minutes, or until soft, stirring regularly. Tip in the beans, juice and all, then half-fill each empty tin with water, swirl and pour into the pan. Simmer until the time is up on the squash and peppers, then stir both into the pan. Trim, finely slice and add the okra, and simmer for a further 20 minutes, or until the feijoada is dark and delicious, loosening with an extra splash of water, if needed. Meanwhile, cook the rice according to the packet instructions, then drain.

To make a quick salsa, deseed the tomatoes, then finely chop with as much chilli as you like and most of the coriander leaves. Scrape into a bowl with the reserved finely chopped onion and toss with the lime juice, then season to perfection. Remove 4 portions of feijoada, bag them up and once completely cool, freeze for a rainy day, when you'll be really grateful it's there. Serve the remaining feijoada with the rice and salsa, a spoonful of yoghurt and a sprinkling of the remaining coriander leaves.

CALORIES	FAT	SAT FAT	PROTEIN	CARBS	SUGAR	FIBRE	
532kcal	7.9g	1.9g	19.9g	93.6g	17.6g	20.1g	1 HOUR 5 MINUTES

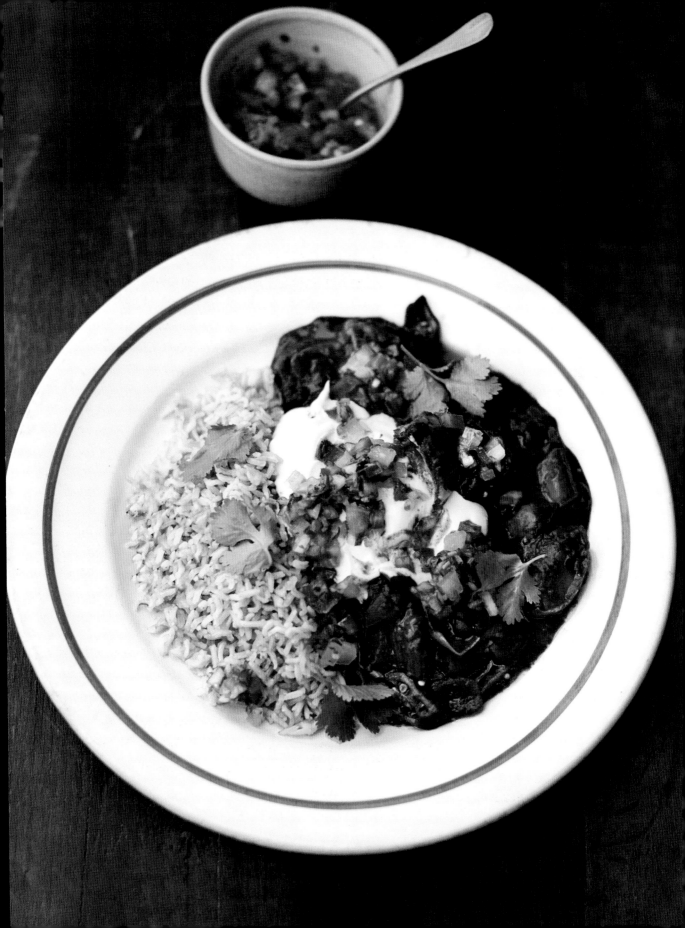

CRUMBED PESTO FISH
ROASTED CHERRY VINES, SPUDS & GREENS

— Juicy cherry tomatoes are high in vitamin C – protecting our cells, helping us to think properly, and really usefull here as it helps us to absorb iron from the spinach —

SERVES 2

200g ripe cherry tomatoes on the vine

1 slice of wholemeal bread

½ a bunch of fresh basil (15g)

½ a clove of garlic

15g pine nuts

1 lemon

20g Parmesan cheese

extra virgin olive oil

2 x 120g fillets of firm white fish, such as cod, haddock, hake, pollock, skin off, scaled and pin-boned

250g baby new potatoes

100g each of green beans, tenderstem broccoli, baby spinach

1 tablespoon balsamic vinegar

Preheat the oven to 200°C/400°F/gas 6. Lay the tomato vines in one side of a baking tray and pop in the oven for 10 minutes while you whiz the bread into crumbs in a food processor, then tip into a shallow bowl. Pound up the basil leaves in a pestle and mortar. Peel the garlic and add with a pinch of sea salt and the pine nuts, and keep pounding until you have a green paste. Squeeze in half the lemon juice, finely grate in the Parmesan, add 1 tablespoon of oil and muddle together. Divide and pat the pesto all over the fish fillets, then pack on the breadcrumbs. Pull the tray out of the oven and sprinkle any spare crumbs next to the tomatoes, then sit the fish on top. Halve the remaining lemon and add the wedges to the tray, then roast for 15 minutes, or until the fish is golden and cooked through.

Meanwhile, cut any larger potatoes in half, place in a large pan, just cover with boiling salted water and cook for 15 minutes, or until tender. Place a colander above the pan, with a lid on. Trim just the stalks off the green beans, halve the broccoli spears lengthways and add both to the colander to steam for the last 5 minutes, adding the spinach for the final 2 minutes.

In a tray, mix the balsamic with 1 tablespoon of oil, then season to perfection. As soon as the veg are done, toss them in the tray of dressing, then drain the potatoes and add, lightly squashing and mixing them in. Serve with the fish, roasted tomatoes and lemon wedges, with an extra drizzle of balsamic.

CALORIES	FAT	SAT FAT	PROTEIN	CARBS	SUGAR	FIBRE	30 MINUTES
518kcal	23.2g	4g	37.5g	42.1g	12.5g	7.7g	

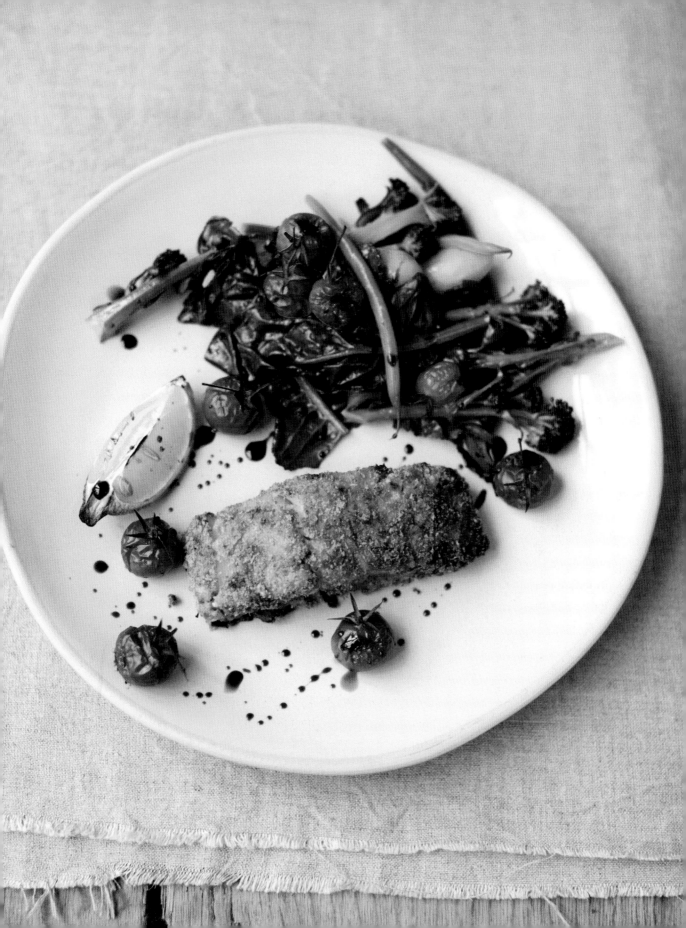

HARISSA ROASTED AUBERGINE
POMEGRANATE, PISTACHIOS, OLIVES, RICE

— With vitamin C-packed cherry tomatoes and comforting aubergine, this dish gives us two of our 5-a-day, plus good unsaturated fat from the pistachios for happy cholesterol —

SERVES 2

1 red onion

2 cloves of garlic

olive oil

½ teaspoon cumin seeds

150g brown rice

800ml really good veg stock

1 large aubergine (300g)

2 teaspoons harissa

1 teaspoon rose water

6 olives (stone in)

200g ripe cherry tomatoes

1 tablespoon balsamic vinegar

2 tablespoons fat-free natural yoghurt

½ a pomegranate

30g shelled pistachios

4 sprigs of fresh coriander

Peel and finely slice the onion and garlic and place in a large shallow casserole pan on a medium-high heat with 1 tablespoon of oil, the cumin seeds and a splash of water. Cook for 5 minutes, or until softened, stirring regularly. Stir in the rice, pour in the stock, bring to the boil, then cover and simmer for just 10 minutes. Halve the aubergine lengthways, lightly score a criss-cross pattern into each cut side and sprinkle with a pinch of sea salt. Loosen the harissa with the rose water then spread over each scored aubergine half and lay them on the rice, harissa side up. Cover the pan again and simmer on a medium-low heat for 20 minutes. Preheat the oven to 180°C/350°F/gas 4.

Meanwhile, destone the olives and tear into a bowl. Halve and add the cherry tomatoes, then toss both with the balsamic vinegar. When the time's up on the aubergine, remove the cover and sprinkle the dressed olives and tomatoes in and around the pan. Transfer to the oven, uncovered, for 30 minutes, or until the rice is cooked through, the liquid has evaporated and the aubergine is beautifully gnarly and looks delicious.

To serve, spoon over the yoghurt. Hold the pomegranate half cut side down in your fingers and bash the back so the sweet jewels tumble over the top, chop and scatter over the pistachios, pick over the coriander leaves and enjoy.

CALORIES	FAT	SAT FAT	PROTEIN	CARBS	SUGAR	FIBRE	
552kcal	21.2g	3.5g	15.6g	79.2g	16.5g	8g	1 HOUR

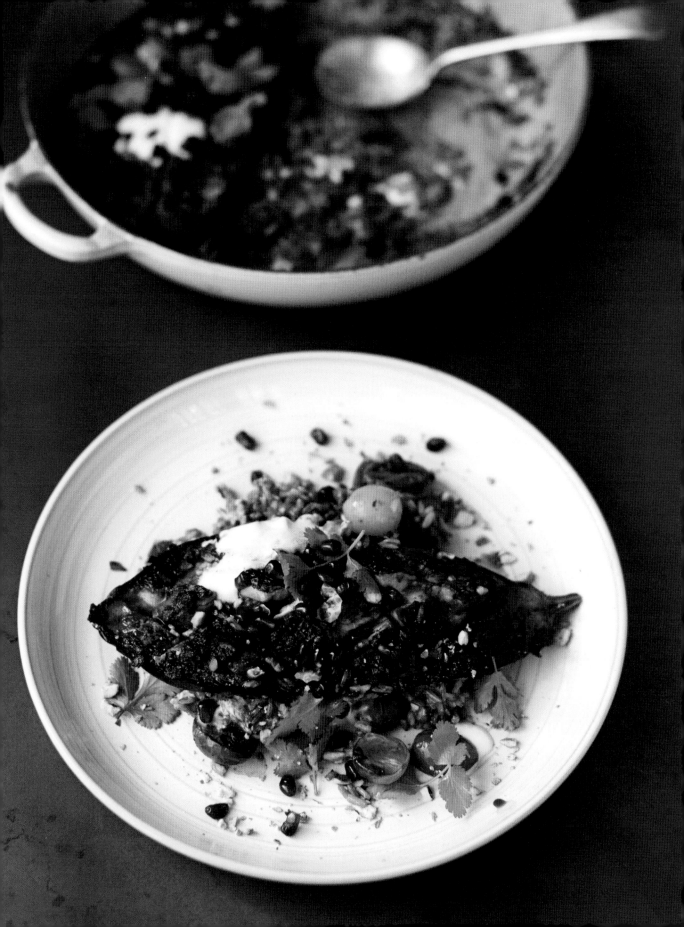

TASTY SAMOSAS
BEEF, ONION & SWEET POTATO

— Unlike potato, sweet potato is a non-starchy carbohydrate, which means it counts towards our 5-a-day. It's also a source of other nutrients, including our forever friend vitamin C —

SERVES 4

50g brown rice

olive oil

100g lean beef mince

medium curry powder

1 onion

2 cloves of garlic

1 sweet potato (250g)

1 fresh red chilli

8 sprigs of fresh coriander

4 large sheets of filo pastry

optional: 1 level tablespoon
    black onion seeds

½ a cucumber

½ a lemon

4 tablespoons natural yoghurt

hot chilli sauce

Cook the brown rice according to the packet instructions, then drain and cool. Meanwhile, put 1 tablespoon of oil, the beef and 1 level tablespoon of curry powder into a casserole pan on a medium heat. Stir regularly while you peel the onion, garlic and sweet potato, then finely chop with the chilli (deseed if you like) and coriander stalks. Add it all to the pan and fry for about 15 minutes, stirring often. Pour in 350ml of water, then simmer for 20 minutes. Crush the sweet potato with a spoon, season the mixture to perfection and leave to cool. Stir through the rice and there's your filling.

Preheat the oven to 200°C/400°F/gas 6. Normally, filo sheets are about 25cm x 48cm so cut each sheet in half lengthways. Lightly brush each with a little water and evenly sprinkle over the black onion seeds (if using). Spoon an eighth of the filling at the base of each sheet. Fold and turn up the pastry to create a triangular samosa shape, using a little water to seal and stick down any overhang at the end. Place on a non-stick baking tray and cook for 20 minutes, or until crisp and golden, turning halfway.

Scoop out and discard the watery core from the cucumber, then finely dice it and dress in the lemon juice. Serve 2 samosas per person with a spoonful of yoghurt, a swirl of chilli sauce and a spoonful of refreshing cucumber. Pick over the coriander leaves, add a pinch of curry powder and tuck right in!

CALORIES	FAT	SAT FAT	PROTEIN	CARBS	SUGAR	FIBRE	
338kcal	6.9g	1.8g	15.7g	54.7g	10g	4g	1 HOUR

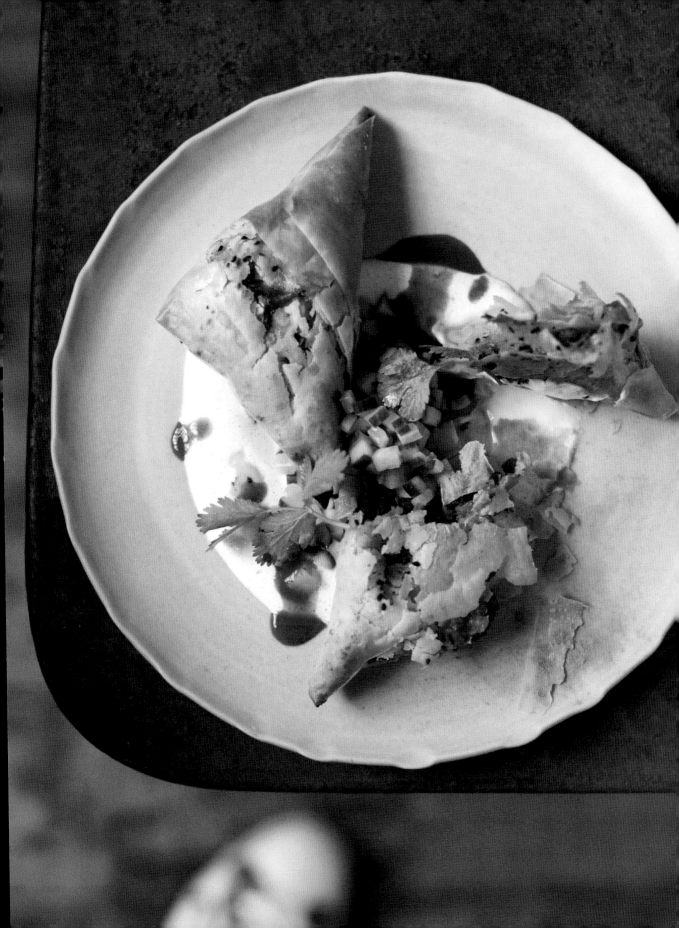

VEGGIE RAMEN
WALNUT MISO, KIMCHEE & FRIED EGGS

— Wonderful walnuts are packed with vitamin E, which acts as an antioxidant and helps protect our cells, helps us maintain healthy skin and eyes, and strengthens our immune systems —

SERVES 2

¼ of a Chinese cabbage (180g)

1 teaspoon hot chilli sauce

2 limes

20g shelled walnuts

1 tablespoon miso paste

300g mixed green veg, such as green beans, tenderstem broccoli, mangetout

150g brown rice noodles

sesame oil

2 large eggs

½–1 fresh red chilli

Put 1 litre of water on to boil in a large pan with a pinch of sea salt. Cut yourself a lengthways quarter wedge of Chinese cabbage. Very finely slice the top leafy half, then mix and scrunch it really well with the chilli sauce and the juice from 1 lime to make a great cheat's kimchee. Cut the bottom part of the cabbage wedge in half through the stalk. Crush the walnuts in a pestle and mortar until fine, then muddle in the miso paste and put aside.

Trim just the stalks off the green beans and place the beans in the boiling water. Trim the ends off the broccoli, then add to the water with the mangetout and cabbage chunks, as well as the noodles to cook according to the packet instructions. Pop the lid on until the veg are just cooked through but still vibrant in colour and the noodles are tender. Meanwhile, put a non-stick frying pan on a medium heat with 1 teaspoon of sesame oil, crack in the eggs and cover with a lid to set them on top while they fry to your liking.

Use a slotted spoon to divide the veg and noodles between your bowls. Mix the walnut miso into the greens water, bring to the boil, and spoon over the veg. Divide up the kimchee, then top with the eggs and a sprinkling of fresh chilli. Serve with lime wedges for squeezing over and tuck right in.

CALORIES	FAT	SAT FAT	PROTEIN	CARBS	SUGAR	FIBRE	
360kcal	16.9g	3.1g	16.9g	35.7g	7.1g	5.6g	20 MINUTES

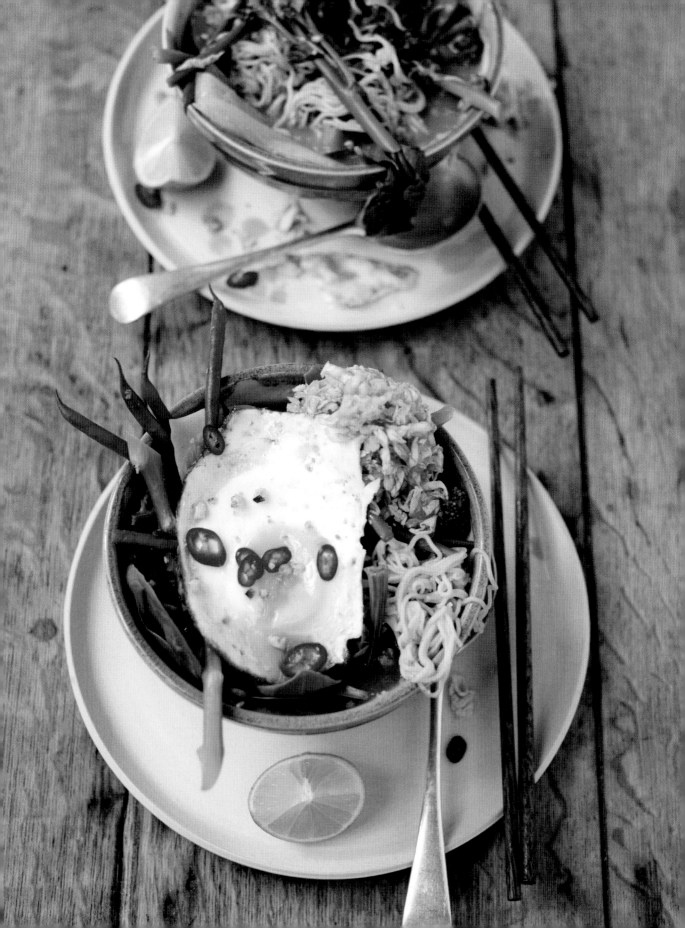

INDIAN ROASTED CAULIFLOWER
PINEAPPLE, CHILLI, CORONATION DRESSING

— Our humble but super-tasty friend cauliflower is really high in vitamin C and folic
acid, both of which aid psychological function, helping us to think properly —

SERVES 4

2 large heads of cauliflower,
  ideally mixed colours
  (1.2kg each)

½ a medium pineapple (600g)

olive oil

1 heaped teaspoon each of fennel
  seeds, black mustard seeds

30g flaked almonds

1 x 400g tin of chickpeas

1 level teaspoon ground turmeric

2 level teaspoons medium
  curry powder

½ a bunch of fresh coriander
  (15g)

3cm piece of ginger

1 lemon

2 teaspoons mango chutney

200g natural yoghurt

1 fresh red chilli

4 wholemeal chapattis

Preheat the oven to 200°C/400°F/gas 6. Chop the cauliflowers into large florets, leaving any nice-looking outer leaves attached. Cook in a large pan of boiling water for 6 to 8 minutes, then drain well and tip into a large roasting tray. Peel and core the pineapple, then chop into 3cm chunks and add to the tray with 1 tablespoon of oil, the fennel and mustard seeds and a pinch of sea salt and black pepper. Toss together, then roast for 30 minutes. Turn everything over then add the almonds and drained chickpeas and cook for another 10 minutes, or until the cauli is charred and gnarly.

Meanwhile, toast the turmeric and curry powder in a dry pan on a low heat for a couple of minutes, or until smelling incredible, then put into a blender with the coriander stalks. Peel, slice and add the ginger, with the lemon juice, mango chutney and half the yoghurt. Blitz until super-smooth, then stir in the remaining yoghurt (you can chuck it all in together, but I find that makes the dressing too thin). Season to perfection and pour over a big platter.

Pile the roasted cauliflower and pineapple mixture on top of the dressing, slice the chilli and scatter over, and sprinkle with the coriander leaves. Toss together and serve with warm chapattis for dipping and dunking.

CALORIES	FAT	SAT FAT	PROTEIN	CARBS	SUGAR	FIBRE	50 MINUTES
569kcal	19.7g	5g	27.4g	71.8g	29.3g	15.2g	

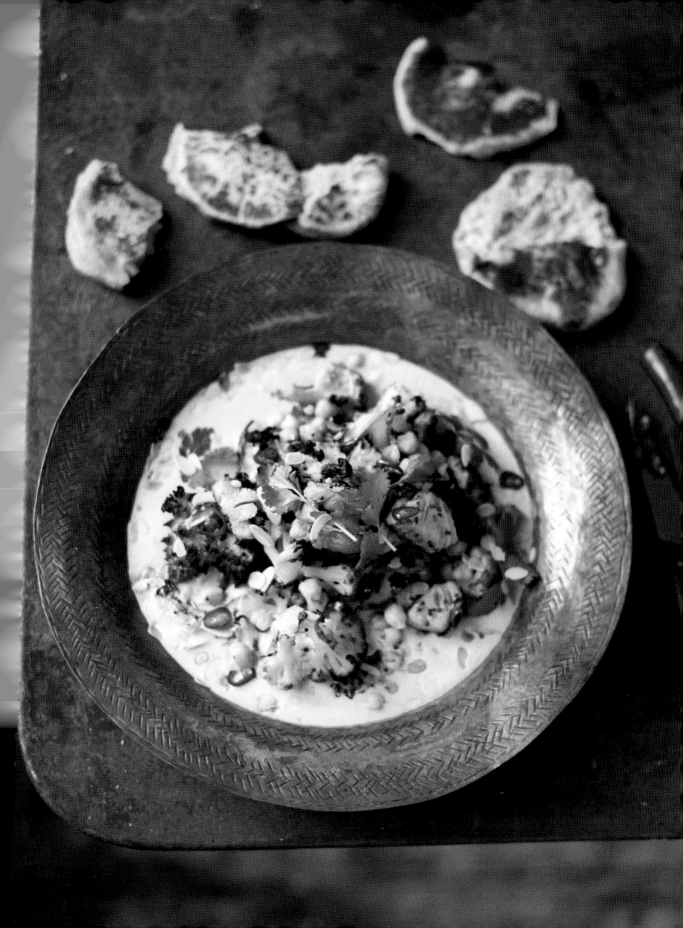

ROASTED CARROT & SQUASH SALAD
MILLET, APPLE, JALAPEÑO & POMEGRANATE

— Millet is super-high in a B vitamin called thiamine, which helps to keep our hearts —
healthy and functioning properly, plus this salad gives us three of our 5-a-day

SERVES 4

½ a butternut squash (600g)

500g carrots

olive oil

300g millet

1 tablespoon white wine vinegar

1 fresh jalapeño chilli

1 handful of radishes

1 eating apple

1 x 290g jar of roasted peeled
   red peppers in brine

4 tablespoons of toasted nut mix
   (see page 228)

1 orange

2 tablespoons natural yoghurt

extra virgin olive oil

½ a pomegranate

20g feta cheese

Preheat the oven to 180°C/350°F/gas 4. Carefully halve then slice just the bulbous seeded end of the squash 1cm thick. Clean the carrots and cut any larger ones in half. In a tray toss both with 1 tablespoon of olive oil and a pinch of sea salt and black pepper. Roast for 50 minutes, or until soft and lightly golden. Meanwhile, cook the millet according to the packet instructions, then drain and place in a large bowl.

Mix the vinegar and a pinch of salt in a bowl. Ideally on a mandolin (use the guard!), finely slice the chilli, radishes and apple, adding them to the bowl as you go, then toss together and pop in the fridge till needed. Drain the peppers, blitz in a blender with the nuts, orange juice, yoghurt and 1 teaspoon of extra virgin olive oil until smooth, then taste and season to perfection.

Add the roasted veg and the pepper dressing to the millet, then use your clean hands to roughly scrunch it all together until everything's vibrant and orange. Sprinkle the crunchy dressed veg on top, then, holding the pomegranate cut side down in your fingers, bash the back of it so the seeds tumble all over the salad. Crumble over the feta and serve.

CALORIES	FAT	SAT FAT	PROTEIN	CARBS	SUGAR	FIBRE	1 HOUR 10 MINUTES
517kcal	27.1g	3.9g	12.3g	56.1g	26.2g	11.1g	

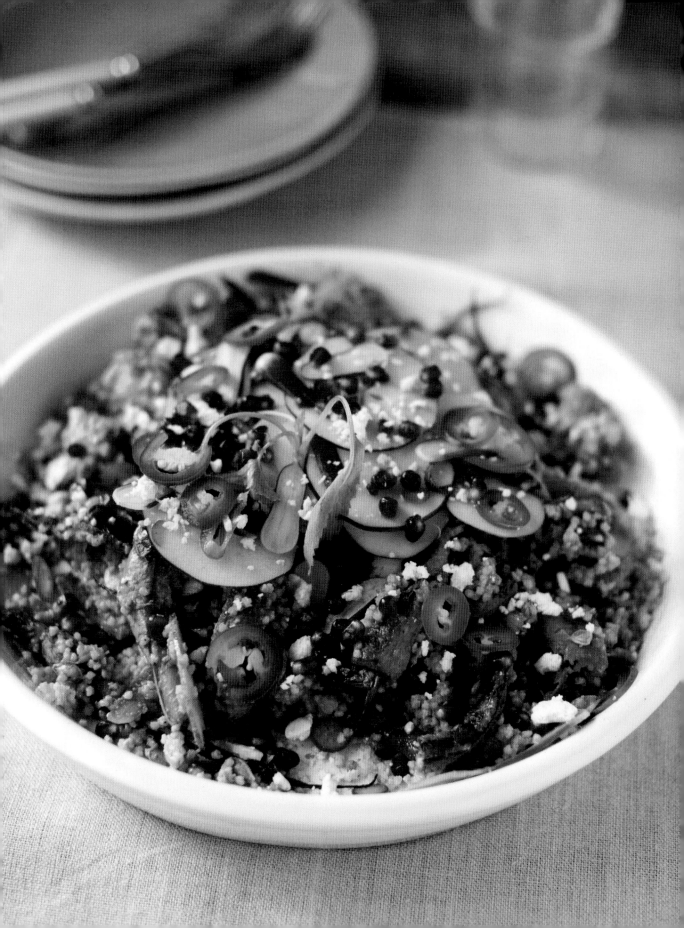

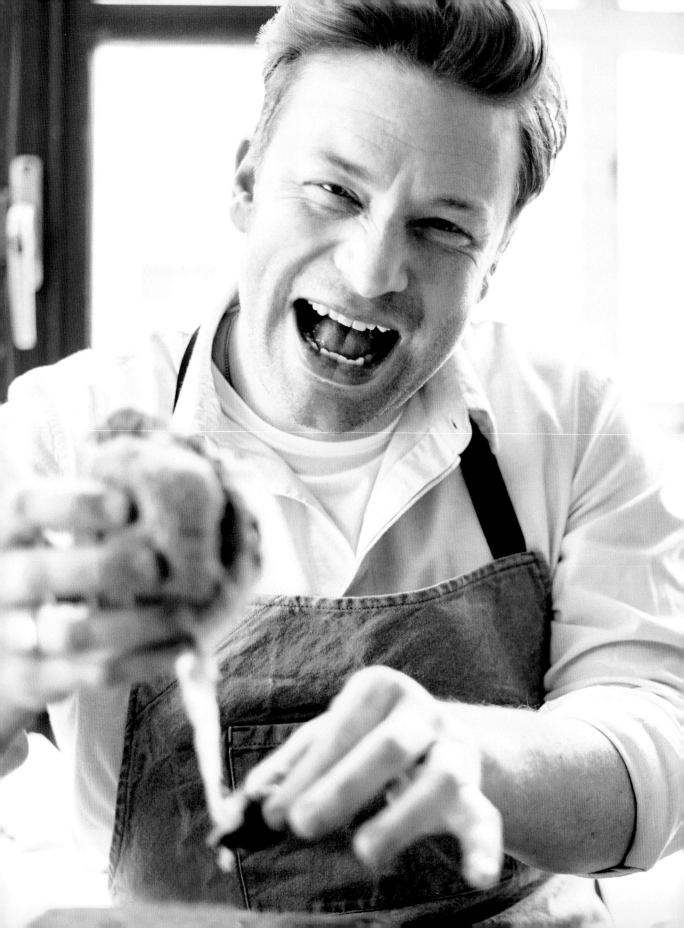

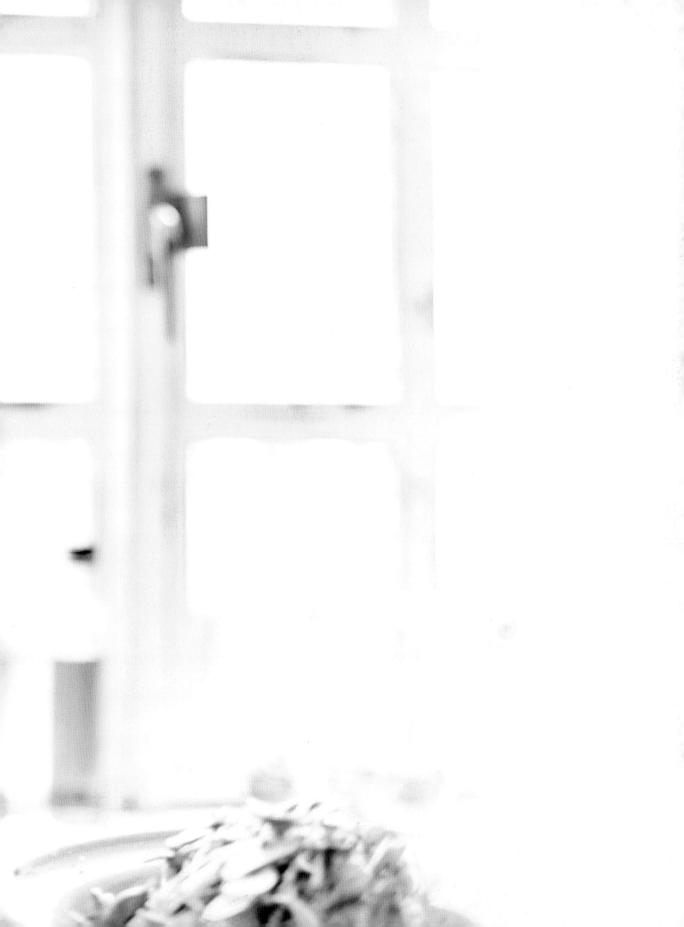

CRISPY SEA BASS
PEA, MINT & ASPARAGUS MASH

— Packed with two of our 5-a-day, this super-simple supper also heroes sea bass, meaning our meal is super-high in vitamin B12, which we need for making healthy red blood cells —

SERVES 2

300g potatoes

1 bunch of asparagus (300g)

100g freshly podded peas

1 bunch of fresh mint (30g)

1 fresh red chilli

2 handfuls of baby spinach

40g strong Cheddar cheese

2 x 120g sea bass fillets, skin on, scaled, scored and pin-boned

extra virgin olive oil

2 lemons

Wash the potatoes, chop into 3cm chunks and put into a medium pan of boiling salted water for 10 minutes. Meanwhile, to make the salad garnish, trim the woody ends off the asparagus. Holding the stalk ends steady, speed-peel just 4 asparagus spears into lovely ribbons, then pop into a bowl with a small handful of the peas. Pick in just the pretty baby mint leaves, finely slice and add the chilli (deseed if you like), then put aside.

Add the remaining asparagus spears and peas to the potato pan to cook for 3 minutes, then drain it all in a colander, steam dry for 1 minute and put into a food processor. Pick in the rest of the mint leaves and add the spinach. Grate in the Cheddar, then pulse to the consistency you like (pulse because blitzing would make it gluey). Have a taste and season to perfection.

Meanwhile, sprinkle the skin of the fish with sea salt and rub all over with 1 teaspoon of oil. Place the fillets skin side down in a cold non-stick frying pan and turn the heat to medium-high. Finely grate over the lemon zest, cover with a scrunched sheet of wet greaseproof paper and cook for around 5 minutes. This is a brilliant method, giving crispy skin and flaky fish, without you having to turn it.

Divide up the mash next to the crispy sea bass, skin side up. Toss the raw peas and asparagus ribbons with the juice from 1 lemon and 1 teaspoon of oil, then pile delicately on top. Serve with lemon wedges for squeezing over.

CALORIES	FAT	SAT FAT	PROTEIN	CARBS	SUGAR	FIBRE	30 MINUTES
424kcal	13.7g	5.5g	40.6g	36.5g	5.9g	7.5g	

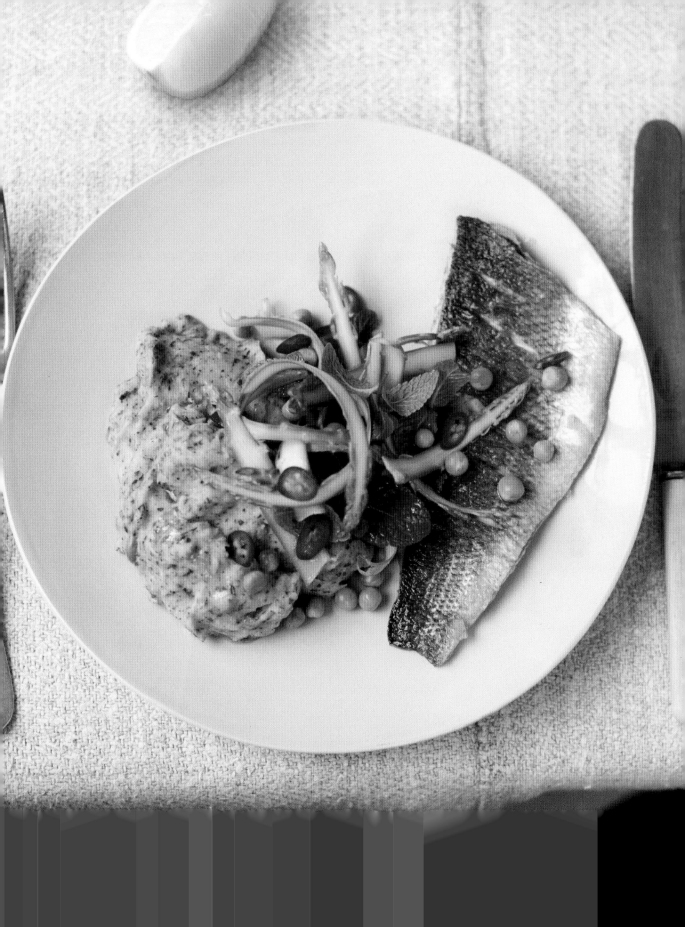

SPRING SQUID
PEAS, ASPARAGUS, BEANS & GREENS

— All the beautiful veg in this recipe gives us three of our 5-a-day plus over a day's worth of vitamin C. Broad beans are high in folic acid, which our bodies use to make protein —

SERVES 2

250g squid tubes (ask your fishmonger to prep them for you)

1 onion

2 sticks of celery

olive oil

100g asparagus

400g potatoes

1 little gem lettuce

100g freshly podded or frozen broad beans

100g freshly podded or frozen peas

500ml really good chicken or veg stock

1 lemon

1 fresh red or yellow chilli

2 sprigs of fresh mint

extra virgin olive oil

Use an eating knife to lightly score the squid at ½cm intervals in a criss-cross pattern, then, with a sharp knife, slice into ½cm-thick strips and put aside.

Peel the onion, trim the celery, then finely chop both and put into a casserole pan on a medium heat with 1 tablespoon of olive oil and a good splash of water. Trim the woody ends off the asparagus, then slice the stalks 1cm thick and add to the pan, reserving the tips. Peel the potatoes and cut into 1cm dice, add to the pan and cook it all with the lid on for around 10 minutes, or until the potatoes have softened, stirring occasionally.

Finely shred the lettuce, then stir into the pan with the broad beans, peas and asparagus tips. Pour in the stock, then bring to the boil. Sprinkle over the squid, pop the lid on, reduce to a low heat and simmer for 3 or 4 minutes, until the squid is brilliantly white and cooked through. Squeeze in half the lemon juice, then taste and season to perfection. Finely slice and scatter over the chilli, pick and tear over the mint leaves and finish with a few drops of extra virgin olive oil. Serve with lemon wedges for squeezing over.

CALORIES	FAT	SAT FAT	PROTEIN	CARBS	SUGAR	FIBRE	35 MINUTES
468kcal	13.1g	2.1g	34.9g	55.8g	11.2g	11.1g	

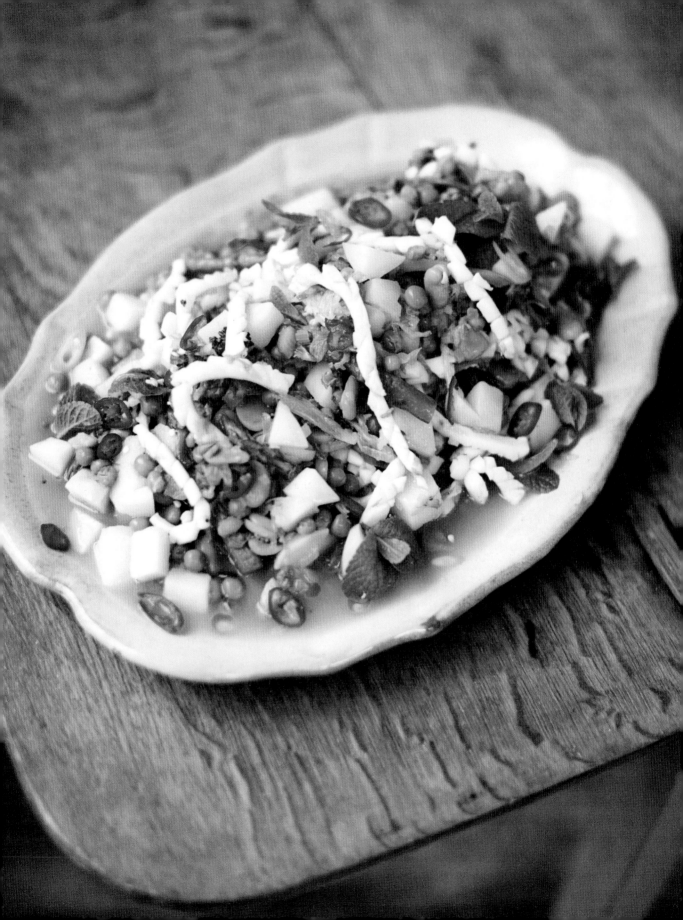

CHICKEN & SQUASH CACCIATORE
MUSHROOMS, TOMATOES, OLIVES, BREAD

_____ This truly comforting one-pan supper contains three of our 5-a-day, and the chicken fulfils _____
half of our daily vitamin B$_{12}$ needs, helping us make healthy red blood cells

SERVES 4

1 onion

1 leek

4 cloves of garlic

2 rashers of smoked pancetta

2 sprigs of fresh rosemary

olive oil

2 fresh bay leaves

½ a butternut squash or sweet
  potatoes (600g)

100g chestnut mushrooms

2 x 400g tins of plum tomatoes

250ml Chianti or other good
  red wine

4 chicken thighs, bone in

8 black olives (stone in)

200g seeded wholemeal bread

Preheat the oven to 190°C/375°F/gas 5. Peel the onion and cut into eighths, trim, wash and slice the leek, peel and slice the garlic. Place a large ovenproof casserole pan on a medium heat. Finely slice the pancetta, pick and finely chop the rosemary leaves, then place both in the pan with 1 tablespoon of oil and the bay leaves. Stir regularly for 2 minutes, then add the garlic, followed by the onion and leek. Cook for 10 minutes, stirring regularly.

Meanwhile, chop the squash or sweet potato (wash first) into bite-sized chunks, leaving the skin on and discarding any squash seeds. I like to cut the stalk and face off the mushrooms because it looks nice – just add the trimmings straight to the pan, along with the whole mushrooms and chopped squash or sweet potato. Remove and discard the chicken skin and add the chicken to the pan. Pour in the wine and let it reduce slightly, then add the tomatoes and break them up with a wooden spoon. Half-fill each tin with water, swirl about, pour into the pan and mix it all together. Destone the olives, then poke them into the stew. Bring to a gentle simmer, then transfer to the oven to cook for 1 hour, or until thick, delicious, the chicken falls off the bone and the squash or sweet potato is lovely and tender. Season to perfection, then serve with bread to mop up that tasty sauce.

CALORIES	FAT	SAT FAT	PROTEIN	CARBS	SUGAR	FIBRE	1 HOUR 20 MINUTES
421kcal	12.2g	2.7g	25.2g	45.1g	17.1g	9.1g	

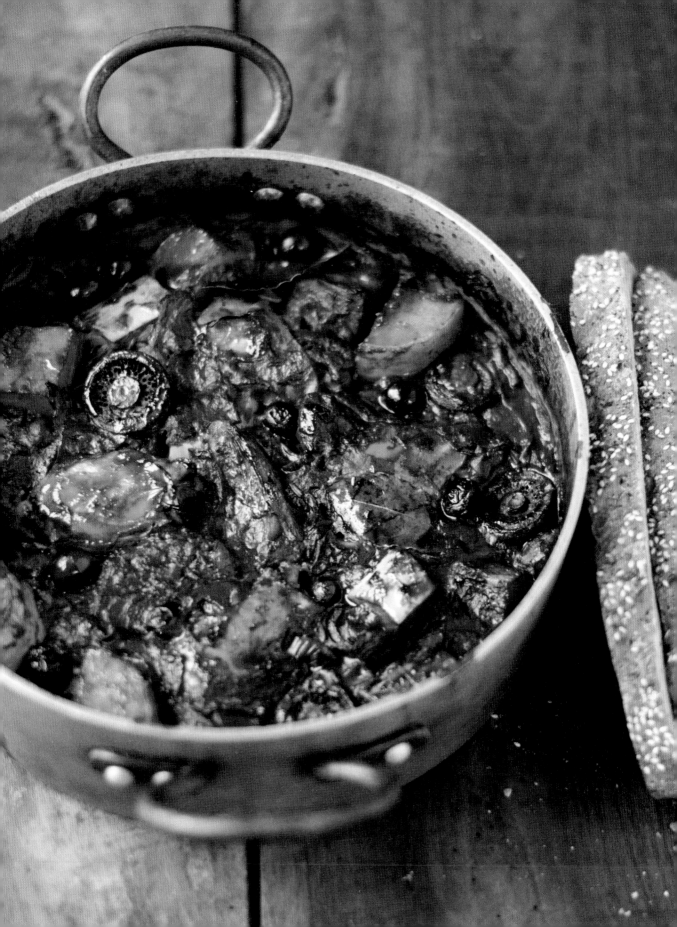

MOREISH FISH SOUP
MACKEREL, MUSSELS, BROTH & COUSCOUS

_ Both mackerel and mussels are super-high in selenium and iodine. The latter helps
our thyroid gland to function, in turn helping to control our metabolism _

SERVES 2

2 x 120g mackerel fillets, skin on,
scaled, scored and pin-boned
(ask for the head and bones too)

cayenne pepper

1 heaped teaspoon fennel seeds

1 heaped teaspoon coriander
seeds

2 cloves of garlic

1 sprig of fresh rosemary

1 lemon

500ml really good veg stock

1 x 400g tin of plum tomatoes

100g wholewheat couscous

2 small potatoes

2 carrots

200g mussels, scrubbed
and debearded

½ a bunch of fresh flat-leaf
parsley or basil (15g)

Put a large pan on a medium-high heat, place the mackerel head (gills removed) and bones in to brown for 5 minutes. Add a good pinch of cayenne, and the fennel and coriander seeds. Crush in the garlic, pick in the rosemary leaves and strip in the lemon zest with a speed-peeler. Stir and fry for 3 minutes to release all that wonderful flavour, then cover with the stock and add the tinned tomatoes. Bring to the boil, then simmer for 15 minutes.

In a bowl, just cover the couscous with boiling water, pop a plate on top, and leave to fluff up. Wash the potatoes and carrots, cut into 1cm dice and place in a casserole pan. Sit a coarse sieve on top and pour the broth through it into the pan, using the back of a ladle to really squash and push everything through, discarding what remains. Cook the potatoes and carrots in the broth for 15 minutes, or until tender. Add 300ml of boiling water and the mussels (tap any that are open and if they don't close, discard). Cover and cook for 5 minutes, or until the mussels open (throw away any that remain closed). When in season, I like to chuck a handful of freshly podded peas in too.

At the same time, place the mackerel fillets skin side down in a dry non-stick frying pan on a medium heat with a sprinkle of cayenne. Cook for 4 minutes, or until crispy – don't move them until the time's up. Flip over for 30 seconds more, then serve on top of your couscous in large warm soup bowls. Finely chop the leafy part of the parsley or basil and stir through the soup with the lemon juice, then season to perfection and divide between your bowls.

CALORIES	FAT	SAT FAT	PROTEIN	CARBS	SUGAR	FIBRE	
583kcal	22.9g	4.4g	39.6g	58.3g	12.2g	8.7g	45 MINUTES

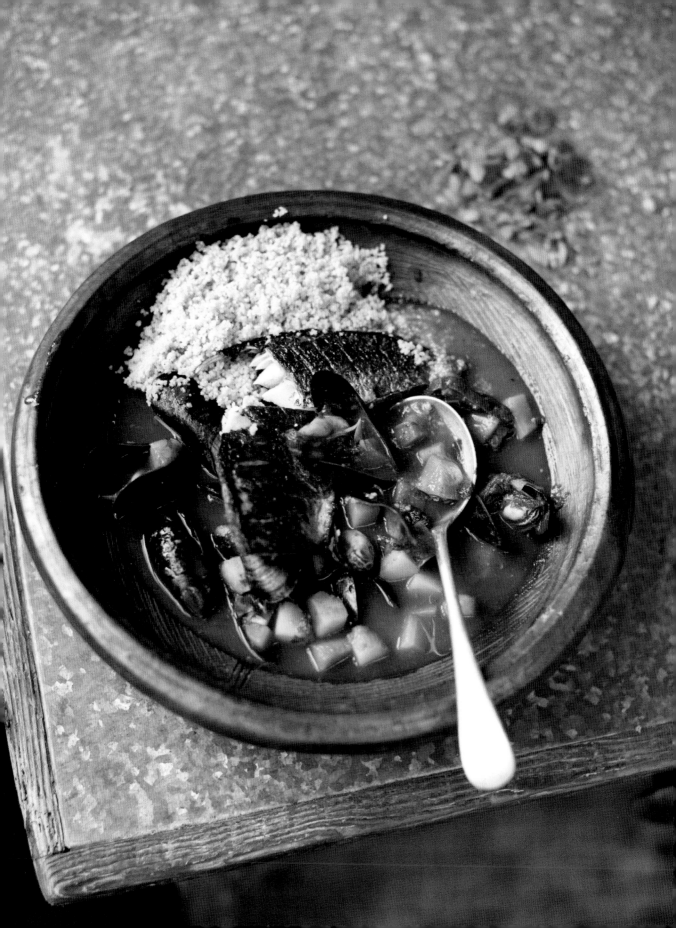

FAGIOLI FUSILLI
SWEET LEEKS, ARTICHOKES & BAY OIL

Protein-rich cannellini beans as well as all the micronutrient-packed tasty veggies in this comforting dish give us three of our 5-a-day, making this a great meat-free meal

SERVES 4

2 cloves of garlic

2 carrots

2 leeks

olive oil

8 fresh bay leaves

1 x 400g tin of cannellini beans

1 x 400g tin of artichokes
 in water

500ml really good veg stock

300g wholewheat fusilli

20g Parmesan cheese

4 sprigs of fresh flat-leaf parsley

Peel and finely chop the garlic. Peel the carrots and chop into ½cm chunks, then trim, wash and slice the leeks ½cm thick. Place a large casserole pan on a medium-high heat with 1 tablespoon of oil. Stir in the garlic and, a minute later, the carrot, leek and 2 bay leaves. Add a splash of water, cover, reduce the heat and cook for 15 minutes, or until softened, stirring occasionally.

Drain and add the beans, then drain, quarter and add the artichokes. Pour in the stock, bring to the boil, then simmer for 15 minutes to let the flavours infuse. Meanwhile, cook the pasta in a large pan of boiling salted water according to the packet instructions. Add 2 ladlefuls of the pasta cooking water to the veg pan, then drain and stir in the pasta. Season to perfection, then leave for a couple of minutes to suck up all that flavour.

Meanwhile, to make a quick bay oil, strip and tear the remaining bay leaves off their stalks into a pestle and mortar with a pinch of sea salt. Pound really well, putting some good effort in, until you have a fine green mush. Muddle in 150ml of oil, then decant into a jar to keep for future use. Serve each portion of pasta with a delicate grating of Parmesan, a sprinkling of black pepper and chopped parsley leaves and 1 teaspoon of your homemade bay oil.

CALORIES	FAT	SAT FAT	PROTEIN	CARBS	SUGAR	FIBRE	40 MINUTES
496kcal	11.2g	2.4g	23.4g	74.8g	8.7g	17.8g	

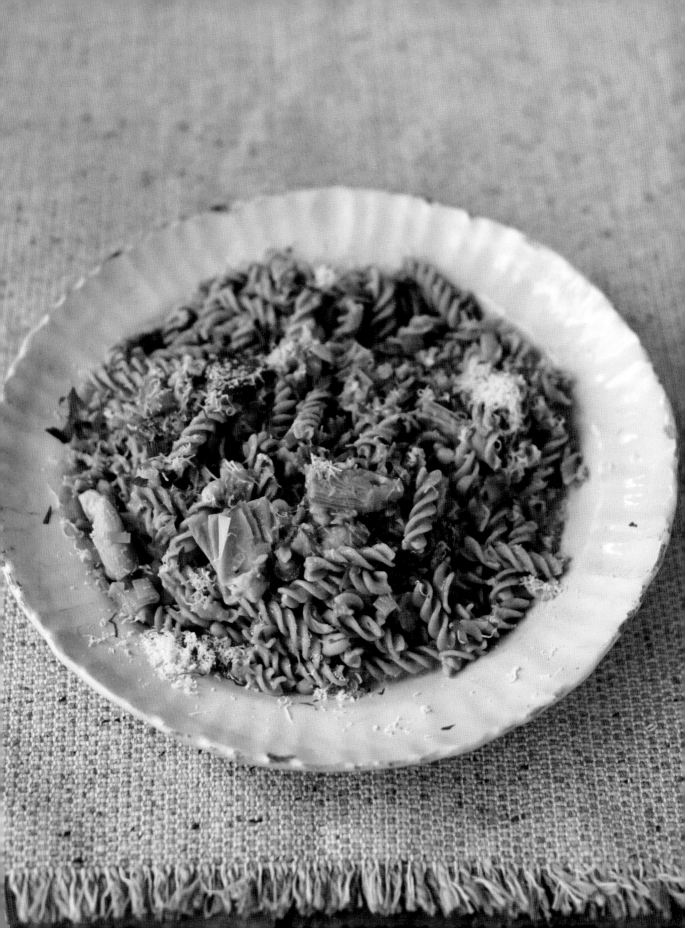

SUPER-TASTY MISO BROTH
CHICKEN, MUSHROOMS & WILD RICE

— Mixed wild rice is much more nutritious than regular rice and is a good source of both —
magnesium and phosphorus, which are good for maintaining healthy teeth and skin

SERVES 2

150g mixed brown and wild
  or brown rice

20g dried porcini mushrooms

1 red onion

sesame oil

5cm piece of ginger

1 heaped teaspoon miso paste

800ml really good chicken stock

6 radishes

rice or white wine vinegar

1 x 200g skinless chicken breast

1 handful of colourful curly kale

1 sheet of nori

150g mixed exotic mushrooms,
  such as enoki, chestnut, shiitake

Cook the rice according to the packet instructions. Put the porcini in a small bowl and just cover with boiling water to rehydrate them.

Meanwhile, peel the onion and cut into eighths, then place in a medium pan on a medium-high heat with 1 teaspoon of sesame oil. Cook for a few minutes, or until dark golden, stirring occasionally, while you peel and matchstick the ginger. Reduce the heat to medium-low, then add the ginger, miso paste and stock, along with the porcini and soaking water, leaving the last gritty bit behind. Cover and simmer gently for 20 minutes. Halve the radishes, put them into a bowl, toss in a splash of vinegar and a small pinch of sea salt and leave aside to quickly pickle.

Finely slice the chicken and tear the kale and nori into small pieces, removing any tough stalks from the kale. Break up the mushrooms, leaving the cute ones whole, and stir it all through the broth. Re-cover and cook for 4 minutes, or until the chicken is cooked through. Drain and divide the rice between your bowls, followed by the radishes. Season the broth to perfection, ladle it into the bowls, then serve.

CALORIES	FAT	SAT FAT	PROTEIN	CARBS	SUGAR	FIBRE	
522kcal	8.1g	1.9g	45.1g	70.4g	5.3g	5.5g	40 MINUTES

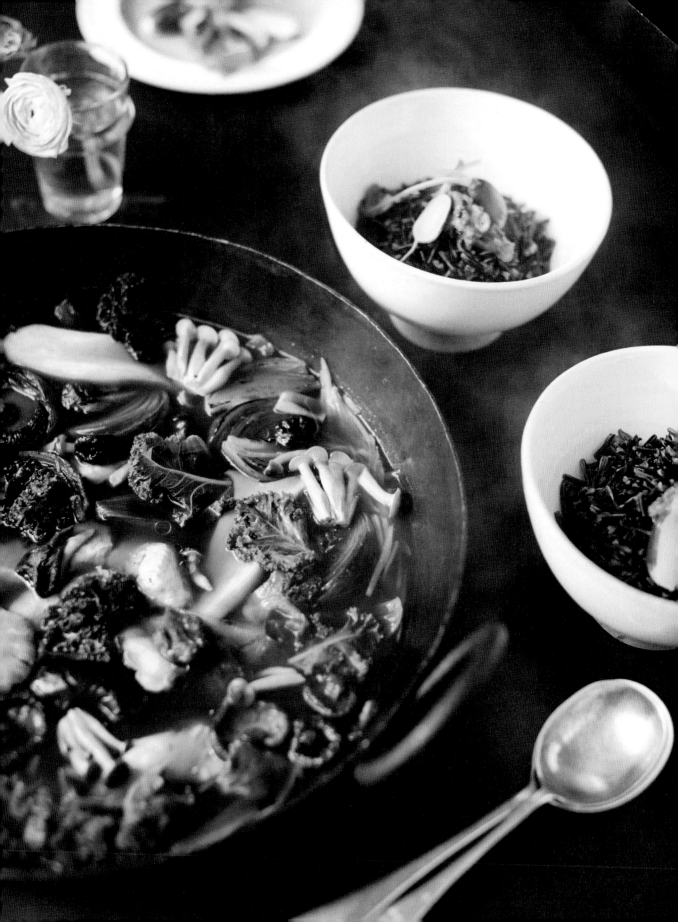

LEMON SOLE & OLIVE SAUCE
SWEET COURGETTES & JERSEY ROYALS

Courgettes and spinach contain folic acid and vitamin C, helping us to think properly, plus one lemon sole fillet gives us our daily selenium requirement for strong skin and nails

SERVES 2

2 large mixed-colour courgettes

4 cloves of garlic

extra virgin olive oil

250g Jersey Royal or baby new
  potatoes

6 black olives (stone in)

1 spring onion

1 fresh red or green chilli

½ a bunch of fresh mint (15g)

2 lemons

150g baby spinach

2 x 120g lemon sole fillets,
  skin off

Quarter the courgettes lengthways, trim away and discard the fluffy core, then slice them at an angle around 2cm thick. Peel and finely slice the garlic. Put a large casserole pan on a medium heat with 1 tablespoon of oil. Add the garlic, followed a minute later by the courgettes. Stir well, then pop the lid on and cook for 15 minutes, stirring occasionally. Remove the lid, reduce the heat a little and cook for another 5 minutes, or until sweet and delicious.

Meanwhile, halve any larger potatoes, cook in a pan of boiling salted water for 15 minutes, or until cooked through, and drain. Squash the olives and tear out the stones, trim the spring onion, then finely slice both with the chilli (deseed if you like). Pick and finely chop the mint leaves. Toss it all in a bowl with the juice of 1 lemon and 1 tablespoon of oil to make a sauce.

Lightly squash the potatoes, then fold them into the courgettes with the spinach and lay the lemon sole fillets on top of the veg. Put the lid back on and leave to steam for 7 minutes, or until the fish is brilliantly white and cooked through – it's super-quick to cook. Plate up, spoon the olive sauce over the fish, and serve with wedges of lemon.

CALORIES	FAT	SAT FAT	PROTEIN	CARBS	SUGAR	FIBRE	40 MINUTES
374kcal	16.3g	2.5g	30.2g	27.9g	7.3g	5.3g	

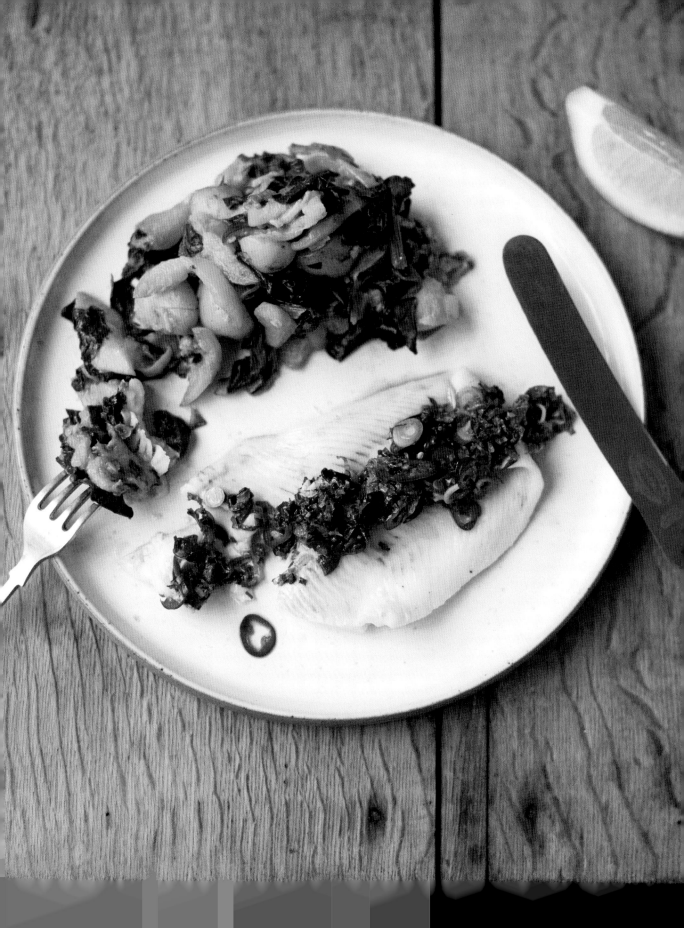

MIGHTY MUSHROOM CURRY
RED LENTILS, BROWN RICE & POPPADOMS

— Mushrooms are a great source of essential B vitamins, which help our metabolisms —
function so we can utilize the energy and nutrients from the food we eat

SERVES 2

100g brown basmati rice

50g red split lentils

300ml whole milk

1 lemon

2 cloves of garlic

3cm piece of ginger

1 fresh red chilli

1 tablespoon curry leaves

1 teaspoon black mustard seeds

olive oil

1 heaped teaspoon medium
  curry powder

1 onion

400g mixed mushrooms

250g ripe tomatoes

2 uncooked poppadoms

Cook the rice and lentils in a pan of boiling salted water according to the packet instructions (they should cook in about the same time, but there are variants, so check and adjust accordingly). Pour the whole milk (it's important that you use whole here) into a heatproof bowl with a pinch of sea salt and the lemon juice and place over the pan of rice to heat and split the milk into lumps of curds, which is pretty cool – just don't be tempted to stir it.

Peel the garlic and ginger, then finely slice with the chilli and put it all into a large casserole pan on a medium heat with the curry leaves, mustard seeds and 1 tablespoon of oil. Cook and toss for 2 minutes, until lightly golden, then stir in the curry powder. Peel and finely slice the onion and stir into the pan. Halve or quarter the mushrooms, leaving any little ones whole so you get a mix of sizes, then add to the pan with a pinch of sea salt and black pepper and a splash of water. Cook for 10 minutes, or until softened, tossing regularly. Turn up the heat and cook for 5 more minutes, or until lightly golden.

When the milk has split into curds and whey, gently pour it all in and around the mushroom pan. Slice the tomatoes and poke them into the pan, then simmer for another 5 to 10 minutes without stirring but just giving the odd shake, until the liquid has reduced down and the flavour is intense – the curds will break down slightly and become part of the sauce. One-by-one, puff up your dry poppadoms in the microwave for around 30 seconds each and serve with the mushroom curry, rice and lentils.

CALORIES	FAT	SAT FAT	PROTEIN	CARBS	SUGAR	FIBRE	
552kcal	18.1g	5.6g	23.1g	79.6g	18.2g	8.3g	45 MINUTES

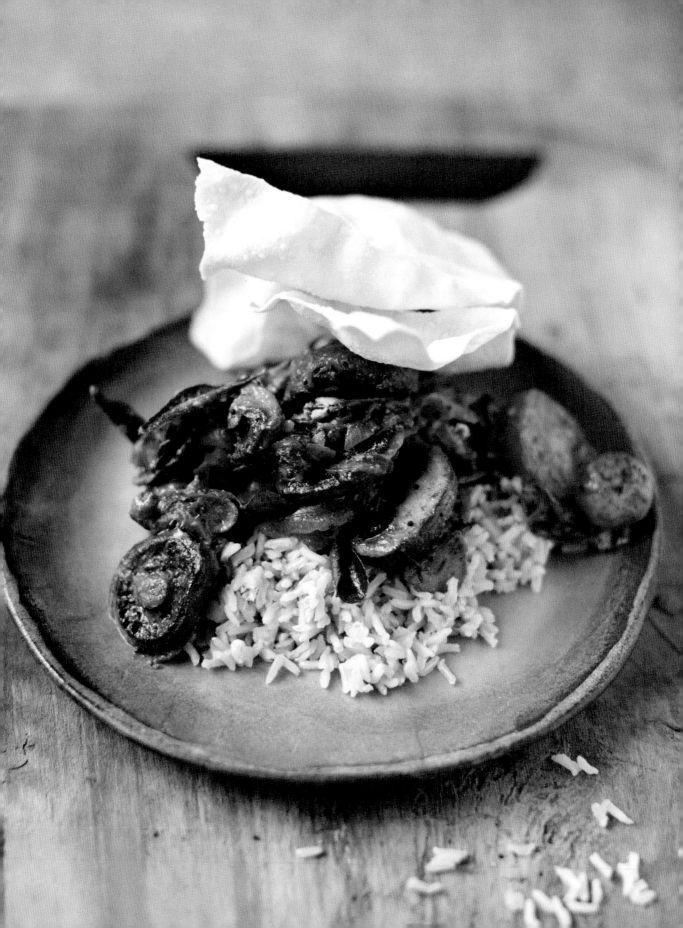

GREEN TEA ROASTED SALMON
GINGER RICE & SUNSHINE SALAD

_ Containing three of our 5-a-day, this recipe uses juicy mango, packed with vitamin C, _
which is important for helping to keep our immune systems in tip-top condition

SERVES 2

150g brown rice

1 x 500g salmon tail, skin on,
   scaled, bone in

1 green teabag

sesame oil

1 clove of garlic

320g mixed salad veg, such as
   carrots, cucumber, tomato,
   chicory

1 small ripe mango

1 lime

low-salt soy sauce

1 fresh red chilli

3cm piece of ginger

1 teaspoon sesame seeds

½ a punnet of cress

Preheat the oven to 180°C/350°F/gas 4. Cook the rice according to the packet instructions, then drain. Meanwhile, score the salmon skin 1cm deep at 2cm intervals and place in a snug-fitting baking dish (use one 300g fillet, if you prefer). Season it with sea salt and black pepper and the green teabag contents, then rub all over with 1 teaspoon of sesame oil, getting it well into the cuts. Peel and finely slice the garlic, then poke a slice into each cut. Bake for 25 minutes, or until cooked through (15 minutes if using a fillet).

Prepare all your salad veg, chopping everything into bite-sized chunks or slices that will be a pleasure to eat. Slice the cheeks off the mango, then peel, slice the flesh and put it into a nice bowl with all the veg. Really squidge and squeeze all the juice out of the mango centre into a separate bowl, then squeeze in the lime juice and season to taste with soy sauce. Deseed, finely chop and add the chilli to make a dressing, then toss with the veg and mango.

Peel and matchstick the ginger and put into a frying pan on a medium heat with 1 teaspoon of sesame oil and the sesame seeds. Fry for 2 minutes until starting to crisp up, tossing regularly, then stir in the rice and season to perfection. Snip the cress over the salad, and serve with the salmon and rice.

CALORIES	FAT	SAT FAT	PROTEIN	CARBS	SUGAR	FIBRE	35 MINUTES
600kcal	21.4g	3.9g	37.8g	70g	6.3g	3.9g	

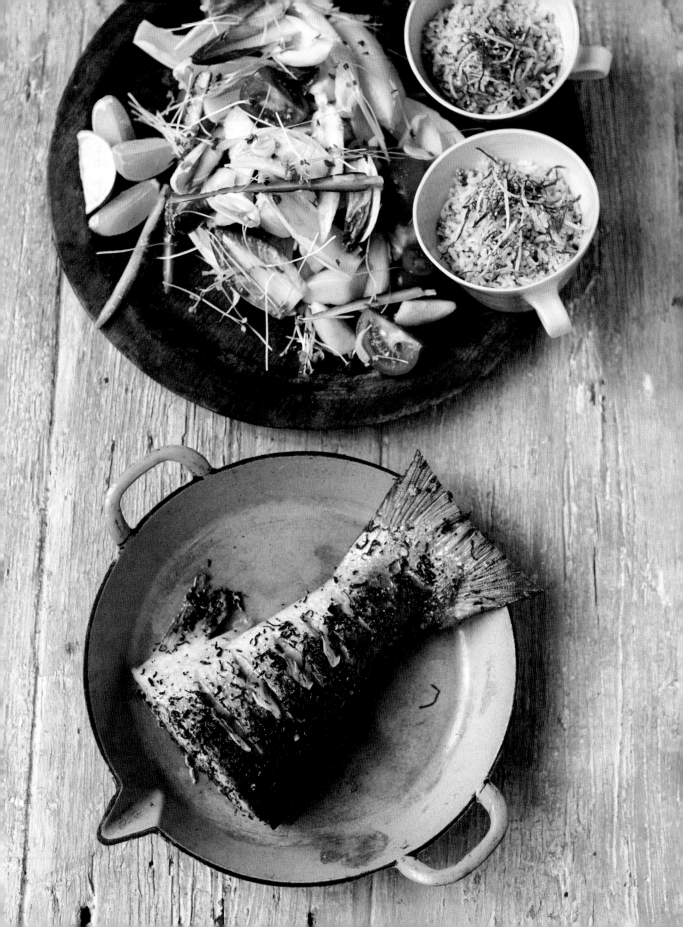

GRIDDLED STEAK & PEPPERS
HERBY JEWELLED TABBOULEH RICE

— Both beef and pomegranates contain lots of B vitamins, which boost our metabolism —
and our nervous and immune system functions, as well as helping us feel less tired

SERVES 2

150g brown rice

½ a bunch of fresh mint (15g)

1 bunch of fresh flat-leaf parsley
(30g)

2 spring onions

1 lemon

extra virgin olive oil

½ a pomegranate

25g shelled unsalted pistachios

200g roasted peeled red peppers
in brine

1 x 200g fillet steak, preferably
3cm thick

10g feta cheese

Cook the rice according to the packet instructions, then drain and put into a bowl. Pick and finely chop the mint and parsley leaves, including any tender stalks. Trim and finely slice the spring onions, then stir through the rice with the herbs, the lemon zest and juice, 1 tablespoon of oil and a pinch of black pepper. Holding the pomegranate half cut side down in your fingers, bash the back of it so the seeds tumble out, stir most of them through the rice, then taste and season to perfection.

Preheat a griddle pan on a high heat, lightly toasting the pistachios while it heats up. Once golden, crush them in a pestle and mortar and stir most of them through the rice. Use a ball of kitchen paper to carefully rub the griddle bars with a little oil. Drain the peppers, open them out and grill on both sides, then remove to a plate. Rub a little oil and a pinch of sea salt and pepper into the steak, then griddle for 2 to 3 minutes on each side for medium-rare, turning every minute, or until cooked to your liking. Rest the steak for a couple of minutes on top of the peppers while you pile the rice on a platter. Toss the steak and peppers in the resting juices, slice up the steak, add both to the platter and crumble over the feta. Scatter over the rest of the pomegranate seeds and pistachios, then serve.

CALORIES	FAT	SAT FAT	PROTEIN	CARBS	SUGAR	FIBRE	30 MINUTES
597kcal	22g	5g	33.7g	69.7g	7.7g	4.1g	

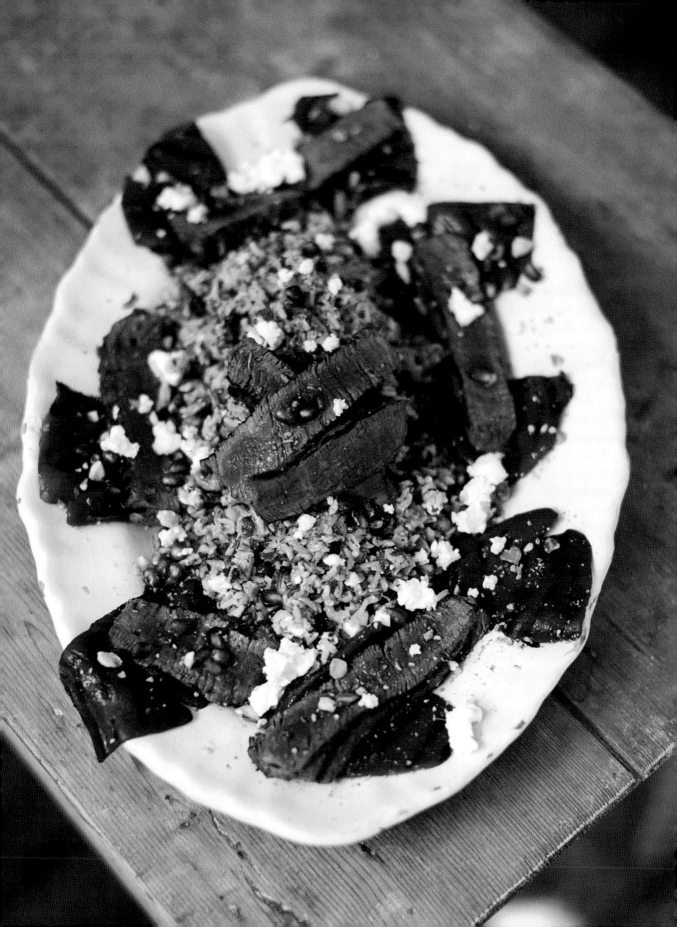

GINGER & CHICKEN PENICILLIN
BROWN RICE, CRUNCHY VEG & SAUCES

— Chicken is a great meat, leaner than most and high in essential B vitamins plus the mineral —
selenium, which among other things puts lead in your pencil, fellas – woop woop!

SERVES 6

1 x 1.4kg whole chicken

4 mixed-colour fresh chillies

3 x 5cm pieces of ginger

1 bulb of garlic

1 bunch of spring onions

½ a bunch of fresh coriander (15g)

1 teaspoon cider vinegar

low-salt soy sauce

2 tablespoons balsamic vinegar

1 teaspoon Worcestershire sauce

hot chilli sauce

400g brown rice

1 cucumber

Place the chicken in your largest pot with the chillies and a good pinch of sea salt. Halve 2 pieces of ginger lengthways. Reserving one clove, cut the garlic bulb in half across the middle. Cut the green tops off the spring onions and trim the bases, putting the whites aside. Add it all to the pan along with the coriander stalks, then top up with water to completely submerge the chicken. Bring to the boil on a high heat, then simmer for 2 hours, skimming away any fat. I sit a smaller pan lid on top of the chicken to help it stay submerged.

For the sauces, peel and finely grate the remaining ginger and the reserved garlic clove, then scrape into a bowl with any juices. Finely slice the end 2cm of each remaining spring onion and mix into the bowl with the cider vinegar and 1 teaspoon of soy. In a separate bowl, mix 1 teaspoon of soy with the balsamic and Worcestershire sauce. Decant some chilli sauce into a bowl too.

Cook the rice according to the packet instructions, then drain. Meanwhile, finely slice the remaining bits of spring onion lengthways. Quarter the cucumber lengthways and cut away the watery core, halve, then slice lengthways again into long strips. Carefully remove the chicken from the broth and discard the skin, then slice or shred all the meat off the bone (wear gloves, if you want). Divide the chicken between your warm bowls with the rice, cucumber and spring onion. Strain the broth, correct the seasoning if needed, and ladle between the bowls. Scatter over the coriander leaves and serve with the bowls of sauces on the side. Mix everything up, then tuck in.

CALORIES	FAT	SAT FAT	PROTEIN	CARBS	SUGAR	FIBRE	2 HOURS 20 MINUTES
442kcal	9.1g	2.5g	31.8g	61.6g	6.4g	2.4g	

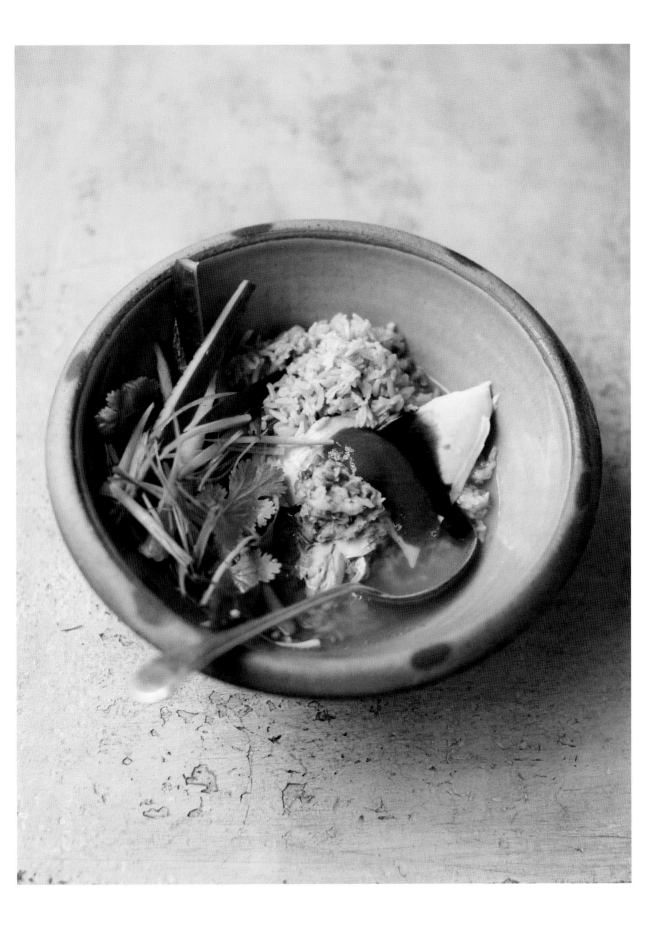

CRAZY FISH
VEG & NOODLE STIR-FRY

— Bream is super-high in phosphorus, helping to keep the cell barriers in our bodies in tip-top condition and ensuring our cells get everything they need to function properly —

SERVES 2

sesame oil

1 heaped teaspoon Chinese
    five-spice

1 x 300g bream, scaled, gutted
    and scored at 2cm intervals

150g brown rice noodles

2 cloves of garlic

5cm piece of ginger

1 fresh red chilli

100g tenderstem broccoli

100g asparagus

100g baby corn

4 spring onions

1 tablespoon balsamic vinegar

1 lime

low-salt soy sauce

Preheat the oven to 180°C/350°F/gas 4. Put a drizzle of sesame oil into an ovenproof pan or roasting tray, then wipe it around with kitchen paper. Rub the Chinese five-spice and a pinch of sea salt all over the bream, inside and out, then place it in the pan – I like to sit the fish upright, as in the picture. Roast for 15 minutes, or until golden and cooked through. The fish will be juicy and flaky, while the skin crisps up and becomes a pleasure to eat.

Cook the noodles according to the packet instructions, then drain. Meanwhile, peel the garlic and ginger, then slice with the chilli. Trim the woody ends off the broccoli and asparagus, then roughly slice the stalks, leaving the tips whole. Halve the corn lengthways, trim and slice the spring onions.

Put a large pan or wok on a high heat. Once hot, add 1 tablespoon of sesame oil, followed by the garlic, ginger and chilli. Stir-fry for 1 minute, then add the veg for a further 2 minutes, tossing often. Toss in the drained noodles and the vinegar for another 2 minutes, allowing the noodles to just start catching. Divide between your plates, and serve with the bream, wedges of lime, and soy sauce so you can season to perfection. Have fun removing the delicious bream from the bone, and get stuck in!

CALORIES	FAT	SAT FAT	PROTEIN	CARBS	SUGAR	FIBRE	
423kcal	12.3g	1.3g	35g	43g	8.6g	4.2g	25 MINUTES

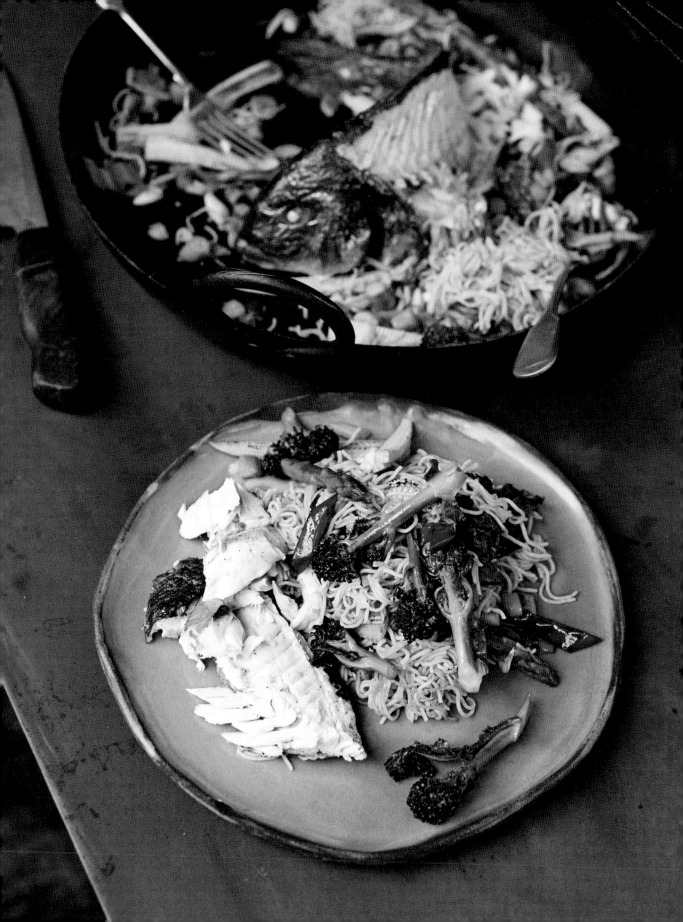

PORK & APPLE SAUCE
GLAZED CARROTS, BROWN RICE & GREENS

Pork is a great source of B vitamins and is especially high in thiamin, which we need for a healthy heart. All the veg here also give us three of our 5-a-day – brilliant!

SERVES 2

2 green eating apples

1cm piece of ginger

150g brown rice

200g small carrots

200g tenderstem broccoli

220g piece of lean pork fillet

1 whole nutmeg, for grating

8 leaves of fresh sage

olive oil

2 oranges

2 tablespoons natural yoghurt

Quarter the apples and remove the cores, peel and finely chop the ginger and place both in a pan with 300ml of boiling water. Boil hard for 10 minutes, stirring occasionally. Tip the contents of the pan into a blender and blitz until smooth. Rinse the pan, return to the heat and cook the rice according to the packet instructions. Steam the carrots in a colander above the rice for 20 minutes with a lid on, then remove them to a plate. Add the broccoli to the colander to steam for the last 5 minutes, then put aside and drain the rice.

Meanwhile, season the pork all over with a pinch of sea salt and black pepper, finely grate over a quarter of the nutmeg, then pick over the sage leaves and really press them into both sides of the pork. Put 1 tablespoon of oil into a large frying pan on a medium heat, then add the pork and steamed carrots. Cook the pork for 4 minutes on each side (depending on its thickness – use your instincts), or until golden and cooked through.

Remove the pork to a board to rest for a few minutes. Reduce the heat to low, squeeze the orange juice over the carrots, shake the pan to coat them and pick up the sticky bits from the bottom, then leave until it becomes a natural syrupy glaze. Slice the pork and serve with the rice, broccoli and carrots. Swirl the yoghurt through half the apple sauce (keep the rest for another day) and serve on the side. Drizzle with any pan and resting juices, and tuck in.

CALORIES	FAT	SAT FAT	PROTEIN	CARBS	SUGAR	FIBRE	50 MINUTES
579kcal	10.6g	3.3g	36.6g	90g	28.3g	9.2g	

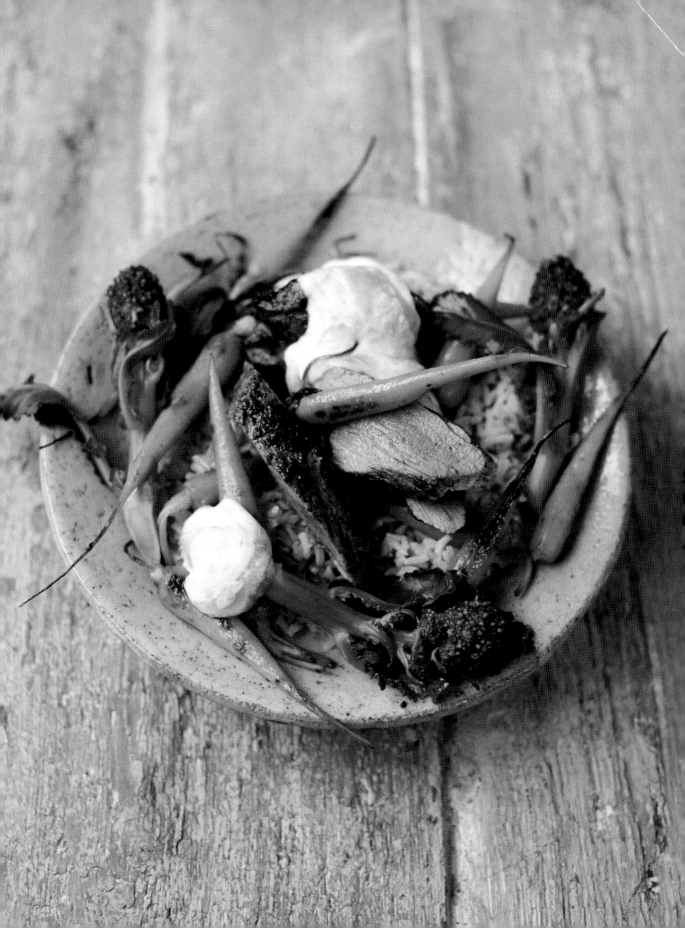

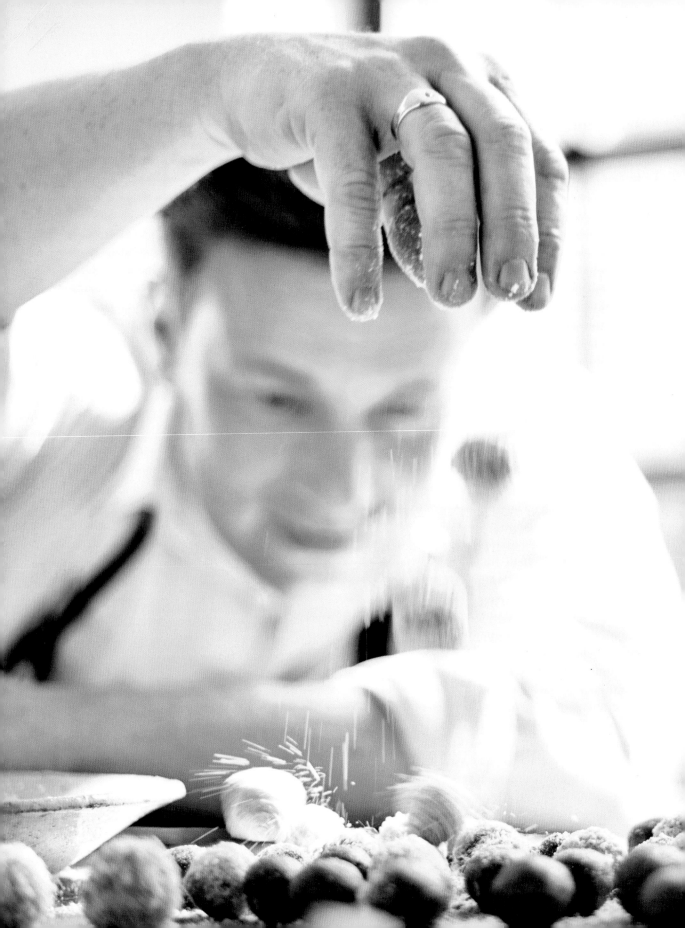

SNACKS & DRINKS

Snacks have that ability to totally tip our daily balance in the wrong direction, without us even realizing – it's very easy to consume a large volume of calories with little nutritional value. As delicious as some naughty treats can be, they should be enjoyed as treats, so this chapter exists to give you some alternatives that you can embrace on a regular basis. I've kept it really simple, with everything coming in at around 100 calories, so that it's super-easy to keep track of the amount you're snacking on throughout the day. Even if you can favour these choices just half the time, I'm sure you'll feel the benefits. I've also had a bit of fun celebrating humble H_2O and some tasty ways to help you enjoy it.

100-CALORIE SALAD SNACK BOWLS
PART ONE

Next time the nibbles strike, instead of hitting the biscuit tin, choose one of these veg-packed salad snack bowls – the high water content of the veg will help fill us up

CREAMY BASIL DRESSING Good for 3 salad portions. Simply blitz **4 tablespoons of natural yoghurt** with **1 tablespoon of white wine vinegar, 1 teaspoon of Dijon mustard,** the leaves from **4 sprigs of fresh basil, ¼ of a fresh red chilli** and a pinch of sea salt and black pepper until super-smooth.

TOASTED SEED MIX Make a batch to use here and as a snack in their own right. Simply toast a mixture of **your favourite seeds, such as sunflower, poppy, sesame, linseed,** in a dry pan until smelling amazing, tossing regularly. Leave them whole or lightly crush them in a pestle and mortar.

EACH SALAD SERVES 1

GEM LETTUCE, RADISH, PEA & CLEMENTINE SALAD Wedge up **1 little gem lettuce** and team it with **2 quartered radishes, 1 small handful of freshly podded peas, 1 segmented clementine,** the smaller leaves from **2 sprigs of fresh basil** and **½ tablespoon of your toasted seed mix.** Toss in **1½ tablespoons of your creamy basil dressing** just before tucking in.

ROUND LETTUCE, FENNEL, BLUEBERRY & CHILLI SALAD Slice **½ a round lettuce,** pick the leafy tops off **¼ of a bulb of fennel** and finely slice it, ideally on a mandolin (use the guard!), and mix with **25g of blueberries, 1 pinch of dried red chilli flakes** and **½ tablespoon of your toasted seed mix.** Toss in **1½ tablespoons of your creamy basil dressing** just before tucking in.

GEM LETTUCE, CUCUMBER, APPLE & MINT SALAD Wedge up **1 little gem lettuce,** slice up a **4cm chunk of cucumber** and **½ a small apple,** preferably with a crinkle-cut knife, and mix with the smaller leaves from **2 sprigs of fresh mint** and **½ tablespoon of your toasted seed mix.** Toss in **1½ tablespoons of your creamy basil dressing** just before tucking in.

CALORIES	FAT	SAT FAT	PROTEIN	CARBS	SUGAR	FIBRE	15 MINUTES
100kcal	4.8g	1.1g	4.8g	11.2g	9.8g	4g	

THESE VALUES ARE AN AVERAGE OF THE THREE SALAD RECIPES ABOVE

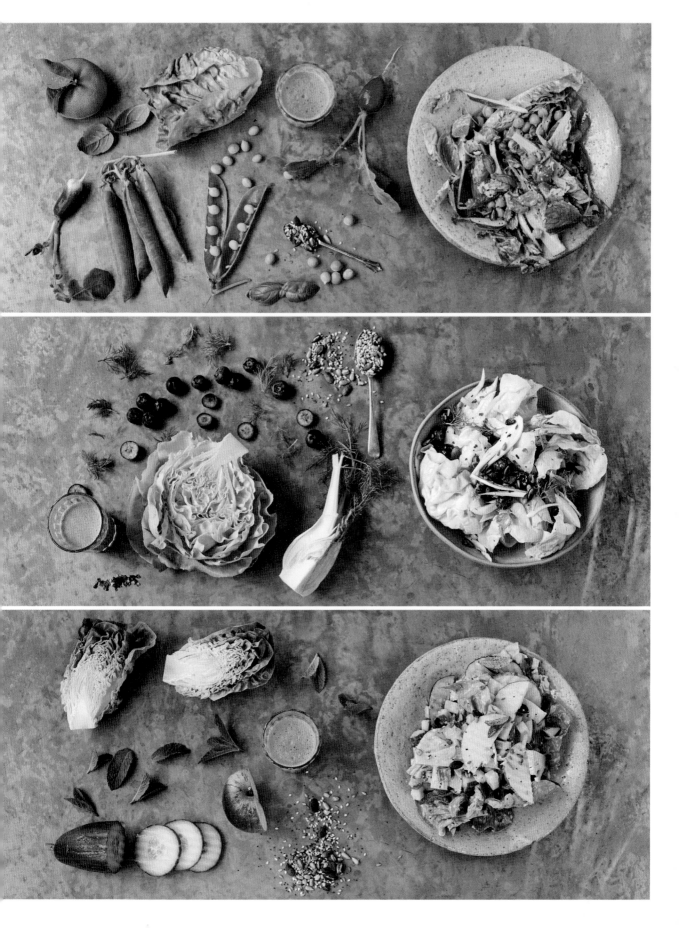

100-CALORIE SALAD SNACK BOWLS PART TWO

These lovely nutritious little salads provide us with a good variety of essential vitamins and minerals, which the fat from the toasted nut mix helps us to absorb

CREAMY MINT DRESSING Good for 3 salad portions. Simply blitz up **4 tablespoons of natural yoghurt** with **1 tablespoon of white wine vinegar**, **1 teaspoon of Dijon mustard**, the leaves from **3 sprigs of fresh mint**, **¼ of a fresh red chilli** and a pinch of sea salt and black pepper until super-smooth.

TOASTED NUT MIX Make a batch to use here and for sprinkling on breakfasts. Simply toast a mixture of **your favourite shelled unsalted nuts, such as walnuts, pistachios, almonds, hazelnuts**, in a dry pan until smelling amazing, tossing regularly, then roughly crush in a pestle and mortar.

EACH SALAD SERVES 1

ICEBERG LETTUCE, COURGETTE, PEAR & DILL SALAD Slice up **¼ of an iceberg lettuce**, speed-peel **2 baby courgettes** into ribbons, finely slice **½ a pear**, and mix with the leaves from **2 sprigs of fresh dill** and **1 teaspoon of your toasted nut mix**. Toss in **1½ tablespoons of your creamy mint dressing** just before tucking in.

ROUND LETTUCE, ASPARAGUS, STRAWBERRY & MINT SALAD Slice up **½ a round lettuce**, halve **5 small strawberries** and speed-peel **3 spears of asparagus** into ribbons, then mix with the smaller leaves from **2 sprigs of fresh mint** and **1 teaspoon of your toasted nut mix**. Toss in **1½ tablespoons of your creamy mint dressing** just before tucking in.

ICEBERG LETTUCE, BROAD BEAN, GRAPE & TARRAGON SALAD Slice up **¼ of an iceberg lettuce** and mix with **1 small handful of freshly podded broad beans**, **6 whole or halved grapes**, the leaves from **2 sprigs of fresh tarragon** and **1 teaspoon of your toasted nut mix**. Toss in **1½ tablespoons of your creamy mint dressing** just before tucking in.

CALORIES	FAT	SAT FAT	PROTEIN	CARBS	SUGAR	FIBRE	
100kcal	4.5g	1.1g	5.1g	10.2g	9g	3.1g	15 MINUTES

THESE VALUES ARE AN AVERAGE OF THE THREE SALAD RECIPES ABOVE

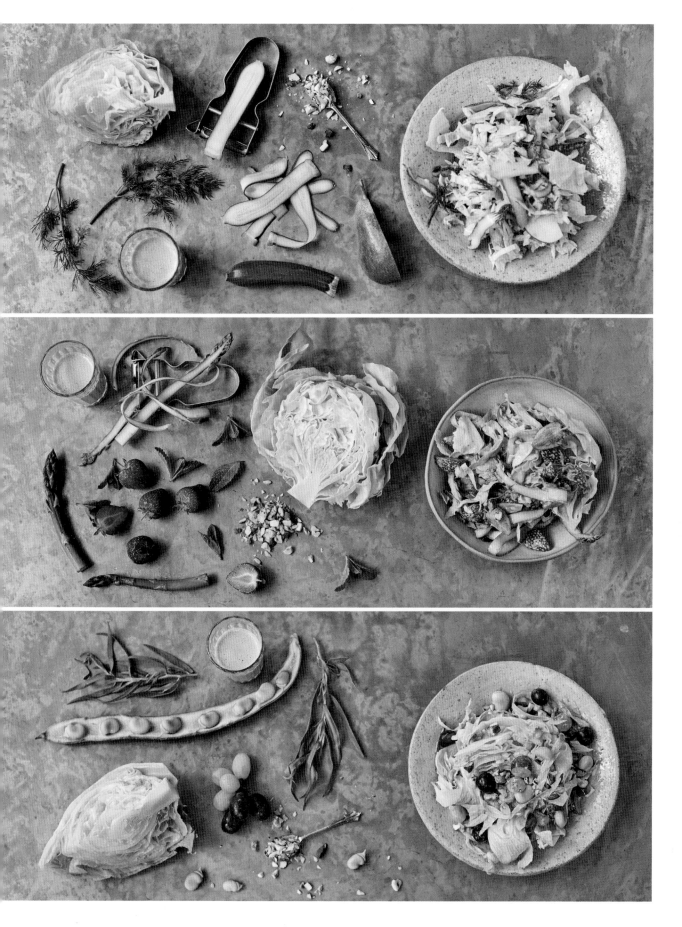

SKINNY HOMEMADE HOUMOUS

Mighty chickpeas are high in protein, fibre and more than ten different micronutrients, including a hefty amount of the mineral copper, keeping our hair and skin nice and healthy

SERVES 8

This recipe requires you to hunt out a jar of really good-quality chickpeas – they have much better flavour, so will guarantee an amazing result. Tip **1 x 660g jar of chickpeas**, juice and all, into a blender. Add **1 teaspoon of tahini**, **2 tablespoons of natural yoghurt**, **½ a peeled clove of garlic**, the **juice of ½ a lemon** and **1 pinch of cayenne pepper**, then blitz until smooth. Taste and season to perfection, then serve with an extra sprinkling of cayenne. Pair a portion of houmous with **80g of raw seasonal crunchy veg crudités** for a great snack.

CALORIES	FAT	SAT FAT	PROTEIN	CARBS	SUGAR	FIBRE	5 MINUTES
99kcal	2.5g	0.5g	5.9g	13.3g	0.8g	4g	

FEISTY BEET & HORSERADISH DIP

Beautiful beets are super-high in folic acid – so they are great for any expectant ladies out there – plus we all need folate to make protein, the building blocks of our bodies

SERVES 4

Roughly chop the contents of **1 x 250g vac-pack of beets**, then put them into a blender, juice and all, with **2 heaped tablespoons of natural yoghurt**, **1 pinch of sea salt and black pepper**, **1 teaspoon of red wine vinegar** and **2 heaped teaspoons of jarred grated horseradish**, or, even better, a **generous grating of fresh horseradish**. Blitz until smooth, taste and correct the balance of flavours, then serve with an extra grating of fresh horseradish, if you dare! Pair a portion of this dip with **80g of raw seasonal crunchy veg crudités** for a super snack.

CALORIES	FAT	SAT FAT	PROTEIN	CARBS	SUGAR	FIBRE	5 MINUTES
60kcal	1.1g	0.4g	1.7g	10.8g	10.1g	3.3g	

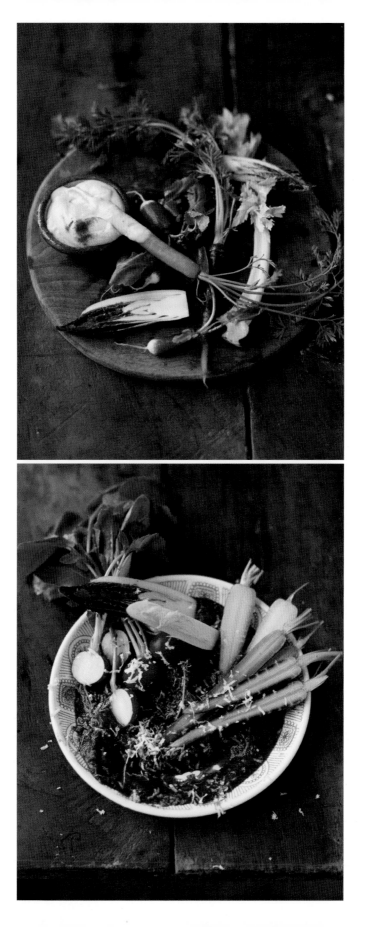

HEALTHY POPPADOM SNACKS
FOUR TASTY TOPPING COMBOS

Gram- or chickpea-flour poppadoms are gluten-free and high in protein, so when teamed
with protein-rich cottage cheese too, this snack is sure to keep hunger pangs at bay

EACH COMBO SERVES 1

CHEESE, CHILLI & SEEDS

Puff up **1 dry poppadom** in the microwave for around 30 seconds. Spoon over **1 tablespoon of cottage
cheese**, **¼ of a very finely sliced fresh chilli** and a little peeled **finely chopped red onion** tossed in
a squeeze of lemon juice. Scatter with **1 teaspoon of mixed poppy and sunflower seeds** and enjoy.

CHEESE, TOMATO & BASIL

Puff up **1 dry poppadom** in the microwave for around 30 seconds. Spoon over **1 tablespoon of cottage
cheese**, chop and add **1 small handful of ripe mixed-colour tomatoes** and pick over **a few fresh baby
basil leaves**. Sprinkle with a pinch of sea salt, drizzle with **a little balsamic vinegar** and enjoy.

CHEESE & MANGO CHUTNEY

Puff up **1 dry poppadom** in the microwave for around 30 seconds. Spoon over **1 tablespoon of cottage
cheese**, then loosen **2 teaspoons of mango chutney** with a splash of water and drizzle over the top. Chop
3 sprigs of fresh coriander, sprinkle over with **1 pinch of sesame seeds** and enjoy.

CHEESE & QUICK PICKLED VEG

Puff up **1 dry poppadom** in the microwave for around 30 seconds. Spoon over **1 tablespoon of cottage
cheese**. Coarsely grate **½ a small carrot** and a **2cm piece of cucumber**, scrunch with **½ a teaspoon each
of white wine vinegar and low-salt soy sauce**, then scatter over with **1 pinch of sesame seeds** and enjoy.

CALORIES	FAT	SAT FAT	PROTEIN	CARBS	SUGAR	FIBRE	5 MINUTES
91kcal	4.6g	1.4g	5.1g	7.9g	3.6g	1.5g	

THESE VALUES ARE AN AVERAGE OF THE FOUR RECIPES ABOVE

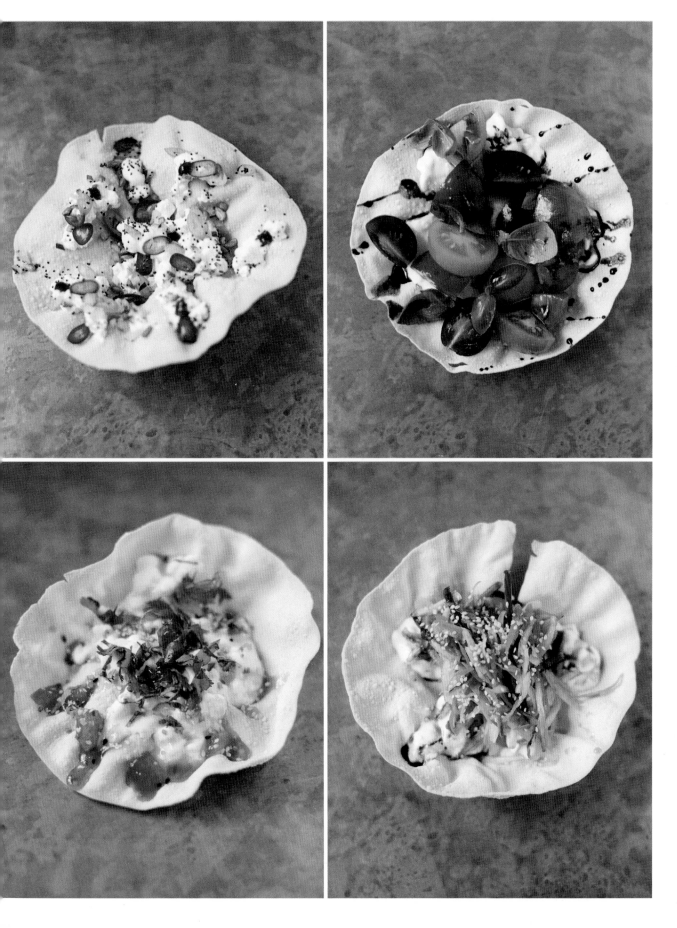

POPCORN FUN
LOTS OF DELICIOUS IDEAS

_ Popcorn cooked this way is super-healthy, fills us up, is a great source of fibre and _
is super-high in vitamin E, helping protect our cells from stress damage

EACH IDEA SERVES 1

We all know popcorn is a delicious snack, but it's often cooked in oil or butter and smothered in lovely caramel and treaty things. That's great – for a treat – but in the spirit of enjoying a super-healthy snack that's also delicious and nutritious, I've tested this really good dry-pan method. I do it all the time now, and the kids love it too! For the best results, I like to cook it just one or two portions at a time.

For a nice portion, like in the picture, put 1 tablespoon of popping corn into a medium non-stick saucepan and place it cold on a medium heat. Starting cold gives you optimum popping conditions. Put a lid on and let it pop, until it stops. As soon as you think it's all popped, turn the heat off – don't overcook it (just avoid eating any kernels that don't pop). If you want to flavour it, apply the flavouring as soon as it's finished popping, shake and serve – just be careful, as the pan will be super-hot.

WORCESTERSHIRE SAUCE / BALSAMIC VINEGAR FLAVOUR

Both of these can really only be successfully distributed if applied with a spritzer (pick one up from a pharmacist – you can use it to add flavour to roast veg and meat too). Spritz about fifiteen times onto your popcorn, and if choosing vinegar, it's helpful to go for a thin one to help it spritz well.

HOT CHILLI SAUCE FLAVOUR

Shake 1 teaspoon of hot chilli sauce all over your super-hot popcorn. Less is more, too much and it will go soggy, but done at the last minute and shaken well, you'll get stunning results with a nice kick.

MARMITE FLAVOUR

Mighty Marmite is particularly good, both in flavour and in the sticky, almost clumpy texture it creates – you'll find 1 teaspoon goes a long way and I find it easiest to apply from a squeezy bottle.

CALORIES	FAT	SAT FAT	PROTEIN	CARBS	SUGAR	FIBRE	15 MINUTES
76kcal	0.9g	0.1g	2.6g	14.3g	0.7g	1.5g	

THESE VALUES ARE AN AVERAGE OF THE FOUR RECIPE IDEAS ABOVE

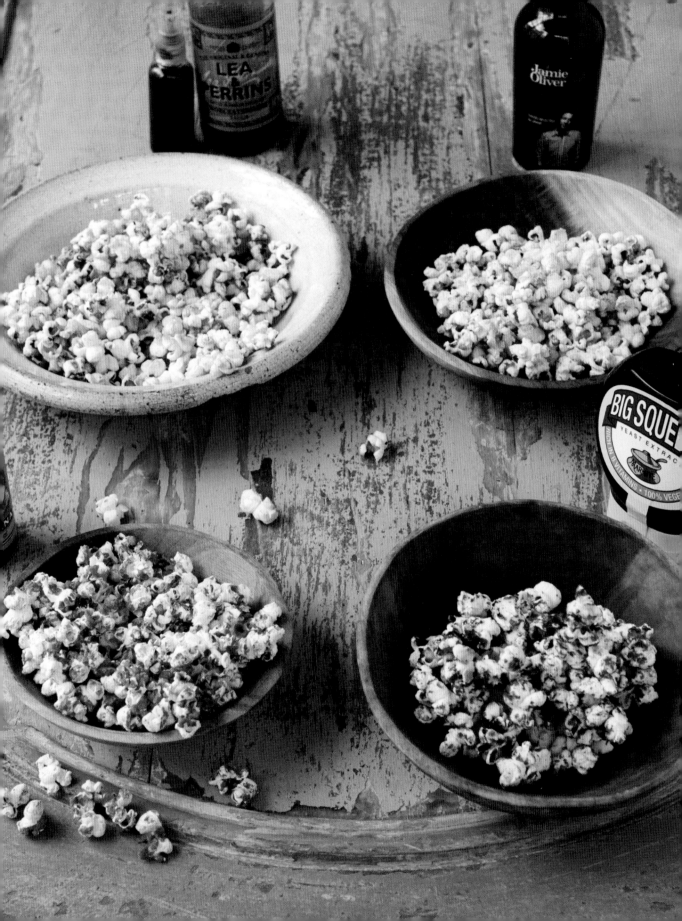

CUCUMBER STICKS
STUFFED WITH LOVELY THINGS

We often mistake hunger for thirst, so enjoying refreshing cucumber as a snack is a great idea because it naturally has a really high water content, so will satisfy us on both counts

EACH SERVES 1

Now this doesn't profess to be cooking – these easy-to-put-together fillings are assembly jobs of staple ingredients that will excite your taste buds. Each stuffed quarter cucumber is under 100 calories, and each recipe uses a whole tub of cream cheese, giving you around 10 portions of filling to keep in the tub, in the fridge, to last a few days.

Halve **1 cucumber** lengthways, scrape away the watery core, then halve across the middle. You need one quarter per snack, so wrap and return any extra to the fridge. Sprinkle your cucumber with a little sea salt and **vinegar.**

TAHINI, SPRING ONION & SESAME

Trim and finely slice **1 spring onion**, then mix half with **180g of cream cheese, 2 tablespoons of tahini** and the **juice of 1 lime.** Spread 1 tablespoon across your **cucumber quarter**, and sprinkle generously with **toasted sesame seeds** and the remaining spring onion.

LIME PICKLE & POPPADOM

Whip **180g of cream cheese** with the **juice of ½ a lemon,** then spread 1 tablespoon across your **cucumber quarter.** Spoon over **little blobs of lime or lemon pickle,** then puff up **½ a dry poppadom** per portion for around 30 seconds in the microwave, crunch and sprinkle over the top like dust.

THE RING OF FIRE

Whip **180g of cream cheese** with the **juice of 1 lemon,** put into a sandwich bag, squeeze it into one corner, then snip the bag and pipe splodges along your **cucumber quarter.** Fill the gaps with **Tabasco chipotle sauce,** then slice and sprinkle over some **fresh chilli.**

SMOKY PEPPERS & SWEET BASIL

In a blender, blitz **100g of jarred peeled red peppers in brine** with **1 teaspoon of Tabasco chipotle sauce** and the **juice of 1 lemon** until smooth. Loosen **180g of cream cheese** with a splash of water, then ripple the pepper mixture through it. Spread 1 tablespoon across your **cucumber quarter** and top with **fresh basil leaves.**

CALORIES	FAT	SAT FAT	PROTEIN	CARBS	SUGAR	FIBRE	5 MINUTES
81kcal	6g	0.9g	3.4g	1.9g	1.8g	0.9g	

THESE VALUES ARE AN AVERAGE OF THE FOUR RECIPES ABOVE

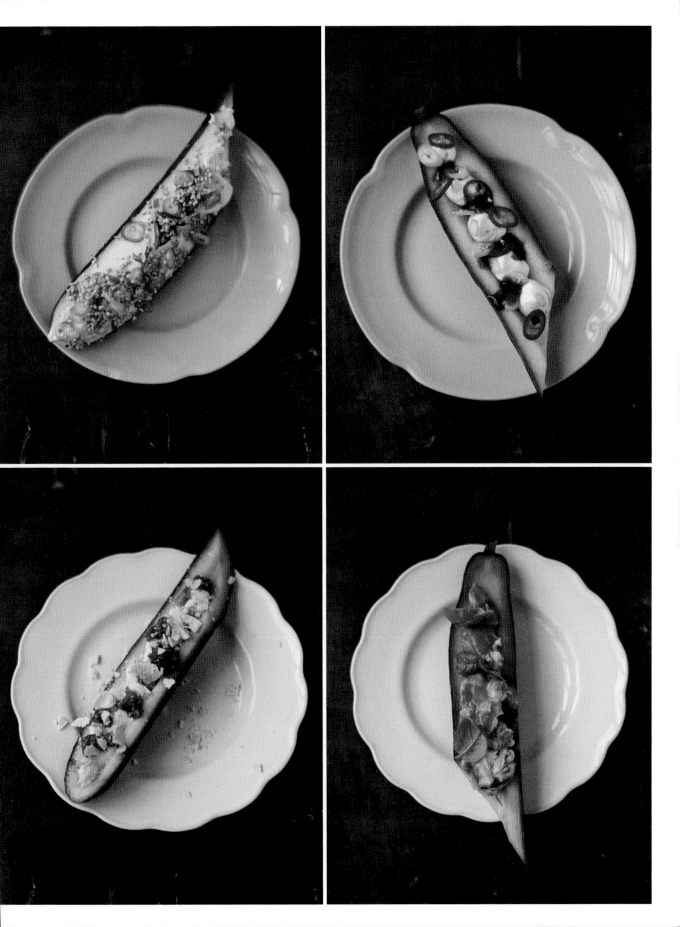

BLUSHING PICKLED EGGS
RED CABBAGE, CLOVES & STAR ANISE

— Brilliant eggs are one of the very few foods that are high in the micronutrient iodine, which our thyroid gland needs for making the hormones that help to control our metabolism —

SERVES 6

6 large eggs

2 star anise

1 teaspoon cloves

½ tablespoon mustard seeds

2 fresh bay leaves

1 tablespoon runny honey

300ml red wine vinegar

½ a small red cabbage (300g)

This is a slightly bonkers one, I admit, but I love it (my wife would hate it). Making delicious pickled eggs and cabbage is fun, and, most importantly, they can be enjoyed in many ways. First up, one blushing egg makes a great, quick protein-boost snack of just 85 calories, but you could also use the eggs and cabbage to pimp up a picnic, antipasti board or ploughman's lunch, a salad niçoise or even a steaming bowl of ramen. This recipe is for 6 eggs, but you can easily double up the ingredients if you want to make a bigger batch.

Gently lower the eggs into a large pan of boiling salted water (a pinch of salt helps to prevent them from bursting). Cook for 10 minutes to hard boil, then place under cold running water. Once cool enough to handle, peel and rinse.

In a large dry casserole pan on a medium heat, toast the star anise, cloves and mustard seeds until smelling amazing, then add the bay leaves and 250ml of boiling water. Simmer for 3 minutes, then stir in the honey, vinegar and 2 heaped teaspoons of sea salt and remove from the heat. Finely shred the red cabbage, then stir it into the pickling liquor and leave for 10 minutes, to let it shrink a little and allow the juices to start exchanging.

Get yourself a 1-litre jar and randomly layer up the cabbage and eggs. Pour in any excess pickling liquor to fill the jar and cover the eggs, then pop the lid on and keep in the fridge until you're ready to tuck in. The eggs are at their most delicious after a week, but perfectly tasty after just 24 hours too. They'll keep happily for 2 weeks, and any leftover liquor is good in salad dressings.

CALORIES	FAT	SAT FAT	PROTEIN	CARBS	SUGAR	FIBRE	25 MINUTES PLUS PICKLING
85kcal	6.3g	1.7g	7.2g	0.5g	0.4g	0.1g	

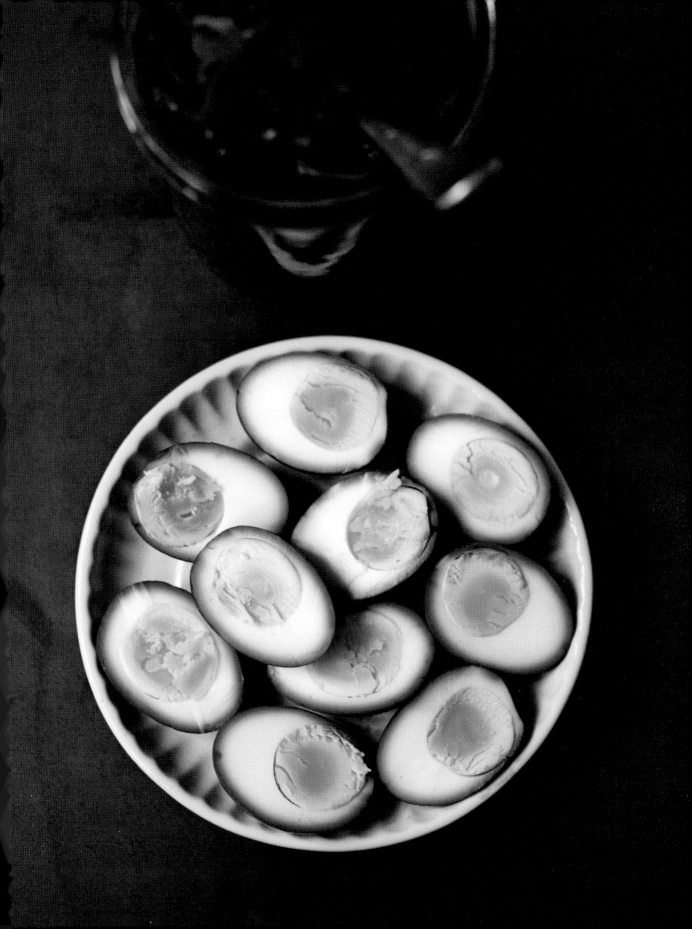

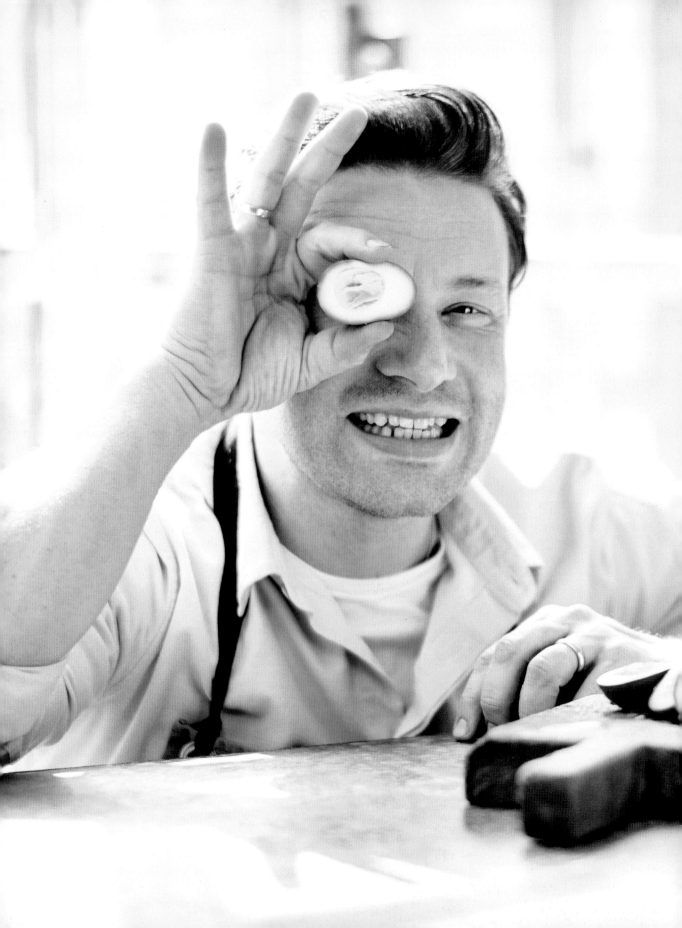

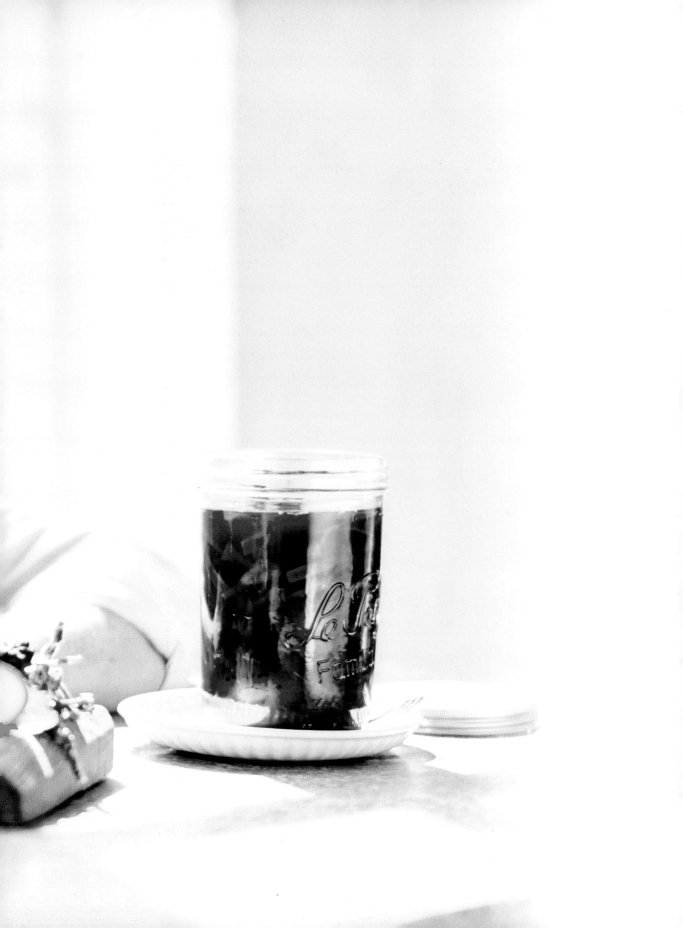

HOMEMADE NUT BUTTERS
FUN, SUPER-TASTY & VERSATILE

— All nuts are generally packed with a good variety of essential vitamins and minerals, and —
are a source of unsaturated fat, which is good for keeping our cholesterol happy

MAKES 1 JAR

200g of your favourite shelled
unsalted nuts, such as Brazils,
almonds, pecans, pistachios,
hazelnuts, cashews, peanuts

Preheat the oven to 180°C/350°F/gas 4. Lay your chosen nuts or nut combo in a single layer on a roasting tray. Roast for 8 to 10 minutes, or until golden and shiny, then remove and leave to cool for 5 minutes. If you prefer, you can make the nut butter without roasting the nuts first, which gives you a purer colour, like the ones at the bottom of this picture. It's still delicious raw, but I find the depth of flavour the roasting brings out is really hard to beat.

Tip the nuts into a food processor or grinder with a small pinch of sea salt – the smaller the receptacle the easier it is to blitz them up. Start blitzing the nuts – they'll quickly go from whole to chopped to finely ground, then they'll take a while longer to turn into nut butter, so be patient and just let the processor do its thing, stopping it occasionally to scrape down the sides and help it along. Blitz to the consistency you like, then decant into a jar.

For a 100-calorie snack, enjoy 1 heaped teaspoon of nut butter with:

+ **80g of raw seasonal veg crudités**, such as fennel, carrots, celery, radishes, baby courgettes, asparagus, cucumber, gem lettuce

+ **1 dry poppadom**, puffed up in the microwave for around 30 seconds

+ **1 apple or pear**, cut into slices to make a fruit and nut butter kinda sandwich

+ **2 tablespoons of natural yoghurt** – swirl them together in a little pot

CALORIES	FAT	SAT FAT	PROTEIN	CARBS	SUGAR	FIBRE	25 MINUTES
91kcal	5.9g	1.1g	3.1g	6.6g	5.1g	2.1g	

THESE VALUES ARE BASED ON 1 HEAPED TEASPOON OF NUT BUTTER WITH 80G OF RAW VEG

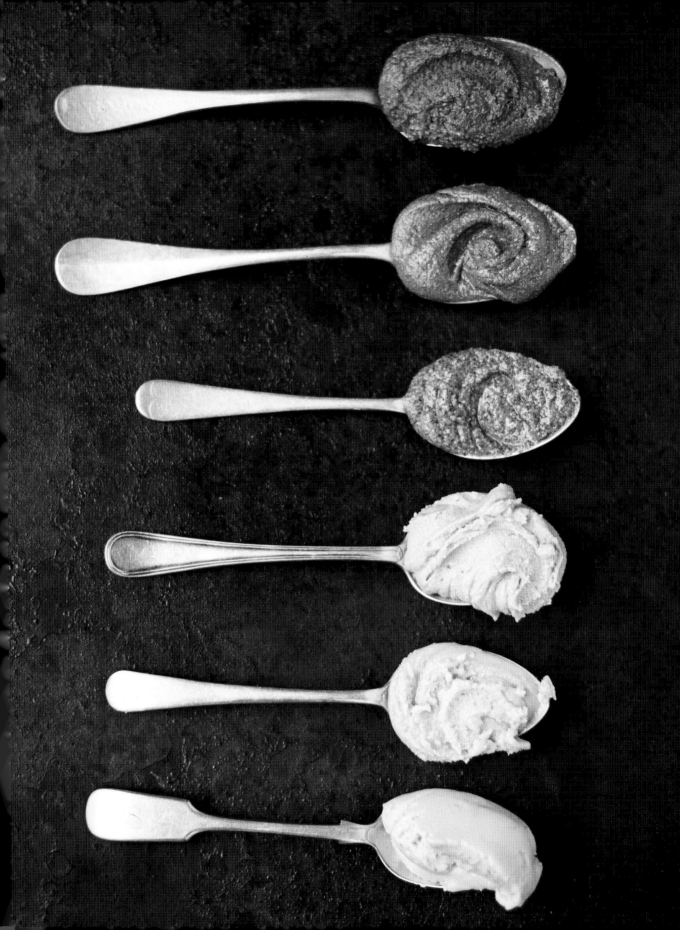

RAW VEGAN FLAPJACK SNACKS
NUTS, SEEDS, DATES, OATS & FRUIT

— These fantastic little pick-me-ups are full of loadsa good stuff, including iron-rich dates – helping us to stay alert – protein-packed seeds and a hit of omega 3 from the nuts —

MAKES 24

100g unsalted pecans

100g unsalted hazelnuts

20g mixed seeds, such as linseeds, chia

180g Medjool dates

100g mixed dried berries, such as blueberries, cranberries, sour cherries

200g porridge oats

2 tablespoons oil (I like walnut oil)

1–2 tablespoons maple syrup

Place the nuts, seeds, dates (destone first) and dried fruit in a food processor and briefly blitz until they're all nicely chopped together. Add the oats, oil and maple syrup and pulse until combined, but still with a bit of texture.

I like to go straight into portion-control mode (my nutrition team will be really proud of me!), and use a 5cm pastry cutter to portion up the 24 flapjacks there and then. For me, the easiest way to do it without getting the scales out is to scrunch and squash the mixture into a rough 75cm sausage, simply cut it in half and into quarters, then divide each piece into 6. One by one, pat and push the portions really firmly into the cutter, pushing down in the centre and squashing the mixture up the sides with your fingers. As you push it down, remove the cutter to give you a nice round flapjack snack.

Place the snacks in an airtight container, where they'll keep happily for up to 2 weeks. Bag up and freeze any you don't need for a later date. If any get bashed or break up, use them as a great breakfast sprinkle.

CALORIES	FAT	SAT FAT	PROTEIN	CARBS	SUGAR	FIBRE	30 MINUTES
100kcal	6.2g	0.5g	2g	10.1g	5.3g	1.7g	

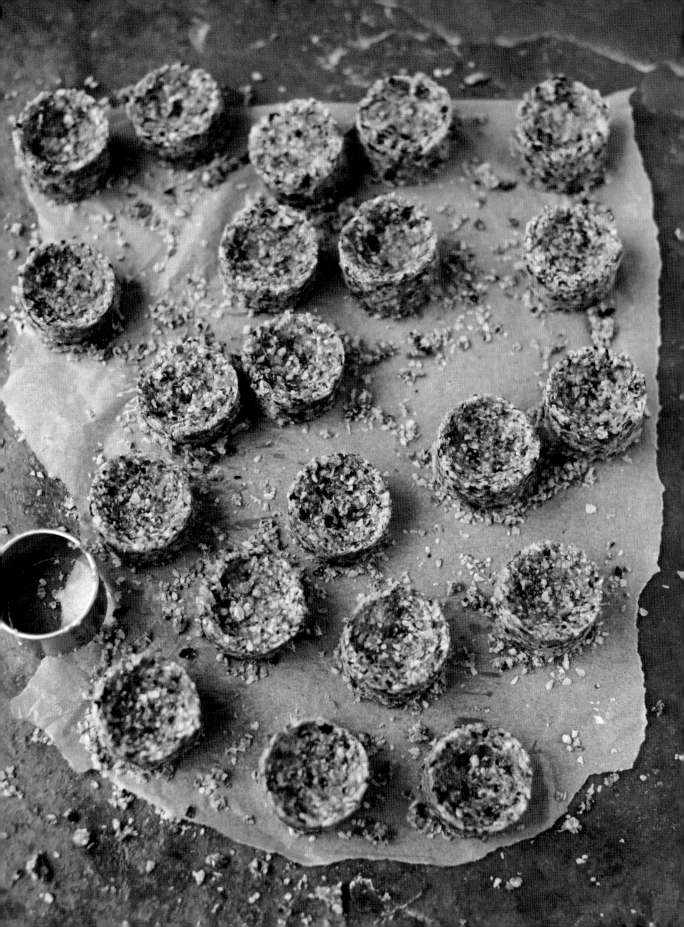

FRO-YO FUN
FRUIT, YOGHURT, NUTS & SEEDS

— These fruity fro-yo treats are packed full of good stuff, and having yoghurt that contains —
live bacteria keeps our gut happy. Look out for unsweetened cones to pair it with

EACH COMBO SERVES 8

RIPE BANANA & BROWN BREAD FRO-YO

In a food processor, blitz **500g of frozen peeled banana slices** (it's convenient to chop and freeze your own), **150g of crustless wholemeal bread** and **1 pinch of ground cinnamon** until finely chopped. Add **200g of natural yoghurt** and blitz again until smooth.

BERRY & BROWN BREAD FRO-YO

In a food processor, blitz **400g of frozen mixed berries, 1 peeled banana, 150g of crustless wholemeal bread** and the leaves from **2 sprigs of fresh mint** until finely chopped. Add **200g of natural yoghurt** and blitz again until smooth.

MANGO, LIME & GINGER FRO-YO

In a food processor, blitz **400g of frozen chopped mango, 1 peeled banana, 150g of porridge oats**, the **zest and juice of 1 lime** and peeled **3cm piece of ginger** until finely chopped. Add **200g of natural yoghurt** and blitz again until smooth.

STRAWBERRY, BALSAMIC & BASIL FRO-YO

In a food processor, blitz **400g of frozen chopped strawberries, 1 peeled banana, 150g of porridge oats, 1 tablespoon of balsamic vinegar** and the leaves from ·**2 sprigs of fresh basil** until finely chopped. Add **200g of natural yoghurt** and blitz again until smooth.

TO SERVE

Serve your fro-yo right away, or you can hold it in a lovely scoopable state in the freezer for up to 40 minutes before it gets too hard. If you want to make it in advance, simply divide between ice cube trays and freeze completely, then tip those into the food processor and whiz up again when you want to serve. Enjoy in a bowl, a cone or a wafer, with a sprinkling of toasted nuts and seeds, and some extra fresh fruit to boost your intake.

CALORIES	FAT	SAT FAT	PROTEIN	CARBS	SUGAR	FIBRE	
83kcal	1.5g	0.8g	3.2g	14.9g	7.5g	2.3g	5 TO 10 MINUTES

THESE VALUES ARE AN AVERAGE OF THE FOUR RECIPES ABOVE

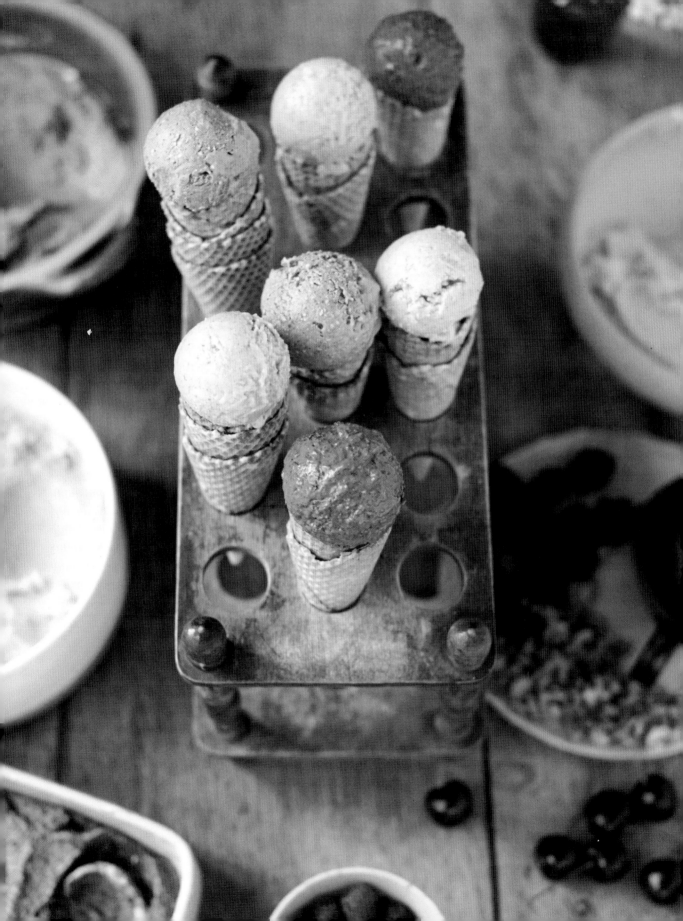

MY TASTY ENERGY BALLS
DATE, COCOA & PUMPKIN SEED

— Medjool dates have the double benefit of being high in both fibre and chloride, a nutrient that helps our digestion, and we get a hit of copper from the pumpkin seeds —

MAKES 12 PORTIONS

70g pumpkin seeds

20g puffed brown rice or puffed quinoa

50g whole almonds

80g Medjool dates

1cm piece of fresh turmeric or ½ teaspoon ground turmeric

½ teaspoon ground cinnamon

1 heaped teaspoon quality cocoa powder

1 teaspoon vanilla extract

½ tablespoon manuka honey

1 orange

Me and my nutrition team have worked hard to create these super-nutritious balanced flavour-packed balls that give us the perfect snack boost to get us through the day – enjoy two balls per snack.

Blitz 40g of the pumpkin seeds into a fine dust in a food processor, then decant onto a plate. Place the remaining pumpkin seeds and the puffed rice or quinoa in the processor with the almonds and dates (destone first), then blitz until finely chopped. Peel and finely grate in the turmeric, if using fresh, or add the ground turmeric, along with the cinnamon, cocoa powder and a pinch of sea salt. Blitz again until finely ground, then add the vanilla, honey and half the orange juice. Blitz for another 1 to 2 minutes, stopping to scrape down the sides a couple of times, and adding an extra squeeze of orange juice to bind, only if needed – it takes a while for the mixture to come together, so be patient and let the processor work its magic.

With wet hands, divide into 24 and roll into balls, dropping them into the pumpkin seed dust as you go. Shake to coat, storing them in the excess dust until needed. They'll keep happily for up to 2 weeks in an airtight container.

CALORIES	FAT	SAT FAT	PROTEIN	CARBS	SUGAR	FIBRE	25 MINUTES
80kcal	5.2g	0.6g	2.7g	6g	4.2g	0.5g	

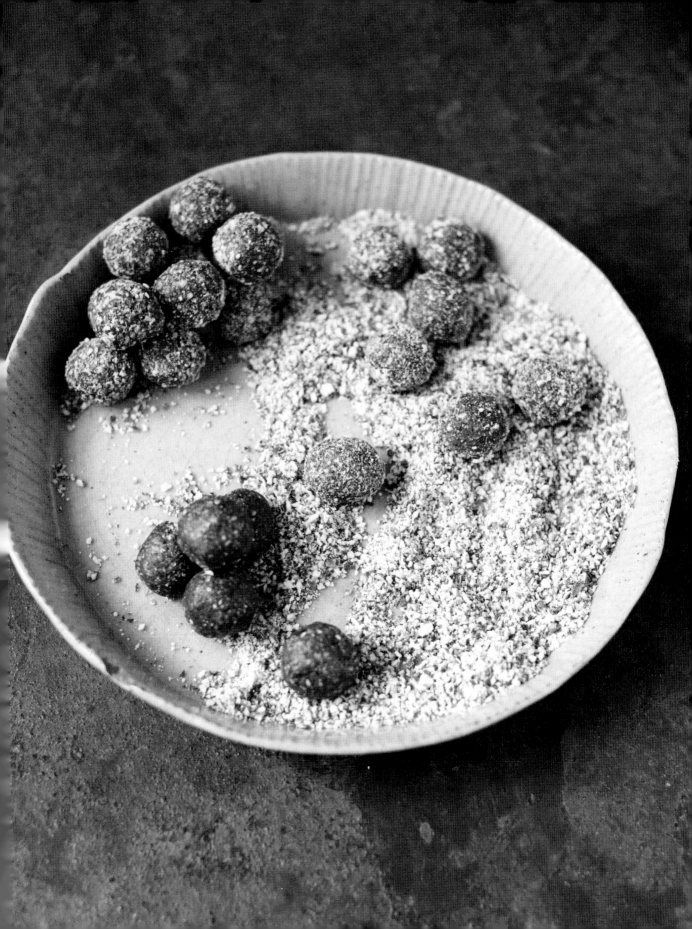

MY TASTY ENERGY BALLS
APRICOT, GINGER & CASHEW

Dried apricots are a brilliant veggie-friendly source of iron and are super-high in potassium, a mineral that our muscles need in order to function properly

MAKES 12 PORTIONS

100g unsalted cashew nuts

20g sesame seeds

80g dried apricots

20g puffed brown rice or puffed quinoa

4cm piece of ginger

½ teaspoon mixed spice

2 tablespoons manuka honey

Me and my nutrition team have worked hard to create these super-nutritious balanced flavour-packed balls that give us the perfect snack boost to get us through the day – enjoy two balls per snack. Toast the cashew nuts and sesame seeds in a dry non-stick pan on a medium heat until lightly golden, tossing occasionally, then tip onto a plate and leave to cool.

Remove 40g of the cashews and blitz into a fine dust in a food processor, then decant on to a separate plate. Place the remaining cashews and sesame seeds, the apricots and puffed rice or quinoa in the processor and blitz until finely chopped. Peel and finely grate in the ginger, and add the mixed spice. Blitz again until finely ground, then add the honey. Blitz for another 1 to 2 minutes, stopping to scrape down the sides a couple of times, and adding an extra squeeze of honey to bind, only if needed – it takes a while for the mixture to come together, so be patient and let the processor work its magic.

With wet hands, divide into 24 and roll into balls, dropping them into the ground cashew dust as you go. Shake to coat, storing them in the excess dust until needed. They'll keep happily for up to 2 weeks in an airtight container.

CALORIES	FAT	SAT FAT	PROTEIN	CARBS	SUGAR	FIBRE	25 MINUTES
86kcal	5.1g	1g	2.4g	8.2g	6.2g	0.9g	

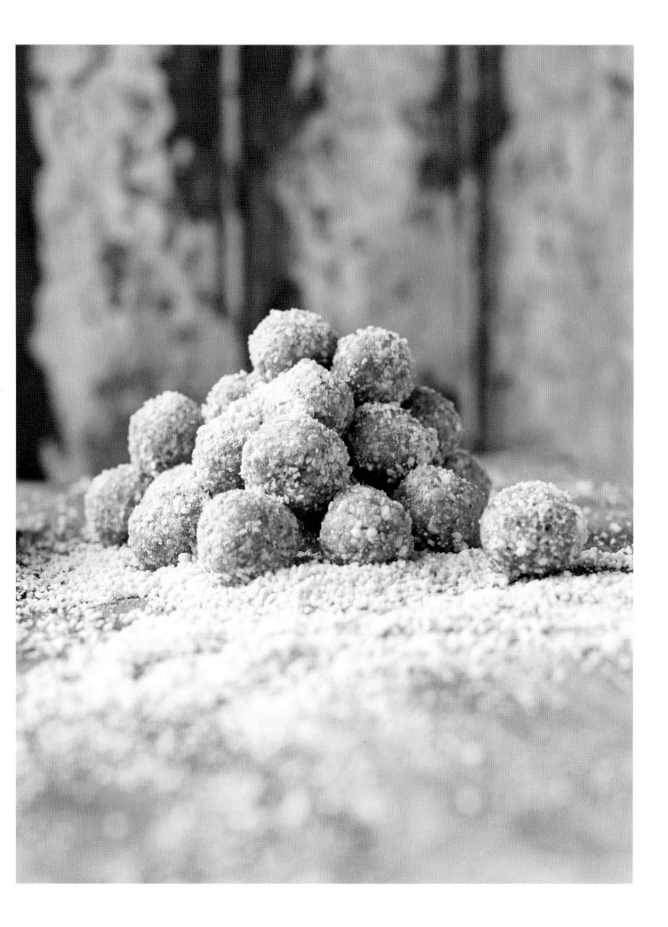

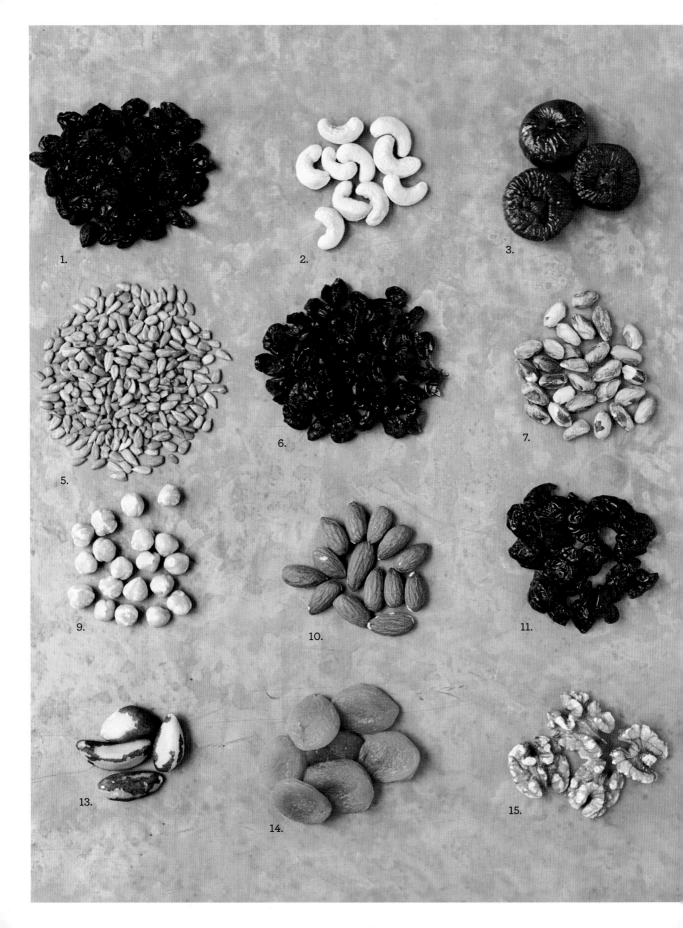

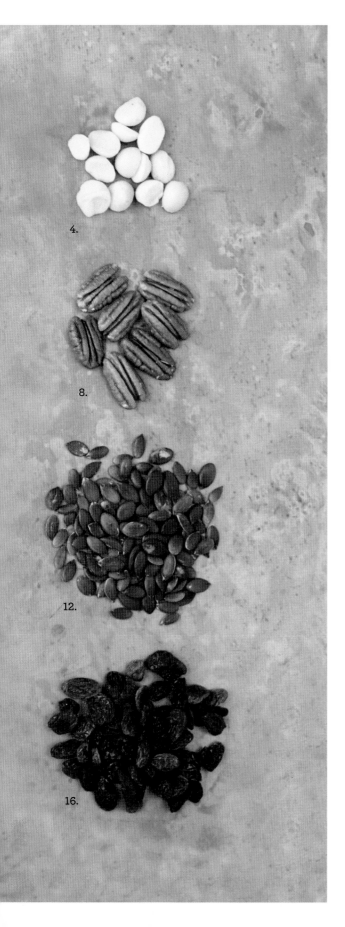

SNACK ATTACK

It's good to have a quick nibble when feeling hungry to keep our energy and focus up, and all these nuts, seeds and dried fruits have lots of lovely nutritional benefits. So – as simple as it may be – each pile on this page shows us roughly what 100 calories really looks like. I hope it will empower you to be a bit more conscious about the amount you're snacking on, and inspire you to mix things up. Just remember to keep an eye on your portion control!

1.	34g raisins
2.	10 unsalted cashew nuts
3.	3 or 4 dried figs
4.	8 unsalted macadamia nuts
5.	16g sunflower seeds
6.	30g dried cranberries
7.	16g shelled unsalted pistachio nuts
8.	7 unsalted pecan nuts
9.	15g unsalted hazelnuts
10.	15 unsalted whole almonds
11.	35g dried blueberries
12.	16g pumpkin seeds
13.	4 unsalted Brazil nuts
14.	7 dried apricots
15.	4 shelled unsalted walnut halves
16.	33g sultanas

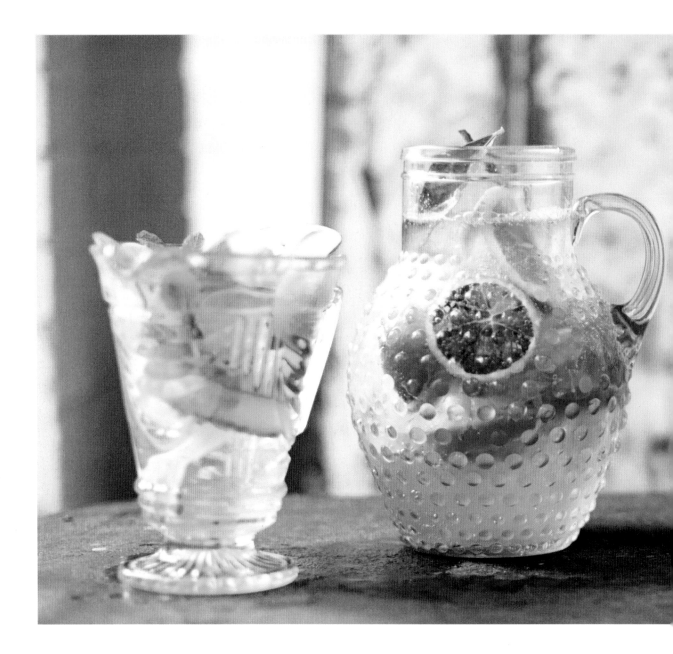

EASY FLAVOURED WATERS

CUCUMBER, APPLE & MINT

Finely slice **1 apple**, ideally on a mandolin (use the guard!). Speed-peel strips of **cucumber** lengthways, then add both to a jug of water over ice. Pick in some **fresh mint leaves**, and stir to get the party started.

ST CLEMENTS

Simply slice up **lemons, oranges** and, if you're lucky enough for them to be in season, **blood oranges**, and add to a jug of water over ice. A few **fresh mint or lemon balm leaves** are also delicious.

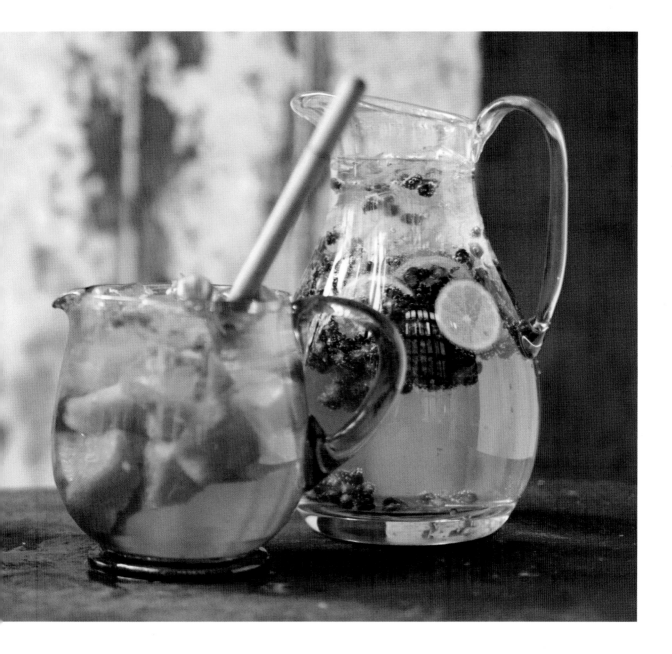

COLOURFUL, BRIGHT & DELICIOUS

WATERMELON & BASIL

Peel and clank up a **wedge of watermelon** and add to a jug of water with lots of ice, then pick in some **fresh basil leaves**. Stir and bash up the watermelon to get the flavours going. Nice with a squeeze of **lime juice**.

POMEGRANATE, GINGER & LIME

Hold half a **pomegranate** cut side down in your fingers and bash the back with a spoon so the seeds tumble into your jug. Finely grate in some **ginger**, slice and add **1 lime** and a **load of ice**, then top up with water.

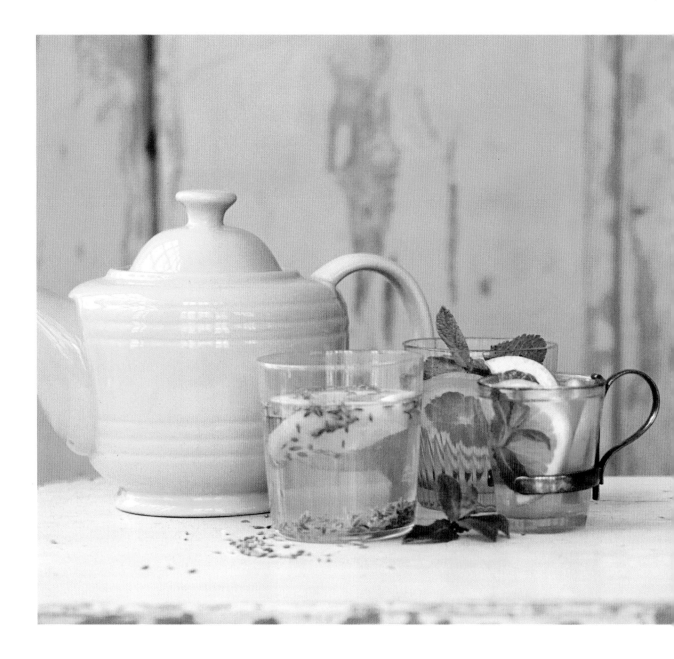

THERAPEUTIC TEAS

FENNEL SEEDS, LEMON & HONEY

Slice **1 lemon** and place in a teapot with **1 teaspoon of fennel seeds**. Stir in 1 litre of just-boiling water, steep for 5 minutes, then strain through a sieve and enjoy hot, sweetening to taste with **runny honey**.

GRAPEFRUIT, ORANGE & MINT

Slice ½ **a grapefruit** (pink if you can get it) and **1 orange** and place in a teapot with **a few sprigs of fresh mint**. Stir in 1 litre of just-boiling water, steep for 5 minutes and enjoy hot, or cool to enjoy as iced tea.

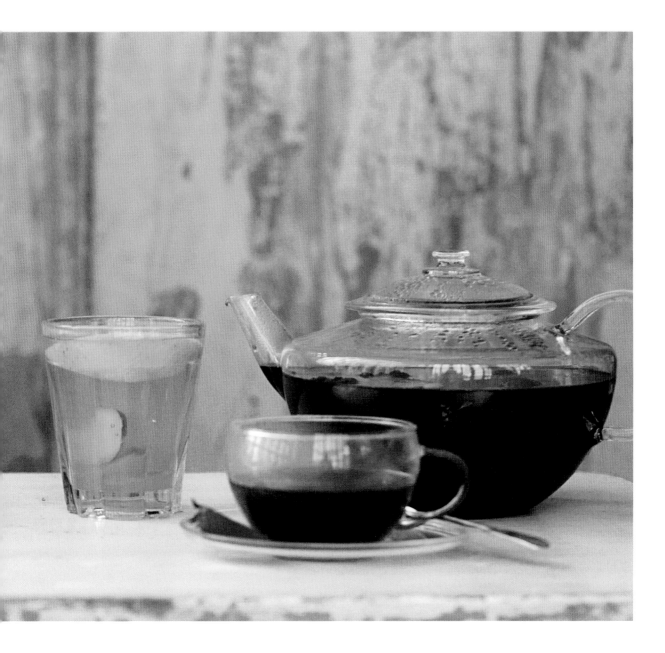

TASTY, VIBRANT & EASY

GINGER, TURMERIC, LEMON & HONEY

Slice **a piece of ginger** and place in a teapot with ¼ **of
a teaspoon of ground turmeric** and **1 sliced lemon**.
Stir in 1 litre of just-boiling water, steep for 5 minutes
and enjoy hot, sweetening to taste with **runny honey**.

STRAWBERRY, HIBISCUS & STAR ANISE

Halve **a few strawberries** and place in a teapot with
2 teaspoons of dried hibiscus flowers and **1 star anise**.
Stir in 1 litre of just-boiling water, steep for 5 minutes,
strain and enjoy hot, or cool to enjoy as iced tea.

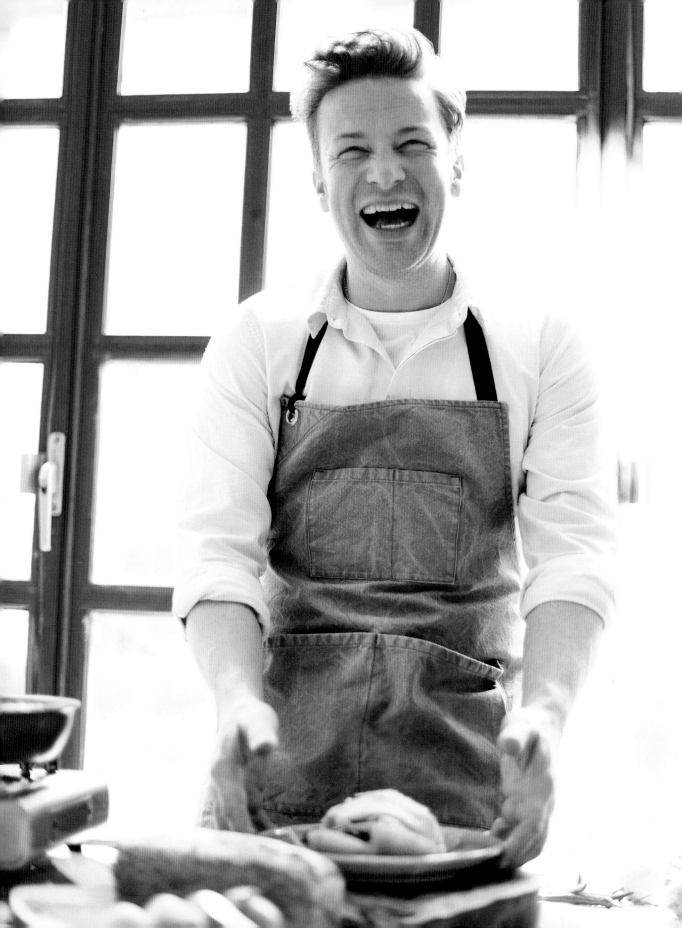

LIVE WELL

A HEALTHIER HAPPIER YOU

While working on this book I've been reading up on nutrition, I've been studying for a nutrition diploma, and I've had the privilege of meeting lots of incredible scientists, professors and experts in their field so that I can share the most useful and accessible info that's out there with you. And it's been the most incredibly inspiring journey, seeing food and lifestyle from a totally different perspective.

So in the pages that follow, I'm going to share what I've learnt around some key areas within health, nutrition and wellbeing. I hope you'll find this information as fascinating as I do, and remember – you really can make positive, sustainable change just by doing the odd thing differently, building on small new habits. I've taken into account everything I talk about in these pages in the development of each and every recipe in the book, so if you just pick up your shopping and get cooking, you'll be in a beautiful place. Happy days.

MY PHILOSOPHY IN THIS BOOK
THE BALANCED PLATE

We all know that balance is absolutely key – but what does it really mean? This page exists to make that super-clear, because if you can get your balanced plate right and keep your portion control in check – which I've done for you with all the recipes in this book – you can be confident that you're giving yourself a really great start on the path to good health.

One of the most useful things you can remember is that you don't have to be spot-on every day – just try to get your balance right across the week. Mix up your choices within the chapters to ensure you're having a varied diet and a wide range of nutrients, and you'll be getting everything you need. As a general guide for main meals, if you eat meat and fish you're looking at at least two portions of fish a week, one of which should be oily (such as salmon, trout or mackerel), then splitting the rest of the week's main meals between brilliant meat-free plant-based meals, some poultry and a little red meat. An all-vegetarian diet can be perfectly healthy too.

WHAT IS THE BALANCED PLATE?

Bear with me on this one – it's going to get a little technical – but it's important to register the facts up front about how to approach putting a meal together. Just look at the table below and you'll get the gist – it's easy really.

THE FIVE FOOD GROUPS (UK)	PROPORTION OF YOUR BALANCED PLATE
Vegetables and fruit	One-third of your plate
Starchy carbohydrates (bread, rice, potatoes, pasta)	One-third of your plate
Protein (meat, fish, eggs, beans, other non-dairy sources)	Around one-sixth of your plate
Dairy foods and milk	Around one-sixth of your plate
Fat/sugar-high foods	Try to only eat a small amount of food high in fat and/or sugar

HOW DOES THAT WORK IN THIS BOOK?

Working closely with my lovely nutrition team and following UK guidelines, I've structured all the recipes in a really clear and easy-to-follow way:

+ All the breakfast recipes are less than 400 calories per portion and contain less than 4g of saturated fat and less than 1.5g of salt

+ All the lunches and dinners are less than 600 calories per portion and contain less than 6g of saturated fat and less than 1.5g of salt – so all of these recipes are interchangeable across the two chapters

I've also included snacks of up to 100 calories, giving you the freedom to enjoy a few tasty energy-boosting snacks a day, with some calories left for drinks.

WHAT DOES THAT MEAN IN REAL LIFE?

In general, the average woman needs about 2,000 calories a day, while the average man can have about 2,500. I'm sure you're aware that these figures are just a guide, and what we eat always needs to be considered in relation to factors like age, build, lifestyle and activity levels. The good news is that all food and drinks can be eaten and drunk in moderation as part of a healthy, balanced diet, so we don't have to completely give up anything that we really enjoy, unless we're advised to do so by a doctor or dietitian.

My grandad's philosophy on life was simple – everything in moderation and a little bit of what you like, and that still stands very true today. Even nutritionists eat cake!

BRILLIANT BEAUTIFUL BREAKFAST

Here's one super-easy thing that I want you to take from this book: eat breakfast! Simple as that. This mighty meal is often overlooked, but it's so important in setting you up for the day. Not only will it fill you up and help prevent you snacking on foods high in fat/sugar, it can kick you off with a boost of micronutrients, such as iron, fibre, the B vitamins and vitamin D. It's been shown that when you miss breakfast you're unlikely to make up on those missed nutrients throughout the rest of the day, so get into good habits and build it into your daily routine from the outset.

CELEBRATING H_2O

Drinking water is absolutely essential. Although it's not – for obvious reasons – part of the balanced plate, it is totally integral to a balanced diet. It keeps us hydrated and alert and keeps our bodies functioning properly. Often when we think we're hungry we're actually dehydrated, so drinking plenty of water can also help prevent us over-eating! Like anything, our requirements vary depending on factors such as age, gender, build, lifestyle and activity levels, as well as things like humidity and the temperature around us. As a general rule, women should aim for at least 1.6 litres per day, while men need at least 2 litres. Embrace it, celebrate it, and enjoy humble H_2O every day. Read more about the wonderful world of hydration on page 278

ILLUSTRIOUS VEG & FRUIT

To live a good healthy life, veg and fruit need to be right at the heart of your diet. The wide bounty of incredible vitamins and minerals we get from the array of veg and fruit out there is honestly astounding.

And by the way, you'll notice I'm referring to veg and fruit, not fruit and veg. It's a great philosophy I picked up from Professor Julie Lovegrove about how we should think about our natural friends: fruit is brilliantly nutritious and we should definitely embrace it, but veggies shouldn't be thought of as second best. Veg and fruit are at the core of the best diets in the world, and why all the recipes in this book are so colourful, vibrant and exciting.

EAT THE RAINBOW

Veg and fruit come in all kinds of shapes, sizes, colours, flavours and textures, and help us to navigate the seasons in a wonderful way. There's no denying their nutrient value, so the best thing we can do to take advantage of this nutritious bounty is to eat the rainbow, enjoying as wide a variety as possible.

HOW MUCH SHOULD WE EAT?

We've all heard about 5-a-day, but I'm here to tell you that we should all be aiming for at least 5-a-day, ideally more. I think five is a compromise because here in the UK we're not doing too well on our consumption, so this lower target dumbs down our expectations. The reality is we should be trying to get seven or eight portions a day. Look at other countries with higher targets – Australia advocates five veg and two fruit portions every day! Plant-based diets are also more prevalent in many of the communities around the world with the highest proportion of centenarians (see page 292).

THE KNOWN HEALTH BENEFITS

Things we know for sure about these nutritional powerhouses are that veg and fruit can help us maintain a healthy weight and a healthy heart, as well as reducing the risk of strokes and some cancers. They are also packed with dietary fibre, keeping us regular (which is a good thing!) and helping reduce the risk of strokes and some cancers. They really should be embraced at every meal and they make great snacks, too.

THE UNKNOWN HEALTH BENEFITS

The brilliant thing about veg and fruit is that there's loads of hidden stuff we're yet to uncover too. For example, I can tell you that broccoli is high in folic acid and vitamin C, but nutritionists are looking at lots of other stuff on top of that, more nutrients, vitamins, minerals and trace elements that are beneficial to the body in many, many ways. Sounds pretty amazing, right – veg and fruit is where it's at! And this is why it's so important to eat the rainbow to get maximum goodness.

+ 80g of fresh, frozen or tinned veg or fruit is considered a portion – that's what I've worked to in the recipes in this book. Because we should be eating a wide variety of veg and fruit, we can only count each variety as one portion, so even if you eat 160g of carrots, for example, it would still only count as one portion of your 5-a-day

+ 30g of dried fruit is considered a portion. I only count one portion a day. Dried fruit is natural, but the sugar is more concentrated

+ 150ml of unsweetened veg or fruit juice can be counted as one portion only each day. A lot of nutrients and fibre are lost when veg and fruit are juiced, which is why it only counts as one of your 5-a-day – personally, I don't count juice at all in my tally. Smoothies are a better choice

+ 80g of beans or pulses – about 3 big tablespoons – can be counted as one portion only each day, and also give us protein

+ And for all you spud lovers out there, I have to point out that our humble potatoes don't count towards our 5-a-day as they're a starchy food so go into our carb tally instead (see page 266). Non-starchy sweet potatoes, on the other hand, do count

GROWING YOUR OWN

In the areas of the world where people live the longest, many of them grow their own food. If you've never tried, I recommend giving it a go. It's the best hobby – it'll keep you fit and save you cash; your relationship with planet earth will become more meaningful (I challenge anyone not to be inspired by watching stuff grow); and best of all, you get to eat the veg, and fruits, of your labour! Plus, if you've got kids, it will get them engaged in food in the most fun, dynamic way. You don't need a garden or a field to get involved – a window box, flat roof, allotment, balcony, pot, grow-bag or bucket all work fine – I've even grown stuff in a gutter pipe!

KEEPING IT FRESH

When you pick stuff straight from the ground it's at its freshest and most nutritious. I get a geeky buzz about turning something into a meal that's been in the ground just minutes before. If you've got a farmer's market nearby and you know stuff's been picked that morning, take advantage of it. As soon as veg are picked, their nutrient levels start to deplete, so eating them as fresh as possible – even raw, if you like – is going to give you more goodness per mouthful.

SHOULD WE GO ORGANIC?

Buying local, seasonal organic produce is always going to be optimal for our health (read more on page 284).

In the Nicoya Peninsula, Costa Rica, I met a community of some of the oldest people on the planet. They cite the humongous amount of fruit they eat as one of their secrets to longevity. But, variety is key. Many of us eat the same type of fruit, week in, week out, but each fruit contains a different cocktail of vitamins, minerals and elements our bodies love and need, so to get the most benefit, mixing up our choices is crucial.

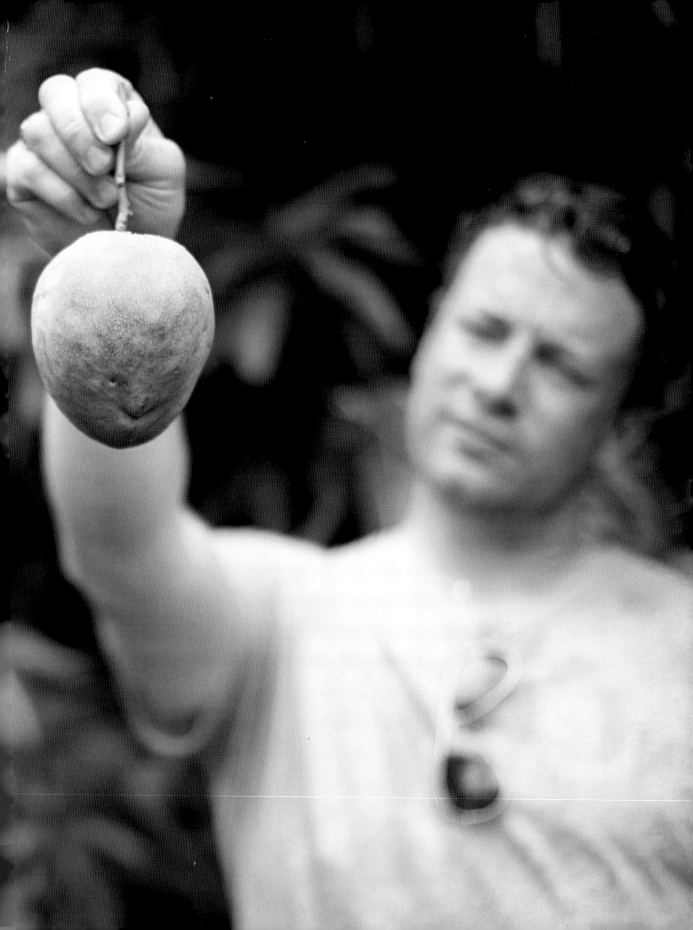

CELEBRATING GOOD CARBOHYDRATES

Starchy carbohydrates are a wonderful thing – they make us feel happy, satisfied and energetic, and quite simply, we need carbohydrates in our diet as they provide a large proportion of the energy we need to move our bodies, and the fuel our organs need to function.

Plus, we all crave and enjoy them. This page exists to help you understand what carbohydrates are, which ones we should be eating, and to dispel all those myths that are giving carbs a bad name. If you know how carbohydrates both work within and affect our bodies, and just why we need them, you can have a much healthier attitude towards them and not buy into a faddy no-carb diet that I'm sure you'll end up crashing out of.

WHAT ARE CARBOHYDRATES?

It's important to recognize that not all carbs are equal – this is where I think the confusion lies. Carbohydrates are either sugars, starch that will eventually be broken down into glucose (a form of sugar) in the gut, or dietary fibre, which we can't break down. So, it's the type and how we consume them that has most impact.

Let me break it down how I see it. Foods that are rich in carbs fall into four main categories:

+ Simple sugars – white and brown sugar, honey, maple syrup

+ White complex carbohydrates – bread, pasta, rice, flour, cereal

+ Wholemeal and wholewheat complex carbohydrates – bread, pasta, rice, flour, cereal

+ Vegetables and fruit – root veg in particular, such as carrots, sweet potatoes, swede, turnips, parsnips

WHAT CARBS SHOULD WE BE EATING?

Simple carbs, such as white refined sugar or sugary processed foods and drinks, can be digested really quickly and are empty calories, giving us a blood sugar spike followed by an energy low that can leave us feeling sluggish. Eating more complex carbohydrates is key – they take longer to break down, are slow-releasing and give us a more sustained level of energy. Even better, choose wholemeal and wholewheat varieties, as these also contain more fibre and other nutrients that our bodies can use and take even longer to digest, helping to keep us feeling fuller for longer. I tend to trade up to wholemeal and wholewheat at least 7 times out of 10 – not only are you upping the nutritional value of what you're eating, you're also getting some really delicious flavours and textures and that drip-feed of energy is more useful. While veg and fruit are often rich in carbs too, because they have such high nutrient values they go into our veg and fruit tally instead (see page 262).

WHY DO CARBS HAVE A BAD REP?

So when people are criticizing carbs, it's generally our excessive sweet tooth that's the problem. It's a huge sweeping statement to say that carbs make us fat. Obviously, like anything, if we consume more than we need that excess is going to be stored as fat in the body, but if we eat the right type of carbs we should all be in a happy place. I'm sure you're aware that many sugary foods also tend to be high in saturated fat, often don't contain any other useful nutrients, and can have a very detrimental effect on our health if consumed too often.

WHY DO WE NEED CARBS?

If we don't get enough carbohydrates and our bodies don't get the energy they need, they have to get it from elsewhere and break down fat and protein instead. Protein (see page 268) is essential to the growth and repair of our bodies, so using it up for energy is inefficient and could eventually lead to muscle wastage. Eating complex carbohydrates is the best way to maintain our blood sugar levels, which helps us to concentrate and carry out our daily chores. So forget that fear of carbs and include them in your diet in the right way, every day.

WHY I LOVE CARBS

Let's just pause from the science for a minute to acknowledge what an integral part of the wonderful world of ingredients carbohydrates are. They are some of the most incredible flavour carriers on the planet – pasta paired with insane sauces, delicious breads and grains, rice in all its guises (stir-fries, risottos, paellas, with curries, stews, in soups), noodles, I could go on . . .

HOW MUCH CAN WE EAT?

What I will say is, because these complex carbohydrates come in so many wonderful different shapes and forms it can be easy to double up and have too much without realizing, so portion control and, frankly, restraint – AKA four roast potatoes, not nine – is the name of the game. Carbs should be about one-third of your balanced plate, and ultimately it's what you pair those with that'll get you on or off the right track. The average adult can have around 260g of carbohydrates a day, with up to 90g coming from total sugars.

FANTASTIC FIBRE

Fibre is also classed as a carbohydrate, and is found mainly in plant-based foods. We should be aiming for about 30g of fibre each day – I've included it in the nutrition box on the recipe pages so you can start to get an idea of how much you get from different meals. We consume two different types:

+ Insoluble fibre – largely found in wholemeal and wholewheat foods, we can't digest this, so its important function is to help other food and waste pass through the gut, keeping our insides happy

+ Soluble fibre – found in foods such as amazing oats, pulses, beans, veg and fruit. We can't digest this but the good bugs in our colon can, which keeps them happy. Also, oats have a proven health claim to reduce blood cholesterol, so we love, love, love them

THE POWER OF PROTEIN

So let's talk about protein. First up, as a chef I must say the word protein is kind of annoying, as the term doesn't give any romance to all the incredible plants, legumes and animals it refers to.

At the same time, there are a lot of misconceptions around protein and its benefits, with some fad diets hailing it as the answer to everything. While protein is definitely an integral part of our diet, it does – like everything else – need to be eaten in the right amounts. I'm going to focus here on what protein does, what it actually is, how much we need, and what my beliefs around welfare and standards are when it comes to different protein sources.

WHAT DOES PROTEIN DO?

Protein is mighty – think of it as the building blocks of our bodies. It is absolutely essential for the growth and repair of muscle tissue, as well as building hormones, enzymes that build and break down substances in our bodies, and antibodies in our immune systems. This list, as I'm sure you'll recognize, is basically everything that's important to how we grow, repair, feel, break down and absorb things, and how we fight disease and infections. Whether you're a seasoned carnivore, a pescatarian, a veggie or a vegan, protein really is your best friend and should be enjoyed in the right way.

WHAT IS PROTEIN?

I think it's important for me not to get too technical here, but basically, proteins are made up of a cocktail of 20 different amino acids. A lot are made in our body, but we have to get the rest from the food we eat.

Just like carbohydrates (see page 266), not all protein sources are equal. Let me break it down:

+ Complete proteins – meat, fish, eggs, milk, cheese

+ Incomplete proteins – beans, nuts, seeds, lentils, cereals, quinoa, oats, peas, tofu, bread, flour, corn

That's not to say that the complete sources are superior, they're just different – think of them as a one-stop shop. What's important is to eat a wide range of different proteins across the week, and that way you've got a really good chance of getting it right. You might have also heard the term 'complementary proteins'. This refers to mixing up your incomplete protein sources with each other in order to build up your volume of amino acids – baked beans on toast or rice and peas are perfect examples of this, and as well as being a match made in heaven on the taste front, are great combos to give you a high amino acid level.

Generally, the optimal amount of protein to aim for is 45g a day for women aged 19–50 (which varies with factors such as pregnancy and breast-feeding), and 55g a day for men in the same age bracket. In the UK we usually get enough, but we do need to be mindful that we're not having too much. About one-sixth of our balanced plate should be made up of protein.

Your balance across a week in terms of meat and fish consumption should generally be at least two portions of fish, one of which should be oily (such as salmon, trout or mackerel), then you want to split the rest of the week between meat-free, poultry and a little red meat.

Some diets advocate high protein consumption, particularly for weight control or building muscle mass, but this can have a whole cascade of negative effects, especially if combined with low carb intake. If you're not an athlete, nor have been advised by a doctor to up your protein levels, excessive consumption isn't a good idea – it can increase our risk of osteoporosis, too much red meat increases the risk of bowel cancer, and we can only metabolize a certain amount of protein anyway, so excrete the excess through our urine.

For me, there's no point in eating meat unless it's been raised well and the animal was at optimal health. Choosing grass-fed animals where possible, that are free to roam and haven't lived in a stressful environment is essential – it makes total sense to me that what we put into our bodies should have lived a good life, to in turn give us goodness. It's about quality over quantity, so please choose organic, free-range or higher-welfare meat and responsibly sourced fish whenever you can.

I'm aware – as journalists often mention – that it does cost more to trade up. This isn't because anyone's being ripped off, but normally because the animal has lived a better-quality, longer life. Remember that you can trade up to higher-welfare meat and still buy the cheaper cuts, such as chicken thighs and minced meat. With clever buying skills and a slight reduction in your overall meat consumption, which is no bad thing, you can afford to improve on quality – double the pleasure.

I feel even more passionate about organic or free-range eggs, and organic milk, yoghurt and butter – the trade-up cost is less, the welfare comparisons are dramatic and we use them a lot, so it makes sense (see page 274).

VEGGIE & VEGAN DIETS

Interestingly, these are looking really rather successful in health terms. Although meat and fish proteins are complete and robust in so many micronutrients, following a vegetarian or vegan diet just means you have to be a bit cleverer about your protein sources. Brilliant veggie options kick off with black beans, the highest source of bean protein, plus all the other beans, pulses, legumes, lentils, tofu, quinoa and chia. Vitamin B12, which is prolific in meat, can often be deficient in vegans. We need it to aid growth, for good digestion, to keep our nerves healthy, produce energy and maintain healthy blood cells. You can get it through supplements if you want, or by eating some forms of algae, so maybe supplements are looking good!

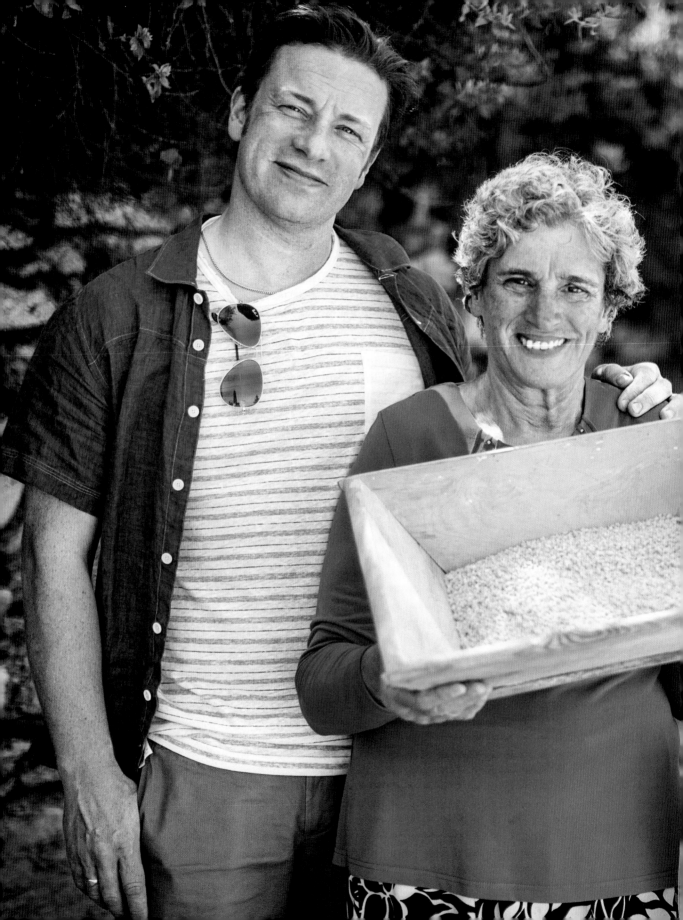

In Ikaria, Greece – which I'm told has more 90-year olds than anywhere else on the planet – I learnt how to make trahana, a cracked wholewheat and goat's milk mixture, with the lovely Maria. Embracing grains and choosing wholemeal and wholewheat foods is one really simple, positive change we can all make. Not only do they taste amazing and have great texture, they're full of fibre, which can lower cholesterol, helping to prevent heart disease. High-fibre foods also help to keep our bowels healthy and keep us feeling fuller for longer.

FAT IS ESSENTIAL

Let's bust a myth right off – there's no need to be afraid of fat, it's not the enemy it's been portrayed as.

Of course, our fat consumption needs to be controlled, at 9 calories per gram it's the nutrient with the highest calorific value, but just because you eat fat doesn't mean you'll get fat. Fat is found naturally in our bodies and some fats we can only get from the food we eat, so it is an essential part of our diet – without it, we'll die.

WHY DO WE NEED FAT?

Its main role is to provide energy, and fat is the way we store excess food energy. This is what allows us to draw on our reserves when food is in short supply – think of it as our natural battery. Adding fat to a meal is the most effective way of increasing the energy content – we also get energy from carbohydrates (see page 266). What's worth remembering is that if we are massively over-consuming fat, and our body doesn't need that much, we will put on weight as our stores build up.

WHAT DOES FAT DO?

Fat provides insulation and protection to our internal organs, and a certain amount of body fat is needed to support fertility for all you ladies out there. What's really crucial is that it supplies some fat-soluble vitamins and essential fatty acids, such as omega 3 and 6. In our weird and wonderful bodies many nutrients need the presence of fat to be properly absorbed. For example, having a little oil-based salad dressing is better than no dressing at all – it means we're able to absorb more vitamin A, in the form of beta-carotene, from the veg.

TYPES OF FAT

+ Unsaturated fats – these are generally the healthier type of fats to consume, where the dominant fatty acid is either monounsaturated or polyunsaturated. They're found in olive oil and other liquid vegetable oils (see right), as well as nuts, legumes, avocados and omega-3 rich oily fish. Some oils help lower bad cholesterol and raise the good stuff – we like that

+ Saturated fats – animal fats (butter, lard, suet, meat fat) tend to contain more saturated fatty acids, but also contain monounsaturated fatty acids. These fats are usually solid at room temperature. Because saturated fats raise cholesterol levels, we should be mindful of our consumption of them. They have also been linked with an increased risk of heart disease

HOW MUCH FAT DO WE NEED?

All fats should be eaten in moderation. In the UK, it's recommended that the average woman gets no more than 70g of fat per day, with less than 20g of that from saturated fat, and the average man no more than 90g a day, with less than 30g coming from saturates.

THE HEALTHIEST OILS

One of the easiest ways to get good fats into your diet is to use a little oil in your cooking. Keep a range in your pantry for different purposes. Here's my top five:

+ Olive & extra virgin olive oil – super-high in omega 9, use cheaper, lighter olive oil for lower-temperature cooking, and save extra virgin olive oil for dressings and finishing. Worth a special mention is cold-pressed new season's extra virgin olive oil – if you can get your hands on some each year, and only use it over that year while it's at its best, you'll be very happy

+ Rapeseed oil – a good source of omega 3, 6 and vitamin E, this contains half the saturated fat of olive oil. It has a fairly neutral flavour, so is great in all sorts of dishes and probably the most affordable healthy oil option out there. Look for cold-pressed varieties

+ Walnut oil – a good source of omega 3 and 6, this oil is brilliant for dressings, marinades and finishing and can be used to great effect in baking

+ Avocado oil – with the natural goodness of avocados, this is super-high in monounsaturated fats, omega 9 and vitamin E, and is useful for lower-temperature cooking, dressings, marinades and finishing

+ Sunflower oil – an excellent source of omega 6 and vitamin E, this is a great, cheap oil to have in stock for higher-temperature cooking

Other oils I use are omega-3 rich hemp oil, omega-9 rich almond oil, groundnut or vegetable oil for higher-temperature cooking, and sesame oil for Asian-style cooking, dressings and marinades.

OMEGA FATTY ACIDS

We need omega-6 fatty acids for many functions, including growth and development, and to maintain healthy skin – we generally get plenty of these in the diet. Omega-3 fatty acids are needed in smaller amounts to help keep our brains and hearts in tip-top condition, as well as helping to reduce our risk of heart attacks and strokes. Omega-3 sources are more limited – oily fish and vegetable oils are our best bet. Both of these essential polyunsaturated fatty acids can't be made in the body, so we have to get them from food. We can, however, make omega-9 fatty acids in the body, but it's still beneficial to use oils rich in them rather than saturated fats to help lower cholesterol and prevent heart attacks.

THE COCONUT OIL MYTH

There are so many health gurus shouting about the health benefits of coconut oil, so I spoke to the leading fat specialist in the UK, Professor Tom Sanders, and others, and they all have the same opinion on this. Now I'm not anti coconut oil, but I am anti its overuse and the fictitious benefits being bandied around it. It's absorbed and turned into energy more quickly, which is perceived as helpful, but it's still the highest saturated fat on the planet and very low in essential fatty acids. If you consume too much it will nudge you in the direction of heart disease. My advice is to use it in moderation and only in dishes where it adds appropriate flavour, such as curries.

DIPPING INTO DAIRY

Dairy is a really interesting food group. Global nutritionists have given it its own slice of the balanced plate because it offers an amazing array of nutrients and is a really good natural food source.

So – unless you're a vegan – this is a lovely area. Milk, yoghurt, cheese, butter, cream – sounds good to me. Though of course, it's worth remembering that it's milk, yoghurt and small amounts of cheese we should be favouring as the portion of dairy in our meals – butter and cream are very high in fat and saturated fat and don't provide the full package of nutrients milk, yoghurt and cheese give us so, butter and cream don't count towards our dairy portion.

WHAT IS DAIRY?

Produced primarily by cows, dairy products can also come from sheep, goats and even buffalo. Being just a small part of the balanced plate, around one-sixth of our meals should be made up of dairy.

EASY DAIRY CHOICES

Embracing the balanced-plate philosophy, you'll find a little bit of dairy in the majority of meals in this book. The easiest way to add dairy is to serve your meals with a dollop of yoghurt, or a little bit of cheese. As well as Parmesan and ricotta, you'll see me using a lot of feta and cottage cheese because not only are they great carriers of flavour, but they can be used in really diverse ways and are much lower in fat than most other cheeses. If you've got a meal that doesn't contain dairy, why not have a little glass of milk with or after it to supplement it, or have some yoghurt and fruit as a snack to get your balance back on track.

WHY DO WE NEED DAIRY?

It contains key nutrients to keep us strong and healthy:

+ Protein – crucial for growth and repair

+ Calcium – for strong bones and healthy teeth (especially during childhood and our teenage years, while our bones are still growing and developing)

+ Vitamin A – for good eye health (this is only found in dairy products that also contain fat)

+ Riboflavin – for healthy skin and helping us digest carbs (milk is the main source in our diets)

+ Iodine – helps to regulate our metabolism so our thyroid gland can function efficiently

In order to efficiently absorb calcium from the food we eat, we need vitamin D – we get this naturally from sunlight, and can top up with oily fish and eggs, or even mushrooms that have been left near a window to soak up a couple of hours of sunshine (believe me!).

With those dairy products that we use as staple ingredients – milk, yoghurt, butter – I honestly couldn't endorse more the trade up to organic. It is slightly more expensive, but not vastly so, and every time you buy organic you vote for a better food system (see page 284). In the EU, organic means that the cows have grazed on grass free from chemical fertilizers, pesticides and agrochemicals. They won't have been routinely fed antibiotics, and will have lived a better life with the best welfare standards, meaning they live an average of two years longer! I like the sound of that. It's better for the environment, too. In some parts of the world, non-organic cows may never even get to step on to grass and are kept indoors within 'mega-dairies'. Sad but true.

Around 3% of people in the UK have a food allergy or intolerance, and dairy intolerance has become more common in recent years. It's caused when our bodies lack an enzyme called lactase, which breaks down the natural sugar found in dairy foods. An intolerance to a certain type of protein found in cow's milk also exists. If you think you have an intolerance, chat to your GP or a dietician. As we get better at diagnosis, the number of dairy alternatives in the shops is rising. Even if you're not lactose intolerant, it's nice to mix up your choices to take advantage of the different flavours on offer (see right) – this is something we do in the Oliver household.

It has a super-high nutrient density for most of the key nutrients and, in the grand scheme of things, is pretty low in fat. Milk is actually better at hydrating the body than water or sports drinks after exercise.

+ Cow's milk – whether you enjoy whole, semi-skimmed or skimmed is down to personal preference. All are great choices nutrient-wise, but the calorie and sat fat levels are higher in whole, so watch your consumption

+ Goat's milk – it tastes a little funkier than cow's milk and has similar lactose levels, but the fat globules are typically smaller, so are easier for us to digest

Most alternative milks are fortified with calcium, B vitamins (including B12, which we can't get from plant-based foods), vitamin D2 and E, to mirror the benefits of dairy milk. All those listed here are good for veggies and vegans, too. Choose unsweetened, when you can.

+ Organic soya milk – high in protein and low in sat fat, plus widely available, this is great for all-round use

+ Almond milk – subtly nutty and light in texture, this is great for breakfasts, such as pancakes, porridge and smoothies. It's low in fat, sat fat and sugar

+ Hazelnut milk – with a wonderful nutty flavour this is perfect for smoothies and even baking

+ Oat milk – great for breakfast recipes and naturally low in fat and sat fat, mighty oats are proven to lower blood cholesterol if consumed regularly

Here, I'm out collecting seaweed with Tadashi in Okinawa, Japan, where some of the oldest people on the planet live. I was amazed to learn that seaweed is the most nutritious plant there is – that's crazy! And many people I met in Japan swear that it's one of the things that has kept them going so long. So wherever you are in the world, seaweed is definitely one to look out for. It has more vitamins, minerals and proteins than any vegetable that grows in the soil, is packed with B vitamins, iodine, antioxidants, fatty acids, calcium and fibre – you can't argue with that. You can already pick up dried seaweed pretty easily – simply rehydrate, shred and add to salads or stir-fries.

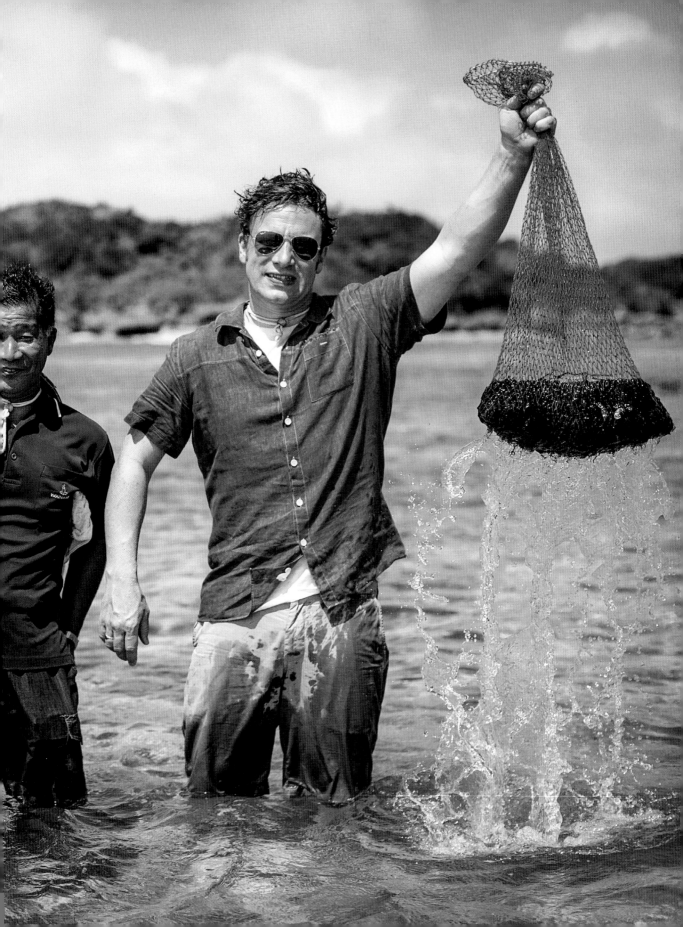

DRINK WATER & THRIVE

If you want to be the very best you can be, staying hydrated is absolutely key. This section is naturally a celebration of one of the most important, calorie-free, life-giving substances on the planet – H_2O.

Most of us are aware of how important it is to stay hydrated – I'm sure it's been drummed into us since we were kids. You might even have been subjected to one of those graded-colour wee charts in the toilet, which in our youth I'm sure we all found funny, but all joking aside, they're actually really useful and this is a serious subject.

WHY IS IT SO IMPORTANT?

It wasn't until I sat down earlier this year, during my nutrition diploma, for a hydration lesson, that I really understood just how integral water is to pretty much every function of the human body. Let's not forget, nearly two-thirds of our body is made up of water! If we're dehydrated, our bodies and brains won't function in the optimal way. This could be how we feel, heal, react, our ability to absorb nutrients from the food we eat or the way our cells and organs function – dehydration really does affect everything we do. Also, our bodies often mistake hunger for thirst, so making sure we keep hydrated throughout the day can help to prevent us from over-eating and consuming calories we don't need. Water is a cheap, obvious, accessible part of the diet that has an immediate and dramatic impact on the way we function and feel. If you take just a handful of things from this book, bigging up H_2O and staying hydrated is one of the most valuable actions you can build into your daily habits.

WHY DO WE FEEL THIRSTY?

As wonderful as the human body is, there is a bit of a lag between our bodies telling our brains that we're actually thirsty and our brains communicating that message. So if you're feeling thirsty, a) you are definitely dehydrated, and b) you were probably dehydrated an hour ago. If you're a parent, it's worth noting that kids are even worse at recognizing when they're thirsty, so it's important to keep reminding them to drink water.

HOW MUCH FLUID DO WE NEED?

The average woman should be getting at least 1.6 litres a day, while the average man is looking at at least 2 litres a day. Like anything, these amounts are a guideline, and our requirements vary depending on factors such as age, build, lifestyle and activity levels, as well as humidity and the temperature around us. Teas and herbal teas, coffee, fruit juice and milk all contribute to our hydration. It's thought that we also get about 20% of our water intake from the food we eat, such as veggies and fruit with a high water content.

KEEP WATER HANDY

My top tip, as ridiculously obvious as it sounds, is to put it in front of you! If you've always got water to hand – a glass at your desk, a jug on the kitchen table, a bottle when you're out and about – you're more likely to pick it up and drink it throughout the day. If you want to naturally flavour it sometimes to keep things interesting, check out the easy ideas on page 254.

TASTY TAP WATER

British tap water goes through loads of checks, so it's safe, clean and should definitely be utilized. It does change in taste regionally – and I know in some places you can taste chlorine – but it's there, it's available, and we're lucky that it's in such free flow. If you don't like the taste, look at getting a filter; and bottled mineral water can be convenient at times too.

SODA & SUGARY DRINKS

In my house, these don't exist and are the enemy. They're a treat, and should be thought of as such. This is why I think they should only be enjoyed at special occasions (if at all, for younger children). Without question they are a fast and simple way to consume humongous amounts of empty calories – they have no nutritional value. The disastrous combination of copious amounts of sugar – often around 12 teaspoons in 500ml – and citric acid, is a nightmare for tooth decay. As people normally sip these drinks, there's no chance for the teeth to defend themselves. Over-consumption of sugar is a huge contributing factor to tooth decay in children, and multiple tooth extraction means they need to be put under general anaesthetic at a really young age. That's no joke.

FRUIT JUICE

If we drink too much, fruit juice can be equally guilty as soda and sugary drinks when it comes to tooth decay, because of the natural sugar and citric acid it contains. But consumed in the right amount, fruit juice is actually beneficial, because it also contains a lovely cocktail of vitamins, minerals and trace elements. So, a few tricks to bear in mind: if you're buying fruit juice, only fill your glass one-quarter full, then top it up with water – this'll save you money too. At lunch and dinner time, squeeze any nice citrus and crush a little soft fruit into a jug then top up with water and ice – we mix it up every day (for more inspiration go to page 254). And remember, juice doesn't have the fibre of the whole fruit, so smoothies are generally going to be more nutritious.

ALCOHOL

There are more than 6,500 preventable alcohol-related deaths in the UK each year. So, bearing in mind that this book is all about optimal health, I thought a page about something that quite a lot of us enjoy, possibly too much as far as government recommendations are concerned, might be helpful.

So I want to share a few facts and some ideas and approaches I've found useful. My aim is that we can still enjoy and consume alcohol responsibly, without letting that enjoyment become detrimental to our health. I know many of you love a drink, just like I do, so let's not patronize each other, but we can always use a few good ideas, right?

LOVING OUR LIVERS

When I met liver specialists Professor Mark Thursz and Professor Gary Frost, what was fascinating to me was that the liver, our largest internal organ, which deals with alcohol and all toxins in the body, is crucial, wonderful and extraordinary. We've only got one, so it's important not to mess it up. The liver breaks down our food and converts it into energy and essential proteins. It's centrally important in our metabolism, and in how we process nutrients and detoxify poisins. The liver also helps to remove waste products, filters toxins from the bowel and plays a role in fighting infections.

Our livers don't like excess alcohol and excess fat – storing too much visceral fat (around our internal organs in the belly area) can increase our risk of type-2 diabetes, and non-alcoholic fatty liver disease. So looking after our liver is absolutely essential, i.e. if you eat unhealthily, don't stay hydrated and drink too much alcohol, it's not looking good. On the food front, all the recipes in this book will help keep your liver happy.

ALCOHOL ISN'T NUTRITIOUS

Regardless of quality, alcohol, as far as your body is concerned, is not nutritious and is toxic. At 7 calories per gram, it's almost up there with fat on the high-calorie scale. It can be addictive, and undoubtedly has been responsible for some of the worst behaviour and decisions on the planet. So let's be responsible about it.

UK GOVERNMENT ALCOHOL RECOMMENDATIONS

+ Men: no more than 21 units a week and 3 to 4 units a day (4 units is just under 1½ pints of lager)

+ Women: no more than 14 units a week and 2 to 3 units a day (3 units is 1 large glass of wine)

So that's a shocker. My first question was: can I save up my Monday to Thursday drinks for the weekend? And of course, government guidelines say NO! Binge drinking isn't advisable for lots of reasons, but what they do like is us having a three-day break from alcohol each week – good to know.

WHAT ARE UNITS OF ALCOHOL?

One unit is 10ml of pure alcohol. A good measure (excuse the pun) of what drinks the liver prefers is the %ABV, that's alcohol by volume. It'll be displayed on packaging as a percentage of the whole drink. The higher the percentage, the more alcohol present.

+ 1 pint of lager or cider (568ml) at 5% ABV is 2.8 units and 215 calories

+ 1 large glass of wine (250ml) at 12% ABV is 3 units and 180 calories

+ 1 shot of spirit/liqueur on ice (25ml) at 40% ABV is 1 unit and 59 calories

+ 1 gin and tonic (1 x 25ml shot and 1 x 250ml tonic) at 40% is 1 unit and 114 calories

So if calories and watching your weight is an issue, then bigging up water as your chosen drink is your biggest weapon. If you are partaking, you can see the calorific value of some of our most common drinks above.

WHAT IS A HANGOVER?

Alcohol is a diuretic, so drinking excessively can make us very dehydrated, which is why we can get a headache or feel nauseous. Crucially, alcohol consumption can disrupt and disturb our sleep. We may sleep for a longer time, but we need quality, not quantity. Excessive alcohol means we get far less deep sleep – that's why we often feel tired after drinking. Regularly hindering our sleep by drinking booze is definitely going to have a negative impact on our overall health.

HOW TO PREVENT A HANGOVER

+ Don't drink on an empty stomach – a carb-based meal can help slow the absorption of alcohol

+ Pairing alcohol intermittently with water is an easy habit to get into and very helpful

+ Two or three days off between drink-ups is much better than consecutive drinking, as it allows your liver time to recover and repair

+ It's suggested that darker spirits are more likely to give you a less clear head the next day

+ Red wines with high sulphite levels are rumoured to cause headaches, but it's more likely dehydration that's the culprit – the tannins in red wine can affect some people, though

HOW TO DEAL WITH A HANGOVER

+ Keep well hydrated in the days after drinking to ensure your body rehydrates properly

+ Paracetamol can help with headaches

+ Avoid 'hair of the dog' or a morning-after drink – this doesn't help, it just prolongs the pain

+ Eat a hearty breakfast – this is one situation where simple carbs can help. Or, enjoy things that will help you to rehydrate, such as soups

+ I always find a nice breath of fresh air helps, so getting outside for a little walk is advisable

+ Take a break from alcohol for a few days after a heavy session to give your liver time to recover

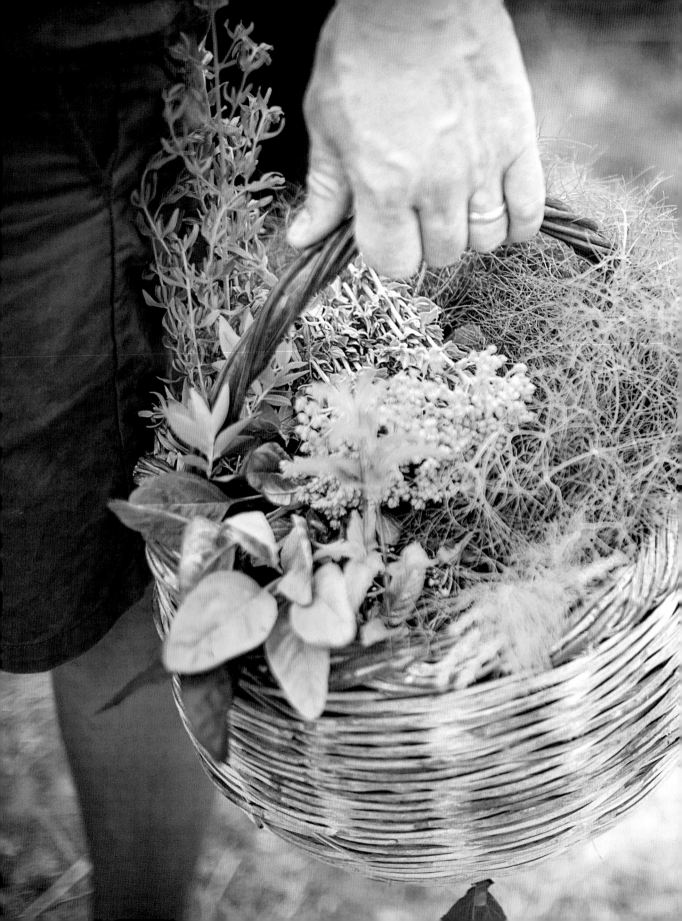

On the island of Ikaria, Greece, they use fresh herbs and wild greens in abundance every day. Both herbs and greens contain loads of amazing vitamins, minerals, trace elements, fibre and a whole other super-long list of reputed medicinal benefits that will only serve us well. Herbs also have that wonderful ability to add big flavour to your food, meaning you can cut down on the salt. One pattern that I witnessed in all the healthy parts of the world I visited was that nearly everyone tended vegetable gardens, keeping them active and giving them food at its freshest. Just grow your own!

VOTE FOR ORGANIC FOOD

I always feel that organic food gets a bit of a bashing in the press because it's a bit more expensive, and is seen as the preserve of the middle classes, foodies, and so-called hippy do-gooders. Let me clarify – organic food is natural food, where nature has been allowed to do its thing, and I'm sure most of us will agree that putting natural ingredients into our bodies is only going to be a positive thing.

I'm talking about the way the planet has been for the whole of time, until, that is, we introduced man-made chemicals, fertilizers and pesticides into our farming system, and stopped proper crop rotation. These things have changed the face of agriculture. Is all non-organic food the devil incarnate? I don't think so, certainly a lot of care and effort has gone into developing certain solutions (such as how to raise animals in more affordable ways), but the simple fact is that often we don't actually need to intervene with nature.

We know so little still about how the body works, but we do know that variety and freshness give us the most nutritional benefits – it makes sense to me that eating organic food, at its freshest, will support that.

Sales of organic and more responsibly produced food are on the rise, and like anything, if we demand more, more will become widely available. Essentially, every time we choose to buy an organic product we're voting for a better food system. I'm not saying we need to be organic all the time – I find it impossible to be 100% organic, but I do trade up whenever I can. If we can all start to re-address

what we buy, cook and eat, gradually buying better and wasting less, that's only going to move our food system forward in a positive and more sustainable way.

When we trade up to organic meat, it will be more expensive, but really at the heart of this book is getting into the habit of eating less meat, and choosing the best when you do. It's all about quality over quantity (see page 269). It's more expensive because it's likely the animal will have lived a much longer, better-quality life. That's what it's all about for me. With organic chickens in the UK in particular, they've lived longer, got there more naturally and are stronger, healthier birds. It makes sense that a healthier bird makes for a healthier food. Plus they taste better too!

The one thing that's super-easy to trade up is the everyday dairy products, such as milk, yoghurt and butter – read why on page 275. Stock cubes are another really easy thing to get into the habit of trading up, choosing organic gives the peace of mind that any meat within it is of a certain standard. Finally worth noting is that when it comes to veg and fruit, sometimes organic doesn't cost any more, especially if you buy seasonally.

A FEW REASONS TO TRADE UP TO ORGANIC

Here are some really interesting facts about organic food and farming that I was really interested to learn from Peter Melchett, Policy Director at the Soil Association, the UK's leading membership charity campaigning for healthy, humane and sustainable food, farming and land use. I wanted to share all this to give you more context about why choosing organic is worth it:

+ Nutritionally, it's been shown that organic crops – veg, fruit, pulses, cereals – are up to 60% higher than non-organic crops in different antioxidants. This is pretty incredible news, and something I hope we'll find out more about in the near future

+ In the UK, think of organic as the gold standard for food production. Having an organic seal of approval lets us know that every stage of production has been carefully inspected to ensure it meets the best standards

+ Organic food comes from trusted sources, and all over the world, food products labelled as organic must meet standards that define what farmers and food manufacturers can and cannot do. All organic farms and food companies are inspected at least once a year, and in the EU the standards for organic food are laid down in European law

+ Organic farming is a modern system, using no fossil fuel-based fertilizers. Farmers instead develop naturally healthy soil, which helps control pests, weeds and disease

+ It's good for nature too – organic farms are more likely to attract wildlife and provide homes for bees, butterflies and birds – we like that

+ Organically managed soils are more resistant to droughts and floods, so in turn are more resilient than other farming methods to the impacts of climate change, which is helpful for farmers

+ On that note, organic farming is looking like it's the best currently available, practical model for reducing greenhouse gas emissions in agriculture, because it stores higher levels of carbon in the soil. To put that into perspective – if organic farming was common practice in the UK, we could offset over 20% of UK agriculture's greenhouse gas emissions, which would be amazing

+ Finally – and pretty powerful info this is too – new research from the United Nations Food and Agriculture Organization is showing that if we reduce food waste and eat a diet with less meat and dairy consumption, organic farming should be able to feed the world without needing any more land

REVOLUTIONIZE SHOPPING

A lot of mistakes in unhealthy diets happen in the shopping basket. Years of research proves that most of us buy the same thing, often the wrong thing, with only tiny variants, week in, week out.

For a lot of people it's a mixture of being trapped on autopilot and feeling a bit lost (and with the makers of bad-quality processed food often on the low-fat, low-sugar diet bandwagon, messages are confusing). Not quite knowing how to make a positive change in our diet, mixed up with being busy, juggling family and work, being over-subservient to kids' likes and dislikes and wanting to please everyone are all contributing factors. The whole shopping experience is deeply psychological and, to make things worse, the kind of hypnotism and positioning of those highly processed, and often discounted, junk foods makes embracing good fresh foods and ingredients a real challenge.

There are a few things that can be done to profoundly change what gets put into the basket. Flexi-planning a weekly menu is probably the best way to go and can be really fun – shop to plan for half the week, then build in meals that are adaptable and can be turned into other things for the remaining days, just in case plans change at the last minute. This allows for focused shopping. Sitting down with a stack of cookbooks or magazines to pick out some meals for the week ahead is a really nice thing to do, and will most definitely bolster your repertoire, as well as your creativity.

Secondly and obviously, because of geography we all have varying food options on our doorstep. Having said that, most of us shop at supermarkets – they're super-convenient and allow us to be flexible and economical with our time, but there are often distractions that can lure us off track, encouraging us to spend more money.

I still religiously use my local butcher, fishmonger and veg and fruit market every week too – shopping around helps you get to know your area and build up local relationships, but also allows you to suss out the best-quality ingredients available, at the best prices, and in a far more strategic way. And if you're lucky enough to have a nearby farmer's market, embrace it, just have a bit of a plan before you go – shopping seasonally will definitely save you money. I also grow some stuff (see page 263), so this, plus a combination of shopping around, almost certainly helps in making healthier choices. Interestingly, if you remove the actual shopping experience and shop online, it can help bring a little more focus, so this might be worth trying, too, if you want a new tack. Home-delivery boxes are a great way of getting more fresh, local, healthy food through your door as well, and they'll often surprise you by including something different.

TIPS FOR A HEALTHIER SHOPPING BASKET

- VEG & FRUIT -

+ Just buy more veg and fruit, more salad, and try something new every week – eat the rainbow

+ Stock up on frozen veg – they're great value, available all year, and are nutritious because they've been frozen at their peak – you can just grab a handful of what you need, when you need it

+ Get lots of herbs and spices in your life – it's a healthy, delicious way to add flavour, can help lower your salt intake, and herbs are easy to grow too

- CARBOHYDRATES -

+ It's easy to swap regular rice, flours, pasta and noodles for wholewheat and wholemeal varieties

+ Exchange regular bread for wholemeal varieties, or even make your own (see pages 44 and 68)

- PROTEIN -

+ When it comes to meat focus on quality not quantity, and trade up on the welfare front whenever you can (see page 268)

+ Be open-minded about the fish you choose (let your fishmonger advise – it'll normally be cheaper)

+ Embrace the wonder of protein-rich eggs, choosing free-range or organic whenever you can

+ Get yourself a range of nuts and seeds and keep them in well-sealed containers ready for adding a delicious crunch and protein boost to your meals

- FAT -

+ Don't buy margarine, buy butter instead, but use it in moderation, and try to use healthy oils whenever you can (see page 273)

- DAIRY -

+ Don't buy sweetened yoghurt, go for really nice, organic natural or Greek yoghurts

+ Trade up to organic when it comes to milk, yoghurt and butter too – it's an easy health investment

- SUGARS -

+ Swap out refined sugars for honey when you can. I use manuka in recipes not exposed to heat; it costs more but the nutritional benefits are much higher

+ Don't buy sugary drinks, just big up jugs of icy cold water with a little squeeze of something – check out the easy flavoured water ideas on page 254

- BREAKFAST -

+ Most cereals are full of sugar, but porridge oats are a nutritional wonder, so embrace those and make your own mixes (see pages 18 and 36). Making your own is also a super-easy way to get nuts, seeds and dried fruit into your diet for added benefit

- DON'T FORGET -

+ Resist buy-one-get-one-free and similar schemes on the stuff you want to limit in your diet – it's only a bargain if you need it!

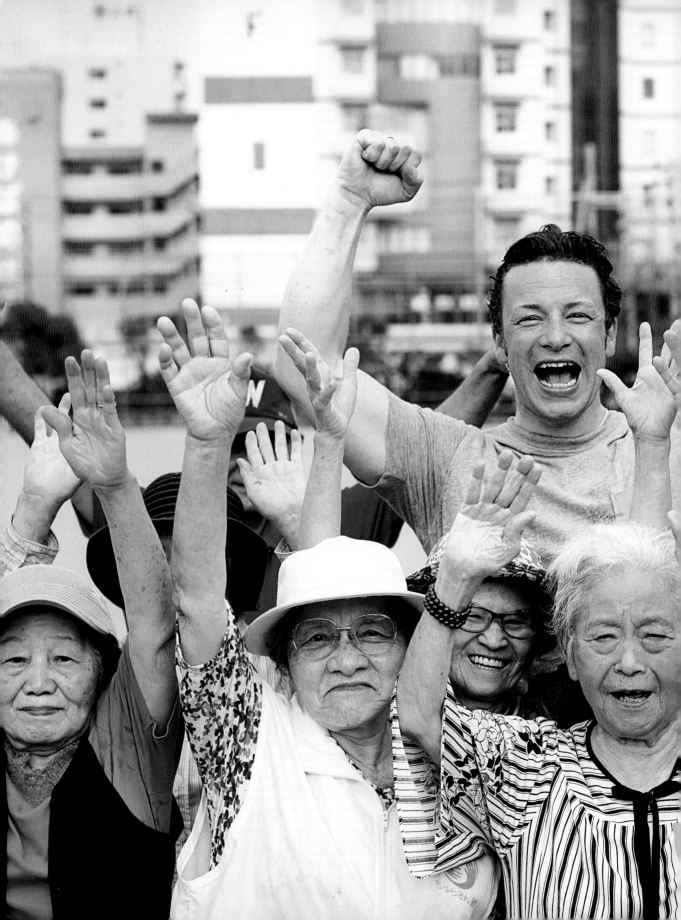

Across the island of Okinawa, Japan, groups like this meet every day at 6.30am to move, stretch, dance and socialize to three songs on the radio. It's called Radio Exercise and has been going on for nearly 100 years. Research shows that staying socially connected means you're three times more likely to live to 100. At the heart of these groups is friendship, community, routine and a sense of daily purpose.

THE BASICS OF SLEEP

It sounds simple, but getting enough sleep is absolutely essential, and really is one of the biggest contributors to good health – it gives our bodies that crucial time they need to grow, heal and repair.

I was getting it all wrong for about five years – only getting three to four hours' sleep a night, which is not good. On average, less than six hours a night or more than nine over a sustained period increases our risk of developing an illness – short sleep has been associated with obesity, type-2 diabetes and cancer, for example. I'm doing really well now, but I literally have to treat sleep like a job, not because I can't sleep once I'm in bed, but because there seem to be a thousand reasons/noises/people/distractions that prevent me from just turning off and getting into bed. I've consciously got myself into a routine that I stick to five or six days a week, and frankly has underpinned all the things I've picked up and tried to express in this book. The following information is fascinating, geeky stuff that I've learnt from super-dude Professor Jason Ellis, one of only a few qualified sleep scientists in the UK.

THE PROCESSES OF SLEEP

We spend every day going through two processes. The first is called process S – it's the drive we all have to go to sleep. It works a bit like being hungry then satiating that feeling by eating. From the moment we wake up, we start developing our drive to go to sleep again – it will increase all day, then drop once we sleep. The second is known as process C, which is our natural body clock – the circadian rhythm. It pretty much works on a 24-hour basis, but weirdly Jason tells me it's actually around 24¼ hours for many of us. This explains why sleep is so fragile – our internal system is constantly fighting an external world, kind of like jetlag. We're always a bit behind or a bit ahead, so regular bedtimes and getting into a good routine is really helpful.

REGULATING SLEEP PROCESSES

There are two hormones that are key to the success of our sleep. Melatonin, a natural hormone, helps us get to sleep. It builds up as it gets dark, reaching a peak at around 4am when it starts to decline. On the other hand is cortisol, the stress hormone. It's got a bit of a bad rep but it allows us to walk, talk, exercise and do what we need to do during the day. It works in the opposite way – we start to produce cortisol in the early hours of the morning to get us ready to wake up. That's the basics – anything that disrupts either of those processes or the intersection between them is a sleep disorder. So, with all that in mind, let's go on to what happens when we're actually asleep, and the repeating cycle we go through every night.

THE 90-MINUTE SLEEP CYCLE

This cycle repeats throughout the course of a night:

STAGE ONE – that warm cosy feeling when we get into bed. Our brainwaves start to slow – about five minutes

STAGE TWO – as we drift off, we get progressively deeper and might experience a jolt, like we're falling off something. This is the 'hypnagogic jerk' and one explanation for it is that we no longer need cortisol, so our muscles tense and jerk to excrete excess quickly. We're at the official onset of sleep – our brainwaves get slower still and more rhythmic, and the majority of our memory consolidation occurs, including black and white dreaming (45–55% of our night)

SLOW WAVE SLEEP – we go into a very deep sleep and it's hard to wake ourselves (or others!) – our brainwaves have spaced out. This stage is the only sleep period where our immune systems work at 100% – we're healing, producing anti-cancer cells, anti-allergens and cleaning the body – this is why we sleep a lot when we're poorly. This is 13–23% of our night

STAGE TWO (AGAIN) – we pop back into stage two, although we don't wake up, we're conscious enough to check our environment is safe, then we move on to . . .

REM CYCLE – this sleep stage is really important for our memory and mind, and clears all the toxins in the brain. It only lasts about five minutes in its first iteration, but is 20–25% of our night. If we don't sleep well, our memory is shot the next day and our problem-solving ability is reduced – good to know. We dream in colour now, and if we don't remember our dreams it just means we're consolidating our memory really well

TIPS FOR A GOOD NIGHT'S SLEEP

Most importantly of all, remember that the quality of your sleep is much more important than the quantity.

+ Avoid bathing in the two hours before going to bed, and don't exercise in that time either – both activities raise the body temperature, not giving it enough time to decrease before trying to sleep

+ Create a cool, dark and quiet environment – we instinctively use light and dark as cues. If it helps, wear ear plugs and an eye mask – I do!

+ Blue light – from electronics – is very unhelpful. If light is essential, go for deep yellow or red, which have long wavelengths and don't interrupt sleep

+ Naps are a good thing, but should be kept to 20 minutes to prevent the body going into a longer sleep cycle, which would mean we wake up groggy, not refreshed, as we've interrupted that deeper cycle

+ Hydrate well throughout the day, and reduce liquid intake slightly from about 5pm onwards, to avoid bathroom trips in the night, disrupting sleep cycles

+ Try not to eat in the two hours before going to bed, or the body will be going through the digestive process as well as trying to get to sleep. Keep it simple!

+ Helpful foods to increase melatonin levels are kiwi fruit (eat two in the evening), cherries, walnuts, unripe bananas, raspberries, tomatoes and jasmine rice

+ Remove clocks from the bedroom – they can create tension and distraction if constantly checked, adding unnecessary pressure. Keep an alarm far enough away from the bed so it can't be reached in the night

DO YOU WANT TO LIVE
TO BE 100 YEARS OLD?

Let's be frank, I don't know about you but I want to live until I'm 100 years old. I want to be fit, healthy, productive and happy, and I want to see my great-grandchildren, heck, my great-great-grandchildren grow up. I've just turned forty years of age, and I definitely want to be here to see another forty at least.

Around the world, people living to be over 100 years old are quite rare, but in a handful of places it does seem to be more common. And it's not just about having a longer life, it's about really living that life – being conscious in each moment, enjoying it and having fun. I want some of that! So, on the journey of creating this book, I went to some of the healthiest places in the world – places where the numbers of exceptionally old, healthy, fit people are unusually high. You'll see some of the incredible characters I met in the images peppered throughout this section of the book. And despite these areas being vastly different in geography and climate, generally there are similarities between all these wonderful old people. Food plays a big part, but there are other factors too.

COMMUNITY & PURPOSE

First of all, the majority of these lovely people are really good fun, and really good company. Now to me, that makes perfect sense, because if you're a miserable old codger, who's going to want to hang out with you and care for you? But in all seriousness, a sense of community, of sustained relationships with the people around you, is really at the heart of these pockets of people. Most have a religion or belief of some sort, all of which vary, but I think the message to be taken is the same – that having a sense of purpose, and having people around you to share that with – family, friends, neighbours, community – is really important. You can live alone, but getting out there, keeping in touch with people, laughing and sharing stories, is key.

MOVEMENT

Movement is pretty interesting too. Exercise as we know it – going to the gym, going for a run – doesn't exist in most places. Instead, movement and being active is simply a natural habit in all aspects of daily life. Generally things are inconveniently got, it sounds daft but people sit on the floor and stand up and down more often, they walk a lot more, tend gardens; I could go on. In the very act of living their lives these wonderful people are probably getting more 'exercise' than you and I do on an average day, without intentionally setting out to do so. It's a great lesson – we've almost made our lives too convenient. Let's all challenge ourselves to be more naturally active each day and quite simply, just move a bit more!

FOOD & WINE

Diet-wise, the key ingredients and habits do vary wildly from place to place, but on the whole, meat consumption is fairly low and plant-based meals are celebrated. Most people have a garden or outdoor area where they grow a few things – giving the opportunity to get outside and keep active, but also to eat food that is the ultimate in seasonality and freshness, picked right from their backyard. A lot of people have a small glass of alcohol each day (that's a small glass, and one, not two, three or four!). And many people share meals when they can with the people around them – rushing less, chewing more, and appreciating their food.

WHAT'S THE SECRET?

I guess what these brilliant folk have taught me more than anything is that the secret to a long, happy, productive life isn't one golden bullet – there's no tablet out there that you can take to give you a longer life. It's about the full package – family, friends, community, keeping stress levels low, the simple act of growing, cooking and eating good food, and sharing that food with the people around you whenever you can, sleeping enough and being nice to people. Remember, there's no such thing as an insignificant healthy choice – they all count, however big or small. It's about joining all the dots together to give yourself the best chance.

Now I don't claim to be an expert on all areas of life, but I can certainly help you out on the food front, and that's why this book exists – to offer a tangible solution to the food part in order to help you live a healthier, happier life. Everything else is up to you – be optimistic, open, and embrace life and all the weird and wonderful challenges it presents us with.

I'm part of a neat little app, called YOU, which is free and totally in the spirit of this book. It's all about completing daily micro actions around food, mindfulness, movement and love. Getting involved and going on that journey only requires one minute of your time each day, and it's a great little tool to help you start making small, achievable, sustainable changes.

This is the youngest daughter of José Guervara, a 106-year-old mega dude I met in Costa Rica who has ten children and over 100 grandchildren! Every day Leonor makes him gallo pinto for breakfast, a wonderfully nutritious meal of herbs, veggies, beans, rice and eggs that he's been enjoying daily since he was a kid. So, the moral of the story for me is don't skip breakfast – this first meal of the day is so important. Choose something nutritious and you're laughing.

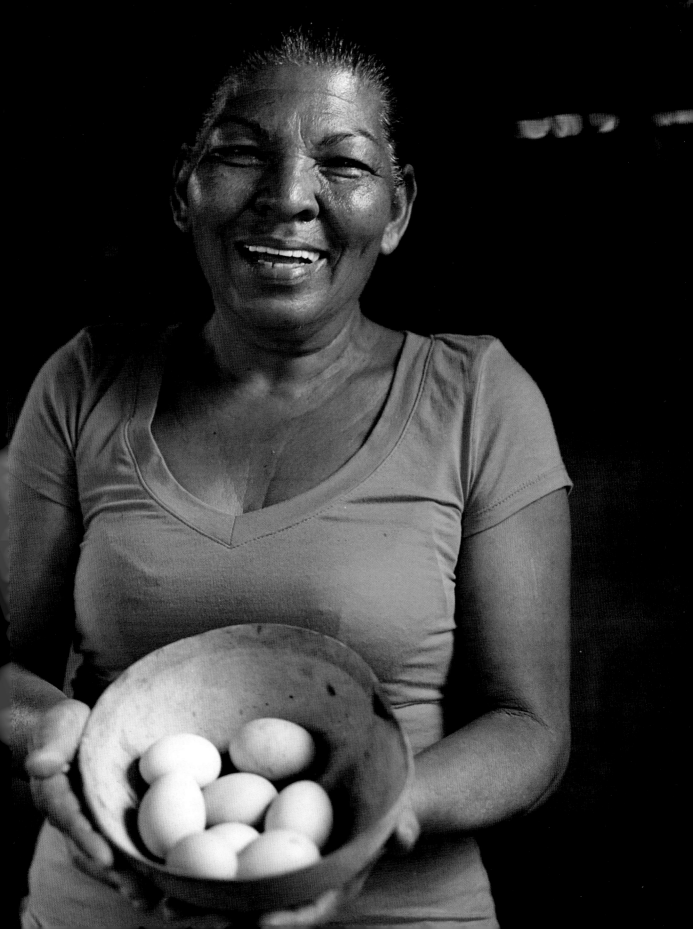

THANK YOU

I've met a lot of wonderfully talented people on the journey of making this book, and I must give a special mention to all these amazing minds who've helped deepen my understanding of health, wellbeing and nutrition. Huge gratitude to: Dr Helen Crawley, Registered Public Health Nutritionist, who manages the charity First Steps Nutrition Trust; Professor Jason Ellis, sleep specialist and Professor in Psychology at Northumbria University and Director of the Northumbria Centre for Sleep Research; Professor Gary Frost, Professor of Nutrition and Dietetics at Imperial College, London; Professor Ian Givens, Professor of Food Chain Nutrition and Head of Food Production & Quality at the University of Reading; Dr Alexandra Johnstone, Senior Research Fellow at the University of Aberdeen, Rowett Institute of Nutrition and Health, who looks at how composition of the diet can affect weight control and how protein can signal satiety; Professor Julie Lovegrove, Professor of Human Nutrition at the University of Reading, who looks at the nutritional influences of cardiovascular health and the development of metabolic syndrome; Peter Melchett, Policy Director at the Soil Association, a UK organic food and farming organization; Professor Tom Sanders, Professor of Nutrition and Dietetics at King's College, London, whose research career has focused on the effects of dietary fat on cardiovascular health; Jamie Sawyer, my incredible trainer; Professor Mark Thursz, Professor of Hepatology at Imperial College, London, whose clinical interests are alcoholic liver disease and fatty liver disease.

Massive dues to the brilliant ladies that have guided me through my nutrition diploma – Nutritionist Ann Kennedy, Academic Director at St Mary's University and sports dietitian Gill Horgan, Programme Director at St Mary's University, and from my old gang, Mary Lynch, a Registered Nutritionist. I never thought I'd go back to school, but you've made every lesson a pleasure.

As always, thank you to my fantastic family and my inspiration, Jools, Poppy, Daisy, Petal, Buddy, my brilliant Mum and Dad, and my good chums Gennaro Contaldo and David Loftus. This book is for all of you.

To the heart of my gang, my incredible food team. The journey on this book has been a little different, so extra thanks to those of you that were beside me as I found my photographer's feet. To my foodie rock Ginny Rolfe, and all her amazing sidekicks, Abigail Fawcett, Georgina Hayden, Christina Mackenzie, Phillippa Spence, Jodene Jordan, Maddie Rix, Elspeth Meston, Rachel Young and Sam Baldwin, as well as Charlie Clapp. To ultimate dude Pete Begg, brilliant Bobby Sebire, and the rest of the wonderful team, Laura James, Joanne Lord, Athina Andrelos, Helen Martin and Daniel Nowland. And of course, lovely Sarah Tildesley and her husband, photographer Sam Robinson, who gave me some friendly advice along the way.

Extra fibre-coated thanks to my outstanding nutrition ninjas, head of nutrition Laura Matthews and Rozzie Batchelar. We've bartered, bantered, laughed and cried, and together we've created this incredible book.

To my girls on words, my editor Rebecca Walker and Bethan O'Connor. Thank you for helping me shape this content in the most accessible yet engaging way, and for considering my drawings (though they didn't make it in!).

Thank you to my publishers at Penguin Random House, for your continued love and support in all that I do. To my main man Tom Weldon and main woman Louise Moore – thank you. To my tattooed brother John Hamilton on the art front, and to lovely ladies Alice Burkle and Juliette Butler in production, as well as Katherine Tibbals. Thank you to the unflappable Ed2 team – to Nick Lowndes and his motley crew: the one and only Annie Lee, Caroline Pretty, Pat Rush and Caroline Wilding.

Huge shout out as well to all the amazing Penguin guys and gals that get the book out there to all of you. On rights to lovely Chantal Noel and her team: Anjali Nathani, Lucy Beresford-Knox, Catherine Wood and Celia Long. On the sales front: Matthew Watterson, Rebecca Cooney, Stuart Anderson, Zoe Caulfield, Martin Higgins, Jessica Sacco, Isabel Coburn, Neil Green, Jonathan Parker, Samantha Fanaken, Claire Bennett and Andrew Sauerwine. And last but definitely not least, the wonderful publicity, comms and brand gang: Clare Parker, George Foster, Jenny Platt, Elizabeth Smith and Bek Sunley.

A massive thanks to James Verity and the team at creative agency Superfantastic on the clear and accessible design. Special mention as well, Jim, for your alter-ego role as my camera assistant – much appreciated.

Big big thanks to Paul Stuart and sidekick Bradley Barnes for capturing the essence of my journey in this book through the portraits you see both on the cover and throughout the chapters. Nice one mate.

And so to the rest of my team. I am constantly blown away by the talented bunch around me – you mean that I look forward to coming to work every day. To Paul Hunt, Claudia Rosencrantz, Claire Postans, Zoe Collins and Louise Holland, for keeping everything in check. To my PR and marketing gang: Peter Berry, Jeremy Scott, Laura Jones, and Katie Bohane, and to Giovanna Milia, Therese MacDermott and Patricio Colombo. To my personal warriors Holly Adams, Amelia Crook, Sy Brighton and Paul Rutherford. And to all the other amazing people around the business, I'd thank you all here individually if I could – you know who you are. Special shout out as well to the office testers who've helped me hone these recipes with great curiosity and enthusiasm.

Lastly to the gang at Fresh One Productions, my TV family, and the team on this series – thank you for making this story come to life. To the unstoppable Jo Ralling, to wonderful Gudren Claire, Sean Moxhay, Susan Cassidy and Lucy Blatch. To the awesome producers and directors – it's been a pleasure, Nicola Pointer, Martha Delap, Chloe Court, Paul Casey, Jess Reid and to Katie Millard – may your enthusiasm never falter. To my old boys on the crew: Luke Cardiff, Olly Wiggins, Dave Miller, Pete Bateson, Mike Sarah, Darren Jackson and Freddie Claire – double pleasure to Freddie for the stunning landscape reportage – and to Louise Harris. Thanks to the guys on the ground: Violeta Grancelli, Manu Tahilramani, Mai Nishiyama and Eleni Fanariotou. Shout out to the super edit team: Jamie Mac, Liam Jolly, Gavin Ames, Kim Boursnell, Russ Peers and Jen Cockburn. And finally of course, to lovely ladies Julia Bell, Julie Akeroyd and Lima O'Donnell for keeping me in check with make-up and clothes, where necessary!

INDEX

Recipes marked V are suitable for vegetarians

A

almonds
Earl Grey banana bread	V	82
figgy banana bread	V	30
sexy stewed prunes	V	76
skinny carbonara		108
super-food protein loaf	V	68

amazing Mexican tomato soup, sweet potato chips, feta & tortilla	V	98

apples
British jam jar salad		104
cucumber, apple & mint flavoured water	V	254
gem lettuce, cucumber, apple & mint salad	V	226
herby pasta salad		116
pork & apple sauce		222
post-gym super salad		72
roasted carrot & squash salad	V	194

apricots
apricot, ginger & cashew energy balls	V	250
my Bircher muesli	V	78

artichokes: fagioli fusilli, sweet leeks, artichokes & bay oil	V	206
Asian crispy beef, brown rice noodles & loadsa salad		88
Asian green salad, tofu, noodles & sesame sprinkle	V	138
Asian steamed fish, black rice, greens & chilli sauce		180
Asian stir-fried veg, crispy sesame noodle omelette	V	144

asparagus
Asian green salad	V	138
Asian stir-fried veg	V	144
crazy fish, veg & noodle stir-fry		220
crispy sea bass, pea, mint & asparagus mash		198
quick homemade tortilla	V	60
round lettuce, asparagus, strawberry & mint salad		228
my Russian salad		148
seared golden chicken, mint sauce & spring veg fest		162
seared tuna, Sicilian couscous & greens		124
spring squid		200

aubergines
happiness pasta	V	90
harissa roasted aubergine	V	186

avocados
grilled corn & quinoa salad		152
magic poached egg	V	22
quick homemade tortilla	V	60
salmon ceviche		142
sesame seared salmon, tahini, avocado & shred salad		150
squash it veg sandwich	V	146

awesome granola dust, nuts, seeds, oats & fruit galore	V	18

B

bacon
grilled corn & quinoa salad		152
healthy cheese & corn pancakes		74
skinny carbonara		108
sprouting seed salad		96
see also pancetta		

baked eggs in popped beans, cherry tomatoes, ricotta on toast	V	16

balsamic vinegar
balsamic vinegar flavour popcorn	V	234
sprouting seed salad		96
strawberry, balsamic & basil fro-yo	V	246

bananas
my Bircher muesli	V	78
Earl Grey banana bread	V	82
figgy banana bread	V	30
healthy cheese & corn pancakes		74
pretty fruit pots	V	34
ripe banana & brown bread fro-yo	V	246
sexy stewed prunes	V	76
smoothie pancakes	V	24

basil
basil & strawberry fruit soup	V	40
cheese, tomato & basil poppadom snacks	V	232
creamy basil dressing	V	226
mega veggie burgers, garden salad & basil dressing	V	158
skinny carbonara		108
smoky peppers & sweet basil cucumber sticks	V	236
strawberry, balsamic & basil fro-yo	V	246
tomato, basil & cheese scrambled eggs	V	58
watermelon & basil flavoured water	V	255

bay oil: fagioli fusilli, sweet leeks, artichokes & bay oil	V	206

beans
baked eggs in popped beans	V	16
fagioli fusilli	V	206
iceberg lettuce, broad bean, grape & tarragon salad	V	228
Mexican pan-cooked brekkie		26
rainbow open wrap	V	54
roasted sweet potatoes	V	110
seared golden chicken, mint sauce & spring veg fest		162
smoky veggie feijoada	V	182
spring squid		200
see also chickpeas; green beans; lentils		

beansprouts: Asian stir-fried veg	V	144

beef
Asian crispy beef		88
British jam jar salad		104
griddled steak & peppers		216
tasty samosas		188
see also bresaola		

beetroot

beets & sardines		112
British jam jar salad		104
feisty beet & horseradish dip	V	230
roasted mustard mackerel, rainbow beets & bulgur wheat		174
my Russian salad		148
sesame seared salmon, tahini, avocado & shred salad		150

berries

berry & brown bread fro-yo	V	246
berry pocket eggy bread	V	52
my Bircher muesli	V	78
raw vegan flapjack snacks	V	244
see also blackberries; blueberries; raspberries; strawberries		

my Bircher muesli, fruit, nuts, yoghurt & seeds	V	78

black beans

Mexican pan-cooked brekkie		26
roasted sweet potatoes	V	110
smoky veggie feijoada	V	182

black rice pudding, mango, lime, passion fruit & coconut	V	28
black-eyed beans: rainbow open wrap	V	54

blackberries

epic fruit salad	V	66
nettle tea & blackberry fruit soup	V	40

blood oranges

chicken & garlic bread kebabs		130
figgy banana bread	V	30
Moroccan jam jar salad	V	106
St Clements flavoured water	V	254
see also oranges		

blueberries

epic fruit salad	V	66
round lettuce, fennel, blueberry & chilli salad	V	226
smoothie pancakes	V	24
toasted oats	V	62

blushing pickled eggs, red cabbage, cloves & star anise	V	238
bok choi: Asian steamed fish		180
Bombay chicken & cauli, poppadoms, rice & spinach		156

bread

beets & sardines		112
berry & brown bread fro-yo	V	246
berry pocket eggy bread	V	52
chicken & garlic bread kebabs		130
chicken & squash cacciatore		202
Earl Grey banana bread	V	82
ripe banana & brown bread fro-yo	V	246
rye soda bread	V	44
silken omelette	V	32
super-food protein loaf	V	68
super-food protein loaf topping ideas	V	70
tomato & olive spaghetti		100
see also crispbreads; croutons; flatbreads; sandwiches; toast		

breakfast popovers, cheese, ham, mushroom & tomato		50
bream: crazy fish, veg & noodle stir-fry		220

bresaola

herby pasta salad		116
orange garden salad		92

British jam jar salad		104

broad beans

iceberg lettuce, broad bean, grape & tarragon salad	V	228
seared golden chicken, mint sauce & spring veg fest		162
spring squid		200

broccoli

Asian green salad	V	138
crazy fish, veg & noodle stir-fry		220
crumbed pesto fish		184
pork & apple sauce		222
quick homemade tortilla	V	60
wholewheat spaghetti, sprouting broccoli, chilli & lemon		132

broths

ginger & chicken penicillin		218
moreish fish soup		204
super-tasty miso broth		208
see also soups		

bulgur wheat

Greek jam jar salad		106
roasted mustard mackerel		174

burgers: mega veggie burgers	V	158

butternut squash

chicken & squash cacciatore		202
cosy squash soup	V	122
delicious squash daal	V	168
roasted carrot & squash salad	V	194
roasted squash laksa bake		170
smoky veggie feijoada	V	182
super squash lasagne	V	176
sweet potato muffins	V	64

C

cabbage

blushing pickled eggs, red cabbage, cloves & star anise	V	238
tasty fish tacos		86
veggie ramen, walnut miso, kimchee & fried eggs	V	190

Caesar salad: healthy chicken Caesar		94

cannellini beans

baked eggs in popped beans	V	16
fagioli fusilli	V	206

carbonara: skinny carbonara		108

carrots

Asian stir-fried veg	V	144
cheese & quick pickled veg poppadom snacks	V	232
fagioli fusilli	V	206
golden salmon steaks, sweet peas & smashed veg		166
harissa waffles	V	42
moreish fish soup		204
Moroccan jam jar salad	V	106
pork & apple sauce		222

post-gym super salad		72
roasted carrot & squash salad	V	194
my Russian salad		148
sesame seared salmon, tahini, avocado & shred salad		150
cashews: apricot, ginger & cashew energy balls	V	250
cauliflower		
Bombay chicken & cauli		156
healthy chicken Caesar		94
Indian roasted cauliflower	V	192
cavolo nero: super green soup		114
ceviche: salmon ceviche		142
chard: seared tuna, Sicilian couscous & greens		124
cheese		
baked eggs in popped beans	V	16
breakfast popovers		50
cosy squash soup	V	122
happiness pasta	V	90
healthy cheese & corn pancakes		74
pan-cooked mushrooms		80
poppadom snacks	V	232
quick homemade tortilla	V	60
silken omelette	V	32
spelt spaghetti, vine tomatoes & baked ricotta	V	160
spinach, Parmesan & chilli scrambled eggs	V	56
squash it veg sandwich	V	146
super squash lasagne	V	176
super summer salad	V	136
sweet potato muffins	V	64
tomato, cheese & basil scrambled eggs	V	58
see also cottage cheese; cream cheese; ricotta cheese		
chia seeds		
fruit soups	V	40
pretty fruit pots	V	34
chicken		
Bombay chicken & cauli		156
chicken & garlic bread kebabs		130
chicken & squash cacciatore		202
ginger & chicken penicillin		218
golden chicken skewers		172
Greek jam jar salad		106
healthy chicken Caesar		94
healthy chicken club		128
post-gym super salad		72
roasted squash laksa bake		170
my Russian salad, golden paprika chicken		148
seared golden chicken		162
seared turmeric chicken		140
super-tasty miso broth		208
chickpeas		
amazing Mexican tomato soup	V	98
cosy squash soup, chickpea salad flatbreads	V	122
Indian roasted cauliflower	V	192
Moroccan jam jar salad	V	106

skinny homemade houmous	V	230
super green soup		114
chillies		
amazing Mexican tomato soup	V	98
Asian crispy beef		88
Asian steamed fish, black rice, greens & chilli sauce		180
Bombay chicken & cauli		156
cheese, chilli & seeds poppadom snacks	V	232
delicious squash daal	V	168
easy curried fish stew		164
happiness pasta	V	90
hot chilli sauce flavour popcorn	V	234
Indian roasted cauliflower	V	192
magic poached egg	V	22
mighty mushroom curry	V	212
the ring of fire cucumber sticks	V	236
roasted carrot & squash salad	V	194
roasted squash laksa bake		170
roasted sweet potatoes, black beans, jalapeño tomato salsa	V	110
round lettuce, fennel, blueberry & chilli salad	V	226
sizzling Moroccan prawns		178
smoky veggie feijoada	V	182
spinach, Parmesan & chilli scrambled eggs	V	56
sweet potato muffins	V	64
tasty fish tacos, game-changing kiwi, lime & chilli salsa		86
tasty samosas		188
tasty veg omelette, raw tomato & chilli salsa	V	120
veggie ramen, walnut miso, kimchee & fried eggs	V	190
wholewheat spaghetti, sprouting broccoli, chilli & lemon		132
Chinese cabbage: veggie ramen, walnut miso, kimchee & fried eggs	V	190
chorizo: super green soup		114
cinnamon		
berry pocket eggy bread	V	52
date, cocoa & pumpkin seed energy balls	V	248
ripe banana & brown bread fro-yo	V	246
clementines		
epic fruit salad	V	66
gem lettuce, radish, pea & clementine salad	V	226
cloves: blushing pickled eggs, red cabbage, cloves & star anise		238
club sandwich: healthy chicken club		128
cocoa		
awesome granola dust	V	18
date, cocoa & pumpkin seed energy balls	V	248
coconut: black rice pudding	V	28
coronation dressing: Indian roasted cauliflower, pineapple, chilli, coronation dressing	V	192
cosy squash soup, chickpea salad flatbreads	V	122
cottage cheese		
breakfast popovers		50
cheese and mango chutney poppadom snacks	V	232
cheese and quick pickled veg poppadom snacks	V	232
cheese, chilli & seeds poppadom snacks	V	232
cheese, tomato & basil poppadom snacks	V	232

healthy cheese & corn pancakes		74
pan-cooked mushrooms		80
quick homemade tortilla	V	60
squash it veg sandwich	V	146
super squash lasagne	V	176
sweet potato muffins	V	64
courgettes		
iceberg lettuce, courgette, pear & dill salad	V	228
lemon sole & olive sauce, sweet courgettes & Jersey royals		210
couscous		
herby pasta salad		116
moreish fish soup		204
Moroccan jam jar salad	V	106
seared tuna, Sicilian couscous & greens		124
seared turmeric chicken		140
sizzling Moroccan prawns		178
crazy fish, veg & noodle stir-fry		220
cream cheese		
lime pickle & poppadom cucumber sticks	V	236
the ring of fire cucumber sticks	V	236
smoky peppers & sweet basil cucumber sticks	V	236
tahini, spring onion & sesame cucumber sticks	V	236
cress		
post-gym super salad		72
sesame seared salmon, tahini, avocado & shred salad		150
crispbreads		
easy Scandi crispbreads		102
orange garden salad		92
crispy sea bass, pea, mint & asparagus mash		198
croutons: healthy chicken Caesar		94
crumbed pesto fish, roasted cherry vines, spuds & greens		184
cucumber		
cheese & quick pickled veg poppadom snacks	V	232
cucumber, apple & mint flavoured water	V	254
cucumber sticks stuffed with lovely things	V	236
gem lettuce, cucumber, apple & mint salad	V	226
ginger & chicken penicillin		218
Greek jam jar salad		106
Mexican gazpacho	V	134
Moroccan jam jar salad	V	106
post-gym super salad		72
salmon ceviche		142
sesame seared salmon, tahini, avocado & shred salad		150
cumin: Bombay chicken & cauli		156

D

daal: delicious squash daal	V	168
dates		
date, cocoa & pumpkin seed energy balls	V	248
Earl Grey banana bread	V	82
raw vegan flapjack snacks	V	244
delicious squash daal, special fried eggs & poppadoms	V	168
dill: iceberg lettuce, courgette, pear & dill salad	V	228

dips		
feisty beet & horseradish dip	V	230
skinny homemade houmous	V	230
dressings		
creamy basil dressing	V	226
creamy mint dressing	V	228
dried fruit		
awesome granola dust	V	18
perfect porridge bars	V	48
snack attack	V	253
drinks		
easy flavoured waters	V	254–5
therapeutic teas	V	256–7

E

Earl Grey tea		
Earl Grey banana bread	V	82
sexy stewed prunes	V	76
easy curried fish stew, prawns, white fish & sweet tomatoes		164
easy flavoured waters, colourful, bright & delicious	V	254–5
easy Scandi crispbreads, pickled herrings, rainbow veg		102
eggs		
Asian stir-fried veg, crispy sesame noodle omelette	V	144
baked eggs in popped beans	V	16
berry pocket eggy bread	V	52
blushing pickled eggs	V	238
breakfast popovers		50
delicious squash daal, special fried eggs & poppadoms	V	168
Earl Grey banana bread	V	82
figgy banana bread	V	30
harissa waffles	V	42
healthy cheese & corn pancakes		74
magic poached egg	V	22
mega veggie burgers	V	158
Mexican gazpacho	V	134
Mexican pan-cooked brekkie		26
mushroom & Marmite scrambled eggs	V	58
rye soda bread	V	44
scrambled eggs		56, 58
silken omelette	V	32
smoked salmon & spring onion scrambled eggs		56
smoothie pancakes	V	24
spinach, Parmesan & chilli scrambled eggs	V	56
super-food protein loaf	V	68
sweet potato muffins	V	64
tasty veg omelette	V	120
tomato, cheese & basil scrambled eggs	V	58
vegeree not kedgeree	V	38
veggie ramen, walnut miso, kimchee & fried eggs	V	190
energy balls		
apricot, ginger & cashew	V	250
date, cocoa & pumpkin seed	V	248
epic fruit salad, delicious natural juices	V	66

F

fagioli fusilli, sweet leeks, artichokes & bay oil   V   206
feijoada: smoky veggie feijoada   V   182
feisty beet & horseradish dip   V   230
fennel: round lettuce, fennel, blueberry & chilli salad   V   226
fennel seeds, lemon & honey tea   V   256
feta cheese
    cosy squash soup   V   122
    super summer salad   V   136
figgy banana bread, blood orange & nut butter   V   30
fish
    Asian steamed fish   180
    beets & sardines   112
    crazy fish, veg & noodle stir-fry   220
    crispy sea bass   198
    crumbed pesto fish   184
    easy curried fish stew   164
    easy Scandi crispbreads   102
    golden salmon steaks   166
    green tea roasted salmon   214
    hot-smoked trout   118
    Italian jam jar salad   104
    lemon sole & olive sauce   210
    moreish fish soup   204
    roasted mustard mackerel   174
    salmon ceviche   142
    seared tuna   124
    sesame seared salmon   150
    smoked salmon & spring onion scrambled eggs   56
    tasty fish tacos   86
    tomato & olive spaghetti   100
    see also seafood
flapjacks: raw vegan flapjack snacks   V   244
flatbreads
    cosy squash soup, chickpea salad flatbreads   V   122
    Mexican gazpacho   V   134
fregola: herby pasta salad   116
fro-yo fun, fruit, yoghurt, nuts & seeds   V   246
fruit
    awesome granola dust   V   18
    berry pocket eggy bread   V   52
    my Bircher muesli   V   78
    black rice pudding   V   28
    Earl Grey banana bread   V   82
    epic fruit salad   V   66
    figgy banana bread   V   30
    healthy cheese & corn pancakes   74
    pretty fruit pots   V   34
    sexy stewed prunes   V   76
    smoothie pancakes   V   24
    toasted oats   V   62
    see also dried fruit; individual fruits

fruit soups, yoghurt & granola dust
    basil & strawberry   V   40
    ginger tea & mango   V   40
    mint & kiwi   V   40
    nettle tea & blackberry   V   40
fusilli
    fagioli fusilli   V   206
    happiness pasta   V   90

G

gazpacho: Mexican gazpacho   V   134
gem lettuce
    gem lettuce, cucumber, apple & mint salad   V   226
    gem lettuce, radish, pea & clementine salad   V   226
    Greek jam jar salad   106
    healthy chicken club   128
    spring squid   200
ginger
    apricot, ginger & cashew energy balls   V   250
    Asian crispy beef   88
    delicious squash daal   V   168
    easy curried fish stew   164
    ginger & chicken penicillin   218
    ginger tea & mango fruit soup   V   40
    ginger, turmeric, lemon & honey tea   V   257
    green tea roasted salmon, ginger rice & sunshine salad   214
    mango, lime & ginger fro-yo   V   246
    perfect porridge bars   V   48
    pomegranate, ginger & lime flavoured water   V   255
    roasted squash laksa bake   170
    super-tasty miso broth   208
golden chicken skewers, yellow pepper sauce, black quinoa   172
golden salmon steaks, sweet peas & smashed veg   166
granola
    awesome granola dust   V   18
    fruit soups   V   40
grapefruit, orange & mint tea   V   256
grapes: iceberg lettuce, broad bean, grape & tarragon salad   V   228
Greek jam jar salad   106
green beans: crumbed pesto fish   184
green tea roasted salmon, ginger rice & sunshine salad   214
greens
    Asian steamed fish   180
    hot-smoked trout   118
    seared turmeric chicken   140
    veggie ramen, walnut miso, kimchee & fried eggs   V   190
    see also asparagus; chard; kale; spinach; sugar snap peas
griddled steak & peppers, herby jewelled tabbouleh rice   216
grilled corn & quinoa salad, mango, tomatoes, herbs, avo, feta   152

H

haddock
    Asian steamed fish   180
    crumbed pesto fish   184
    easy curried fish stew   164
    tasty fish tacos   86
ham: breakfast popovers   50
happiness pasta, sweet tomato, aubergine & ricotta   V   90
harissa roasted aubergine, pomegranate, pistachios, olives, rice   V   186
harissa waffles, sesame fried eggs & carrot salad   V   42
hazelnuts
    black rice pudding   V   28
    homemade nut butters   V   242
    raw vegan flapjack snacks   V   244
healthy cheese & corn pancakes, smoky bacon & caramelized banana   74
healthy chicken Caesar, awesome shredded salad & croutons   94
healthy chicken club, tomato, lettuce, pear & tarragon   128
healthy poppadom snacks   V   232
herby pasta salad, radishes, apples, feta & bresaola   116
herrings: easy Scandi crispbreads   102
hibiscus: strawberry, hibiscus & star anise tea   V   257
homemade nut butters   V   242
honey
    apricot, ginger & cashew energy balls   V   250
    Asian crispy beef   88
    berry pocket eggy bread   V   52
    black rice pudding   V   28
    blushing pickled eggs   V   238
    date, cocoa & pumpkin seed energy balls   V   248
    fennel seeds, lemon & honey tea   V   256
    fruit soups   V   40
    ginger, turmeric, lemon & honey tea   V   257
    perfect porridge bars   V   48
    smoothie pancakes   V   24
    toasted oats   V   62
horseradish
    beets & sardines   112
    feisty beet & horseradish dip   V   230
hot-smoked trout, green lentils, fresh tomato sauce   118
houmous   V   230
    seared turmeric chicken   140
    squash it veg sandwich   V   146

I

iceberg lettuce
    iceberg lettuce, broad bean, grape & tarragon salad   V   228
    iceberg lettuce, courgette, pear & dill salad   V   228
    post-gym super salad   72
Indian roasted cauliflower, pineapple, chilli, coronation dressing   V   192
Italian jam jar salad   104

J

jalapeños
    roasted carrot & squash salad   V   194
    roasted sweet potatoes, black beans, jalapeño tomato salsa   V   110
jam jar salads
    British jam jar salad   104
    Greek jam jar salad   106
    Italian jam jar salad   104
    Moroccan jam jar salad   V   106

K

kale
    super green soup   114
    super-tasty miso broth   208
kebabs
    chicken & garlic bread kebabs   130
    golden chicken skewers   172
kedgeree: vegeree not kedgeree   V   38
kimchee: veggie ramen, walnut miso, kimchee & fried eggs   V   190
kiwi fruit
    mint & kiwi fruit soup   V   40
    tasty fish tacos, game-changing kiwi, lime & chilli salsa   86

L

lasagne: super squash lasagne   V   176
leeks
    chicken & squash cacciatore   202
    fagioli fusilli, sweet leeks, artichokes & bay oil   V   206
lemon sole & olive sauce, sweet courgettes & Jersey royals   210
lemongrass: roasted squash laksa bake   170
lemons
    fennel seeds, lemon & honey tea   V   256
    ginger, turmeric, lemon & honey tea   V   257
    Moroccan jam jar salad   V   106
    St Clements flavoured water   V   254
    salmon ceviche   142
    seared tuna   124
    wholewheat spaghetti, sprouting broccoli, chilli & lemon   132
lentils
    delicious squash daal   V   168
    hot-smoked trout   118
    mighty mushroom curry   V   212
lettuce
    gem lettuce, cucumber, apple & mint salad   V   226
    gem lettuce, radish, pea & clementine salad   V   226
    Greek jam jar salad   106
    healthy chicken Caesar   94
    healthy chicken club   128
    iceberg lettuce, broad bean, grape & tarragon salad   V   228
    iceberg lettuce, courgette, pear & dill salad   V   228
    Moroccan jam jar salad   V   106

post-gym super salad		72
round lettuce, asparagus, strawberry & mint salad		228
round lettuce, fennel, blueberry & chilli salad	V	226
spring squid		200
lime pickle & poppadoms cucumber sticks	V	236
limes		
black rice pudding	V	28
epic fruit salad	V	66
mango, lime & ginger fro-yo	V	246
pomegranate, ginger & lime flavoured water	V	255
salmon ceviche		142
tasty fish tacos, game-changing kiwi, lime & chilli salsa		86
linseeds		
protein porridge	V	36
super-food protein loaf	V	68

M

mackerel		
moreish fish soup		204
roasted mustard mackerel		174
magic poached egg, smashed avo & seeded toast	V	22
mango chutney: cheese & mango chutney poppadom snacks	V	232
mangos		
black rice pudding	V	28
epic fruit salad	V	66
ginger tea & mango fruit soup	V	40
green tea roasted salmon, ginger rice & sunshine salad		214
grilled corn & quinoa salad		152
mango, lime & ginger fro-yo	V	246
pretty fruit pots	V	34
toasted oats	V	62
Marmite		
Marmite flavour popcorn	V	234
mushroom & Marmite scrambled eggs	V	58
super-food protein loaf	V	68
mega veggie burgers, garden salad & basil dressing	V	158
Mexican gazpacho, flatbreads & garnishes	V	134
Mexican pan-cooked brekkie, eggs, beans, tomatoes, mushrooms		26
Mexican tomato soup	V	98
mighty mushroom curry, red lentils, brown rice & poppadoms	V	212
millet: roasted carrot & squash salad	V	194
mint		
creamy mint dressing	V	228
crispy sea bass, pea, mint & asparagus mash		198
cucumber, apple & mint flavoured water	V	254
epic fruit salad	V	66
gem lettuce, cucumber, apple & mint salad	V	226
grapefruit, orange & mint tea	V	256
herby pasta salad		116
mint & kiwi fruit soup	V	40
round lettuce, asparagus, strawberry & mint salad		228
seared golden chicken, mint sauce & spring veg fest		162

miso		
super-tasty miso broth		208
veggie ramen, walnut miso, kimchee & fried eggs	V	190
moreish fish soup, mackerel, mussels, broth & couscous		204
Moroccan jam jar salad	V	106
Moroccan prawns, fluffy couscous & rainbow salsa		178
muesli: my Bircher muesli	V	78
muffins: sweet potato muffins	V	64
mushrooms		
breakfast popovers		50
chicken & squash cacciatore		202
Mexican pan-cooked brekkie		26
mighty mushroom curry	V	212
mushroom & Marmite scrambled eggs	V	58
orange garden salad		92
pan-cooked mushrooms		80
super-tasty miso broth		208
vegeree not kedgeree	V	38
mussels: moreish fish soup		204
mustard		
creamy basil dressing	V	226
creamy mint dressing	V	228
healthy chicken Caesar		94
healthy chicken club		128
roasted mustard mackerel		174
my Russian salad		148

N

nettle tea & blackberry fruit soup	V	40
noodles		
Asian crispy beef		88
Asian green salad	V	138
Asian stir-fried veg, crispy sesame noodle omelette	V	144
crazy fish, veg & noodle stir-fry		220
sesame seared salmon		150
veggie ramen, walnut miso, kimchee & fried eggs	V	190
nuts		
awesome granola dust	V	18
my Bircher muesli	V	78
homemade nut butters	V	242
perfect porridge bars	V	48
protein porridge	V	36
smoothie pancakes	V	24
snack attack	V	253
toasted nut mix	V	228
see also individual nuts		

O

oats		
awesome granola dust	V	18
my Bircher muesli	V	78
easy Scandi crispbreads		102

mango, lime & ginger fro-yo	V	246
perfect porridge bars	V	48
protein porridge	V	36
raw vegan flapjack snacks	V	244
roasted mustard mackerel		174
rye soda bread	V	44
strawberry, balsamic & basil fro-yo	V	246
toasted oats	V	62
okra: smoky veggie feijoada	V	182
olives		
chicken & squash cacciatore		202
Greek jam jar salad		106
harissa roasted aubergine	V	186
lemon sole & olive sauce		210
tomato & olive spaghetti		100
omelettes		
Asian stir-fried veg, crispy sesame noodle omelette	V	144
silken omelette	V	32
tasty veg omelette	V	120
100-calorie salad snack bowls	V	226–8
oranges		
my Bircher muesli	V	78
chicken & garlic bread kebabs		130
figgy banana bread	V	30
grapefruit, orange & mint tea	V	256
Moroccan jam jar salad	V	106
orange garden salad		92
St Clements flavoured water	V	254

P

pan-cooked mushrooms, tomato, pancetta, spinach & cheese		80
pancakes		
awesome granola dust	V	18
healthy cheese & corn pancakes		74
smoothie pancakes	V	24
pancetta: pan-cooked mushrooms		80
paprika: my Russian salad, golden paprika chicken		148
passion fruit		
black rice pudding	V	28
epic fruit salad	V	66
pasta		
fagioli fusilli	V	206
happiness pasta	V	90
herby pasta salad		116
Italian jam jar salad		104
skinny carbonara		108
spelt spaghetti, vine tomatoes & baked ricotta	V	160
super squash lasagne	V	176
tomato & olive spaghetti		100
wholewheat spaghetti, sprouting broccoli, chilli & lemon		132
peaches		
Earl Grey banana bread	V	82
epic fruit salad	V	66

peanuts: roasted squash laksa bake		170
pearl barley: British jam jar salad		104
pears		
healthy chicken club		128
iceberg lettuce, courgette, pear & dill salad	V	228
peas		
Asian green salad	V	138
crispy sea bass, pea, mint & asparagus mash		198
gem lettuce, radish, pea & clementine salad	V	226
golden salmon steaks, sweet peas & smashed veg		166
my Russian salad		148
seared golden chicken, mint sauce & spring veg fest		162
skinny carbonara		108
spring squid		200
tasty veg omelette	V	120
vegeree not kedgeree	V	38
pecans		
Earl Grey banana bread	V	82
homemade nut butters	V	242
raw vegan flapjack snacks	V	244
peppers		
golden chicken skewers, yellow pepper sauce, black quinoa		172
griddled steak & peppers		216
Mexican gazpacho	V	134
seared turmeric chicken		140
smoky peppers & sweet basil cucumber sticks	V	236
smoky veggie feijoada	V	182
tasty veg omelette	V	120
perfect porridge bars, nuts, seeds, fruit & spices	V	48
pesto fish, roasted cherry vines, spuds & greens		184
pickled eggs, red cabbage, cloves & star anise	V	238
pineapples		
epic fruit salad	V	66
Indian roasted cauliflower	V	192
pistachios		
berry pocket eggy bread	V	52
harissa roasted aubergine	V	186
homemade nut butters	V	242
pomegranates		
griddled steak & peppers, herby jewelled tabbouleh rice		216
harissa roasted aubergine	V	186
Moroccan jam jar salad	V	106
pomegranate, ginger & lime flavoured water	V	255
roasted carrot & squash salad	V	194
sizzling Moroccan prawns		178
popcorn: popcorn fun	V	234
popovers: breakfast popovers		50
poppadoms		
Bombay chicken & cauli		156
delicious squash daal	V	168
healthy poppadom snacks	V	232
lime pickle & poppadom cucumber sticks	V	236
mighty mushroom curry	V	212

poppy seeds

    cheese, chilli & seeds poppadom snacks   V   232

    sweet potato muffins   V   64

pork

    pork & apple sauce, glazed carrots, brown rice & greens   222

    see also bacon; chorizo

porridge

    awesome granola dust   V   18

    perfect porridge bars   V   48

    protein porridge   V   36

portable jam jar salads   104-6

post-gym super salad, chicken, quinoa & loadsa veg   72

potatoes

    crispy sea bass, pea, mint & asparagus mash   198

    crumbed pesto fish   184

    golden salmon steaks, sweet peas & smashed veg   166

    lemon sole & olive sauce, sweet courgettes & Jersey royals   210

    moreish fish soup   204

    my Russian salad   148

    spring squid   200

    super green soup   114

    tasty veg omelette   V   120

prawns

    easy curried fish stew   164

    sizzling Moroccan prawns   178

preserved lemons: Moroccan jam jar salad   V   106

pretty fruit pots, trendy chia & nut milk   V   34

protein porridge, blended oats, seeds, nuts & quinoa   V   36

prunes: sexy stewed prunes   V   76

pumpkin seeds: date, cocoa & pumpkin seed energy balls   V   248

Q

quick homemade tortilla, scalded veg, chilli, cheese & avo   V   60

quinoa

    golden chicken skewers, yellow pepper sauce, black quinoa   172

    grilled corn & quinoa salad   152

    post-gym super salad   72

    protein porridge   V   36

    super summer salad   V   136

R

radishes

    gem lettuce, radish, pea & clementine salad   V   226

    herby pasta salad   116

    super summer salad   V   136

rainbow open wrap, salad, feta & spiced crispy beans   V   54

ramen, walnut miso, kimchee & fried eggs   V   190

raspberries

    awesome granola dust   V   18

    berry pocket eggy bread   V   52

    epic fruit salad   V   66

    protein porridge   V   36

smoothie pancakes   V   24

raw vegan flapjack snacks, nuts, seeds, dates, oats & fruit   V   244

rice

    Asian steamed fish   180

    black rice pudding   V   28

    Bombay chicken & cauli   156

    easy curried fish stew   164

    ginger & chicken penicillin   218

    green tea roasted salmon, ginger rice & sunshine salad   214

    griddled steak & peppers, herby jewelled tabbouleh rice   216

    harissa roasted aubergine   V   186

    mighty mushroom curry   V   212

    pork & apple sauce   222

    roasted squash laksa bake   170

    roasted sweet potatoes   V   110

    salmon ceviche   142

    smoky veggie feijoada   V   182

    super-tasty miso broth   208

    vegeree not kedgeree   V   38

rice noodles

    Asian crispy beef   88

    Asian green salad   V   138

    Asian stir-fried veg, crispy sesame noodle omelette   V   144

    crazy fish, veg & noodle stir-fry   220

    sesame seared salmon   150

ricotta cheese

    baked eggs in popped beans   V   16

    happiness pasta   V   90

    spelt spaghetti, vine tomatoes & baked ricotta   V   160

roasted carrot & squash salad, millet, apple, jalapeño & pomegranate   V   194

roasted mustard mackerel, rainbow beets & bulgur wheat   174

roasted squash laksa bake, chicken, lemongrass, peanuts & rice   170

roasted sweet potatoes, black beans, jalapeño tomato salsa   V   110

rocket: Italian jam jar salad   104

round lettuce, asparagus, strawberry & mint salad   228

round lettuce, fennel, blueberry & chilli salad   V   226

my Russian salad, golden paprika chicken   148

rye bread

    beets & sardines   112

    rye soda bread   V   44

    silken omelette   V   32

S

St Clements flavoured water   V   254

salads

    Asian crispy beef   88

    Asian green salad   V   138

    epic fruit salad   V   66

    green tea roasted salmon, ginger rice & sunshine salad   214

    grilled corn & quinoa salad   152

    harissa waffles   V   42

    healthy chicken Caesar   94

herby pasta salad			116
hot-smoked trout			118
Indian roasted cauliflower	V		192
mega veggie burgers, garden salad & basil dressing	V		158
100-calorie salad snack bowls	V	226–8
orange garden salad			92
portable jam jar salads			104-6
post-gym super salad			72
rainbow open wrap	V		54
roasted carrot & squash salad	V		194
my Russian salad			148
salmon ceviche			142
sesame seared salmon, tahini, avocado & shred salad			150
sprouting seed salad			96
super summer salad	V		136

salmon
golden salmon steaks		166
green tea roasted salmon		214
salmon ceviche		142
sesame seared salmon		150
smoked salmon & spring onion scrambled eggs		56

salsas
roasted sweet potatoes, black beans, jalapeño tomato salsa	V		110
sizzling Moroccan prawns, fluffy couscous & rainbow salsa			178
smoky veggie feijoada	V		182
tasty fish tacos, game-changing kiwi, lime & chilli salsa			86
tasty veg omelette, raw tomato & chilli salsa	V		120

samosas: tasty samosas, beef, onion & sweet potato — 188

sandwiches
healthy chicken club		128
squash it veg sandwich	V	146

sardines
beets & sardines	112
tomato & olive spaghetti	100

scrambled eggs
mushroom & Marmite scrambled eggs	V	58
smoked salmon & spring onion scrambled eggs		56
spinach, Parmesan & chilli scrambled eggs	V	56
tomato, basil & cheese scrambled eggs	V	58

sea bass: crispy sea bass — 198

seafood
easy curried fish stew	164
moreish fish soup	204
sizzling Moroccan prawns	178
spring squid	200

seared golden chicken, mint sauce & spring veg fest — 162

seared tuna, Sicilian couscous & greens — 124

seared turmeric chicken, houmous, peppers, couscous & greens — 140

seeds
awesome granola dust	V	18
my Bircher muesli	V	78
perfect porridge bars	V	48
raw vegan flapjack snacks	V	244

snack attack	V	253
super-food protein loaf	V	68
toasted seed mix	V	226
see also individual seeds		

sesame seeds
Asian green salad	V	138
Asian stir-fried veg, crispy sesame noodle omelette	V	144
harissa waffles	V	42
sesame seared salmon		150
tahini, spring onion & sesame cucumber sticks	V	236

sexy stewed prunes, toast, banana, yoghurt, almonds	V	76
silken omelette, spinach, tomato, Parmesan & rye	V	32
sizzling Moroccan prawns, fluffy couscous & rainbow salsa		178
skinny carbonara, smoky bacon, peas, almonds & basil		108
skinny homemade houmous	V	230
smoked salmon & spring onion scrambled eggs		56
smoky veggie feijoada, black beans, squash, peppers & okra	V	182
smoothie pancakes, berries, banana, yoghurt & nuts	V	24
smoothies: awesome granola dust	V	18
snack attack	V	253

soups
amazing Mexican tomato soup	V	98
cosy squash soup	V	122
fruit soups	V	40
Mexican gazpacho	V	134
moreish fish soup		204
super green soup		114
see also broths		

spaghetti
skinny carbonara		108
spelt spaghetti, vine tomatoes & baked ricotta	V	160
tomato & olive spaghetti		100
wholewheat spaghetti, sprouting broccoli, chilli & lemon		132

spinach
Bombay chicken & cauli	156
British jam jar salad	104
chicken & garlic bread kebabs	130
crispy sea bass, pea, mint & asparagus mash	198
crumbed pesto fish	184
lemon sole & olive sauce	210
pan-cooked mushrooms	80
post-gym super salad	72

silken omelette	V	32
spinach, Parmesan & chilli scrambled eggs	V	56
super squash lasagne	V	176
vegeree not kedgeree	V	38

spring onions
crazy fish, veg & noodle stir-fry		220
ginger & chicken penicillin		218
smoked salmon & spring onion scrambled eggs		56
tahini, spring onion & sesame cucumber sticks	V	236

spring squid, peas, asparagus, beans & greens	200
sprouting seed salad, smoky bacon & balsamic dressing	96

squash *see* butternut squash

squash it veg sandwich, houmous, avocado & cottage cheese V 146

squid: spring squid 200

steak: griddled steak & peppers 216

stews: easy curried fish stew 164

strawberries

    basil & strawberry fruit soup V 40

    epic fruit salad V 66

    round lettuce, asparagus, strawberry & mint salad 228

    strawberry, balsamic & basil fro-yo V 246

    strawberry, hisbiscus & star anise tea V 257

sugar snap peas: Asian green salad V 138

sunflower seeds

    cheese, chilli & seeds poppadom snacks V 232

    squash it veg sandwich V 146

    super squash lasagne V 176

    sweet potato muffins V 64

super green soup, chickpeas, veg & smoky chorizo 114

super squash lasagne, spinach, cottage cheese & seeds V 176

super summer salad, watermelon, radishes, quinoa & feta V 136

super-food protein loaf, wheat-free, gluten-free V 68

    & super-tasty topping ideas 70

super-tasty miso broth, chicken, mushrooms & wild rice 208

swede: golden salmon steaks, sweet peas & smashed veg 166

sweet potato muffins, chilli, cheese & seeds V 64

sweet potatoes

    amazing Mexican tomato soup V 98

    chicken & squash cacciatore 202

    roasted sweet potatoes V 110

    sweet potato muffins V 64

    tasty samosas 188

sweetcorn

    Asian stir-fried veg V 144

    crazy fish, veg & noodle stir-fry 220

    grilled corn & quinoa salad 152

    healthy cheese & corn pancakes 74

    Mexican gazpacho V 134

Swiss chard: seared tuna, Sicilian couscous & greens 124

T

tabbouleh: griddled steak & peppers, herby jewelled
tabbouleh rice 216

tacos: tasty fish tacos 86

tahini

    sesame seared salmon, tahini, avocado & shred salad 150

    tahini, spring onion & sesame cucumber sticks V 236

tarragon

    healthy chicken club 128

    iceberg lettuce, broad bean, grape & tarragon salad V 228

my tasty energy balls

    apricot, ginger & cashew V 250

    date, cocoa & pumpkin seeds V 248

tasty fish tacos, game-changing kiwi, lime & chilli salsa 86

tasty samosas, beef, onion & sweet potato 188

tasty veg omelette, raw tomato & chilli salsa V 120

tea

    Earl Grey banana bread V 82

    ginger tea & mango fruit soup V 40

    green tea roasted salmon 214

    nettle tea & blackberry fruit soup V 40

    sexy stewed prunes V 76

    therapeutic teas V 256–7

therapeutic teas, tasty, vibrant & easy V 256–7

toast

    baked eggs in popped beans V 16

    Earl Grey banana bread V 82

    healthy chicken club 128

    magic poached egg V 22

    mushroom & Marmite scrambled eggs V 58

    pan-cooked mushrooms 80

    sexy stewed prunes V 76

    smoked salmon & spring onion scrambled eggs 56

    spinach, Parmesan & chilli scrambled eggs 56

    tomato, basil & cheese scrambled eggs 58

toasted nut mix V 228

toasted oats, mango, blueberries & yoghurt V 62

toasted seed mix V 226

tofu

    Asian green salad V 138

    mega veggie burgers V 158

tomatoes

    amazing Mexican tomato soup V 98

    baked eggs in popped beans V 16

    breakfast popovers 50

    British jam jar salad 104

    cheese, tomato & basil poppadom snacks V 232

    chicken & squash cacciatore 202

    crumbed pesto fish 184

    easy curried fish stew 164

    Greek jam jar salad 106

    grilled corn & quinoa salad 152

    happiness pasta V 90

    harissa roasted aubergine V 186

    healthy chicken club 128

    hot-smoked trout 118

    Italian jam jar salad 104

    magic poached egg V 22

    mega veggie burgers, garden salad & basil dressing V 158

    Mexican gazpacho V 134

    Mexican pan-cooked brekkie 26

    mighty mushroom curry V 212

    moreish fish soup 204

    pan-cooked mushrooms 80

    post-gym super salad 72

    quick homemade tortilla V 60

    roasted sweet potatoes, black beans, jalapeño tomato salsa V 110

salmon ceviche			142
seared tuna, Sicilian couscous & greens			124
silken omelette	V		32
spelt spaghetti, vine tomatoes & baked ricotta	V		160
super squash lasagne	V		176
tasty veg omelette, raw tomato & chilli salsa	V		120
tomato & olive spaghetti			100
tomato, cheese & basil scrambled eggs	V		58
vegeree not kedgeree	V		38
tortillas			
amazing Mexican tomato soup	V		98
Mexican gazpacho	V		134
Mexican pan-cooked brekkie			26
quick homemade tortilla	V		60
trout: hot-smoked trout			118
tuna			
Italian jam jar salad			104
seared tuna			124
turmeric			
Bombay chicken & cauli			156
ginger, turmeric, lemon & honey tea	V		257
perfect porridge bars	V		48
seared turmeric chicken			140

V

vegeree not kedgeree, spiced rice, veg, eggs & yoghurt	V	38
veggie burgers, garden salad & basil dressing	V	158
veggie ramen, walnut miso, kimchee & fried eggs	V	190

W

waffles: harissa waffles	V	42
walnuts		
snack attack	V	253
veggie ramen, walnut miso, kimchee & fried eggs	V	190
water: easy flavoured waters	V	254–5
watercress: British jam jar salad		104
watermelon		
Mexican gazpacho	V	134
super summer salad	V	136
watermelon & basil flavoured water	V	255
wholewheat spaghetti, sprouting broccoli, chilli & lemon		132
Worcestershire sauce flavour popcorn		234
wraps		
quick homemade tortilla	V	60
rainbow open wrap	V	54

Y

yoghurt		
beets & sardines		112
berry pocket eggy bread	V	52
my Bircher muesli	V	78

Earl Grey banana bread	V	82
fro-yo fun	V	246
fruit soups	V	40
sexy stewed prunes	V	76
smoothie pancakes	V	24
toasted oats	V	62
vegeree not kedgeree	V	38

LIVE WELL

alcohol	280–1
balanced plate	260–1
breakfast	261
carbohydrates	266–7, 287
cereals	287
coconut oil	273
dairy	274–5, 287
fat	272–3, 287
fibre	266, 267
fruit	262–3, 287
fruit juice	279
hangovers	281
hydration	261, 278–9
longevity	292–3
milk	275
omega fatty acids	273
organic food	275, 284–5
protein	268–9, 287
shopping	286–7
sleep	290–1
sugars	266–7, 279, 287
vegan diets	269
vegetables	262–3, 287
vegetarian diets	269
water	261, 278–9

For a quick reference list of all the dairy-free, gluten-free and vegan recipes in this book, please visit:

jamieoliver.com/everyday-super-food

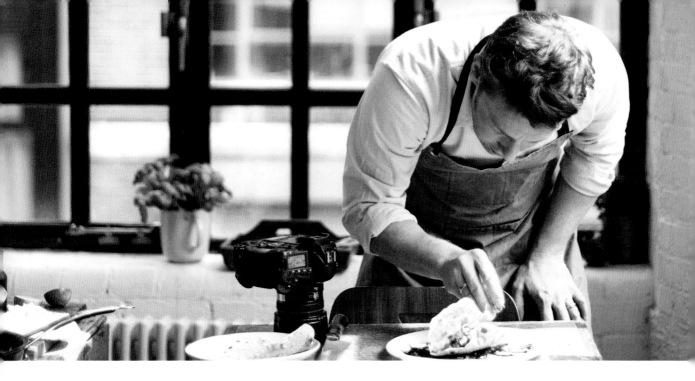

HUNGRY FOR MORE?

For handy nutrition advice, as well as videos, features, hints, tricks and tips on all sorts of different subjects, and loads of brilliant, tasty recipes, plus much more, check out **jamieoliver.com** and **youtube.com/jamieoliver**

JAMIEOLIVER.COM

A NOTE ON NUTRITION

The job of Jamie's nutrition team is to make sure that he can be super-creative with his recipe writing, while also ensuring that all recipes meet the set guidelines.

Every book has a different brief, and Jamie's aim with *Everyday Super Food* was to provide you with lots of delicious, balanced recipes you can cook every day, that just happen to be healthy and that fit within a daily structure of calories (see page 261 – this is based on a woman's daily recommended intake of about 2,000 calories). Remember that these figures are just a guide, and what you eat will always need to be considered in relation to factors such as age, gender, build and physical activity levels. In order for you to be able to make informed choices, we've published the nutritional content for each recipe on the recipe page itself, giving you a really easy access point to understand what you're eating, should you wish to do so. Remember that a good, balanced diet and regular exercise are the keys to a healthier lifestyle.

For more information about our guidelines and how we analyse recipes, please visit: **jamieoliver.com/nutrition**

Laura Matthews – Head of Nutrition, RNutr (Food)

MICHAEL JOSEPH

UK | USA | Canada | Ireland | Australia | India | New Zealand | South Africa

Michael Joseph is part of the Penguin Random House group of companies
whose addresses can be found at global.penguinrandomhouse.com

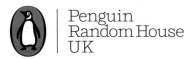

First published 2015

001

Copyright © Jamie Oliver, 2015

Recipe photography copyright © Jamie Oliver Enterprises Limited, 2015

Jacket and studio photography copyright © Paul Stuart, 2015

Reportage photography copyright © Freddie Claire, 2015

The moral right of the author has been asserted

Design by Superfantastic

Photographic post production by The Laundry Room

Colour reproduction by Altaimage Ltd

Printed in Germany by Mohn Media

A CIP catalogue record for this book is available from the British Library

ISBN: 978–0–718–18123–9

penguin.co.uk

jamieoliver.com

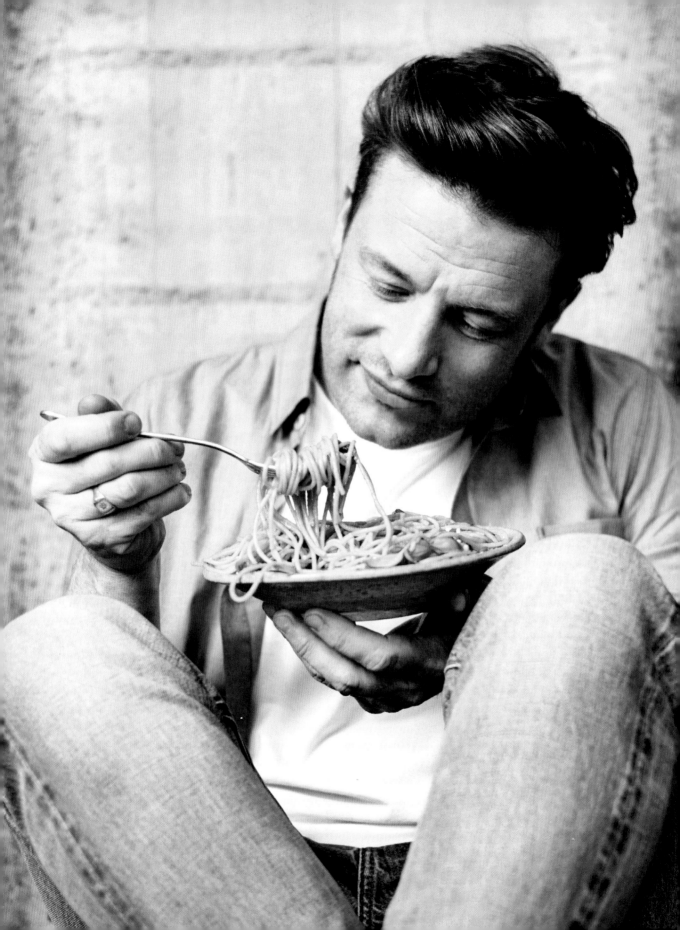